EMERGENCY MEDICINE DECISION MAKING: CRITICAL CHOICES IN CHAOTIC ENVIRONMENTS

NOTICE

Medicine is an ever-changing science. As new research and clinical experience broaden our knowledge, changes in treatment and drug therapy are required. The authors and the publisher of this work have checked with sources believed to be reliable in their efforts to provide information that is complete and generally in accord with the standards accepted at the time of publication. However, in view of the possibility of human error changes in medical sciences, neither the editors nor the publisher nor any other party who has been involved in the preparation or publication of this work warrants that the information contained herein is in every respect accurate or complete, and they disclaim all responsibility for any errors or omissions or for the results obtained from use of the information contained in this work. Readers are encouraged to confirm the information contained herein with other sources. For example and in particular, readers are advised to check the product information sheet included in the package of each drug they plan to administer to be certain that the information contained in this work is accurate and that changes have not been made in the recommended dose or in the contraindications for administration. This recommendation is of particular importance in connection with new or infrequently used drugs.

EMERGENCY MEDICINE DECISION MAKING: CRITICAL CHOICES IN CHAOTIC ENVIRONMENTS

SCOTT WEINGART, MD
Assistant Professor of Emergency Medicine
Elmhurst Hospital Center
Mount Sinai School of Medicine
New York

PETER WYER, MD
Associate Professor of Medicine
Columbia University College of Physicians and Surgeons
New York

The McGraw·Hill Companies

Emergency Medicine Decision Making:
Critical Choices in Chaotic Environments

1 2 3 4 5 6 7 8 9 0 DOC DOC 0 9 8 7 6 5

ISBN: 0-07-144212-X

This book was set in Times Roman by Keyword Group Ltd.
The editor was Marty Wonsiewicz.
The production supervisor was Catherine H. Saggese.
The cover designer was Aimee Nordin.
Project management was provided by Keyword Group Ltd.
R. R. Donnelley was printer and binder.

This book is printed on acid-free paper.

Library of Congress Cataloging-in-Publication Data

Weingart, Scott.
  Emergency medicine decision making: critical choices in chaotic environments / Scott Weingart, Peter Wyer.
     p. ; cm.
  Includes bibliographic references and index.
  ISBN 0-07-144212-X
     1.   Emergency medicine. 2. Evidence-based medicine. I. Wyer, Peter. II. Title.
     [DNLM: 1. Emergency Medicine–methods. 2. Evidence-Based Medicine. WB 105
  W423e 2006]
  RC86.7.W45 2006
  616.02′5—dc22   2005054047

SW
To Dr. Andy Jagoda for making me an Emergency Physician and
Dr. Sabrina Bhagwan for making me extremely happy.

PW
To my wife, Judith Rencoret de Wyer, for her loving support and for
adding many new dimensions to my life.

CONTENTS

FOREWORD

Authors have written a great deal about the process of therapeutic and, particularly, diagnostic decision-making, both from a descriptive and prescriptive perspective. More recently, enthusiasts for evidence-based medicine (EBM) have written an increasing variety of texts introducing the clinical community to an evidence-based framework for clinical decision making. Yet, for the promise of EBM to be fulfilled, trainees must integrate its concepts and precepts as essential elements of how they think. The premise of the book is that educators must combine clinical reasoning, as traditionally taught from the standpoint of principles of logic and logical fallacies, with the precepts of evidence-based medicine to most effectively communicate with entry level clinicians – that is, residents and junior faculty.

The principal author, Scott Weingart, independently synthesized this concept on his own as a resident in emergency medicine. The second author, Peter Wyer, helped define and formulate the approach, in particular distinguishing it from available EBM texts. The authors have done a great job, and the practical integration of clinical reasoning with insights from evidence-based medicine is compelling.

Part of what makes the book so compelling is that the authors have created a format that convincingly penetrates the reality of the intellectual life of a first-year resident in a high-powered emergency medicine training program. The presentation is streamlined, bulleted, and pithy. While an understanding of classical logical syllogisms clearly underlies the presentation, readers are spared the details. The result captures readers' attention; it encourages them to start thinking about thinking. It teaches residents to bring clinical evidence into the clinical process, at the same time as they are advancing their skills in sizing up patients, and developing management strategies, all within the chaos of the emergency department.

One can think of the book as a life raft that an emergency medicine resident might grab hold of as they find themselves subjects of the traditional approach to learning how to swim: you throw the kid into the pool and she either learns to swim or ... she does not. Many of their senior peers and role models may give only lip service to the desirability of evidence-based medicine. This book provides a lucid guide for young clinicians who wish to go beyond the "just tell me what to do" mentality that may easily consume the learner in the emergency medicine environment. It allows clinicians to understand and apply fundamental concepts of evidence-based clinical reasoning to their everyday practice.

The structure of the book reflects, and helps direct, the true sequence in which emergency medicine residents encounter the concepts of EBM in the course of a training program, and the order in which they acquire the relevant skills. The book begins with the resident who has the evidence, and wonders what to do with it. The next part deals with the question: was this evidence any good in the first place? If residents have been satisfied with these aspects of applying evidence-based reasoning, they will be inclined to look for evidence in other situations; the book's third part provides guides for this bit of the process.

The book does not supersede more comprehensive and definitive texts, but rather opens doors that will lead residents to these works. The book represents an inspired response of a gifted resident and an experienced clinician, who has done more than any other individual to bring evidence-based decision-making to the emergency medicine community.

Gordon Guyatt, MD

PREFACE

Before we begin our discussion of making critical decisions in chaotic environments, we wanted to take a moment to explain what inspired us to write this text.

SW

A few years ago, during my residency and fellowship training, I noticed that the physicians I respected most used clear and unfettered clinical reasoning. All of them had a practice informed by evidence, though only a few of them laid claim to the formal use of evidence-based medicine (EBM). Aspiring to one day become as skilled a teacher and clinician as the attendings I admired, I began to study EBM.

I quickly realized that while there are many fine texts and resources for learning EBM, most do not address the way we practice as emergency physicians. Further, I discovered that EBM only informs part of the process of clinical reasoning. There was something more, which allowed skilled emergency physicians to take the evidence and actually use it to make the right decisions in difficult situations.

During my undergraduate years, I studied critical thinking, a branch of cognitive psychology, which teaches self-reflection and clear thought processes to allow good decisions. It occurred to me that good doctors, but especially good doctors in the emergency department, were all critical thinkers, though most of them would never use this term to describe themselves. I began to believe that critical thinking was the path to integrating evidence-based medicine and clear clinical reasoning in emergency medicine. I knew if there was a book on this topic, it would benefit my training, but no such text existed. I asked myself: "Why not just write one yourself?" (Warning – questions like these can lead to a huge loss of free time and a year's worth of bleary eyes and sore fingers.)

When I approached the editors at McGraw-Hill with the idea for this book, it was with a mix of excitement and trepidation. The excitement stemmed from a desire to create a text especially for EM residents with the hope that their practice and training would be enhanced. The trepidation emerged from the fact that I had no idea whether I could actually write such a book. When the editors greeted the idea with enthusiasm and support, I realized I needed the backup of an experienced educator in evidence-based emergency medicine.

PW

Upon initially learning of this endeavor, I muttered to myself: "Oh no, not another introductory book on evidence-based medicine!" After several exchanges and discussions, we found ourselves both excited and relieved to realize that we were not talking about a book on evidence-based medicine per se, but rather one on critical thinking in the era of evidence-based medicine.

I have enjoyed the mixed "blessing" of never undergoing formal residency training (a course I do not recommend to others). Throughout my academic career, I have worried that the EM residency experience may have the ultimate effect of reducing practice for many residents to fixed formulas and uninformed heuristics.

Over the last decade, in the course of many teaching efforts aimed at bringing the fruits of evidence-based medicine, in a fairly rigorous form, into the EM spotlight, I have noticed a cognitive gap among the graduates of such efforts. Despite strong learner motivation and a preliminary exposure to the core concepts of EBM, the content of EBM frequently remains sequestered and remote from the realm of day-to-day activity. As a result, the initial grasp of the concepts and skills decays rapidly and the most motivated learners not uncommonly present themselves as participants in subsequent "introductory" courses and workshops.

The opportunity to present a selected subset of essential EBM concepts in a context in which the focus is on clinical reasoning intrigued me and persuaded me to join in the undertaking.

SW and PW

The result is, we hope, a reasonably concise synthesis of essential precepts of cognitive psychology and evidence-based medicine, presented in a fashion that speaks to the needs, experiences, and stresses of EM residents acquiring knowledge and behavior amidst the chaotic environment of our specialty.

INTRODUCTION: EVIDENCE AND ERRORS

This book is about clinical reasoning. It embraces both *evidence* and *error*: how to use, evaluate, and find the former while simultaneously searching for and avoiding the latter. It is an attempt to enhance the likelihood that we will make good decisions to solve the problems our patients bring to the chaotic environment of an emergency department (ED). Our decisions are among the most critical in medicine; mistakes can cost patients their lives. We make these decisions in one of the most ill-structured domains imaginable. The emergency department is a cognitive proving ground, where errors are inevitable.

There are many excellent and exhaustive texts on evidence-based medicine (EBM), cognitive psychology, critical thinking, and clinical decision-making; we are not aware of another concise text that has attempted to bring the fruits of all of these domains to bear on the practice of emergency medicine. Throughout this book, we have chosen examples that are directly relevant and recognizable to learners and practitioners within our critical and chaotic environment. This concentration allowed us to focus on the areas that would matter most to emergency physicians.

Our Intended Audience

We wrote this book primarily for EM residents. We believe that if you are to achieve true excellence in emergency medicine, the processes of identifying relevant evidence, bringing it to bear systematically on the care of your patients, and routinely examining your own cognitive thought processes, must become intrinsic and automatic parts of your practice. We further believe that for these processes to become intuitive, their development must start during the first formative moments of your training.

The emergency department is a cognitive battlefield. The experience of arriving upon such a scene, with lives immediately at stake, may seem comparable to throwing a deck of cards into the air and then having to instantly conceptualize (at gunpoint) a universal law that accounts for the arbitrary order in which they land. It is during the first hours, weeks, and months of training that the learning behavior of an emergency physician is largely shaped, and it is just at this time that the essential principles of evidence-based critical thinking are most effectively absorbed.

If, as a resident, you integrate the ideas of critical thinking at the same time you are assimilating all of the facts and procedures of our field, your ability to make decisions should be infinitely greater than if you wait until graduation to learn to think and use evidence properly.

For two reasons, EM junior attendings may also find the contents of this book essential. First, if your residency training did not adequately cover EBM and critical thinking, this book will provide a guide to assimilating this information and help to allow decisions that are free from cognitive error. Second, if you are an attending at an academic program, this text can provide a firm foundation for the teaching of EBM and clinical reasoning to your residents. We hope this book can make you a better clinician and a better educator.

Of course, more seasoned emergency physicians may also gain much from this text, if they have not been previously exposed to evidence-based medicine or the cognitive psychology of decision-making.

Anesthesiosologists, intensivists, trauma surgeons, and any other specialist who commonly deals with emergencies, may also find this book applicable to their practice. Many of the critical decisions we make in emergency medicine are also a part of these fields.

The Necessary Environment

We wrote this book to address the immediacy of an EM resident's leaning needs and practice experience, beginning at the outset of specialty training. It is premised on an environment in which the concepts of evidence-based medicine and critical thought have been accepted as desirable goals and in which there is a visible attempt to integrate them into teaching and practice. An environment overtly hostile to these precepts and goals would pose special challenges to residents and junior faculty of a sort we have not attempted to address. Fortunately, we are not aware of very many of these difficult environments still present in our field and suspect that they will become even rarer over time.

Structure of the Book

The layout of this book differs significantly from most dealing with evidence-based medicine. Classically, the order of teaching is:

- Find the evidence
- Evaluate the evidence
- Apply the evidence to make decisions.

We have chosen to discuss these essential steps in just the opposite order. This contrary arrangement is not merely iconoclasm; when the focus is critical thinking in emergency medicine, it makes more sense to start with a discussion of how to make decisions. No matter what our level of training or our desire to parse through the literature primarily, it is our job to make decisions about our patients' care.

Part I: Making Decisions: Incorporating Evidence and Avoiding Error

In the first section of the book, we discuss how to use trusted evidence to assess a patient, determine a plan, and check our thought processes for cognitive error. If learning critical thinking in emergency medicine is a journey, then this is surely the first step.

Part II: Evaluating the Evidence that Informs Decisions

The next step of our journey and the next part of the book deals with the evaluation of the literature. We discuss the art of weighing the value and faults of evidence for ourselves. If we already have an understanding of how we will use this evidence to make decisions, our evaluation is far more pertinent to our practice; therefore, this part of the book naturally follows the first part in which we discuss decision-making.

The ordering of the first two parts does not dictate the actual chronology of teaching EBM in a program. It rather reflects a conceptual sequence. In the nascent stages of training, we may be evaluating literature given to us by our attendings or for journal clubs. As we progress, we will begin to evaluate new evidence on a regular basis to stay current and refine our knowledge base.

Some emergency physicians may choose not to evaluate evidence on their own. They may seek out preappraised evidence and use this form of literature as the basis for their practices. Even these practitioners will benefit from learning the fundamentals of the evaluation of the literature, as it will allow them to understand the terms and concepts of a pre-appraised source.

Part III: Finding the Evidence

It may seem that the search for evidence would be the easiest EBM skill to learn, but without a thorough understanding of the concepts discussed in Parts I and II, it is easy to become bogged down in a mountain of non-pertinent studies. If we already know how to use and evaluate the literature, we will know exactly the type of evidence we wish to find.

This part of the book also deals with the methods for recording evidence and keeping it available for bedside decisions and teaching.

Again, this does not mean that instruction in the use of online resources to find evidence relevant to clinical evidence should be deferred to the late stages of residency training. Placing this part last in the sequence rather reflects a didactic construct.

We offer the schematic in Fig. I-1 as a representation of the interaction of the three parts of the book.

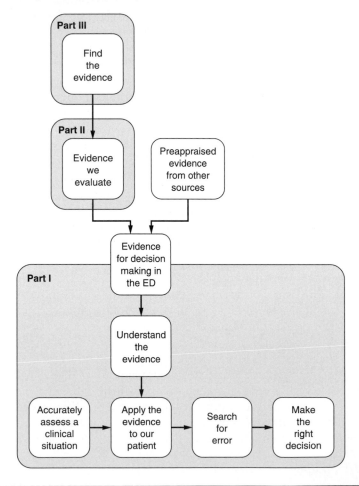

— FIGURE I-1 —   *The structure of this book.*

Feel Free to Choose Your Own Path

Though we have chosen what at first may seem a contrarian ordering for this book, we hope you will find it to be an ideal progression. However, in the spirit of never limiting an individual's learning style, feel free to start with Part II or Part III. To make this option possible, all throughout the text, we have inserted links to previous and future sections, as shown below.

Link to Page XXX

The presence of these links will allow you to start anywhere in the book and still be able to follow the discussion.

Readers who are familiar with traditional presentations of evidence-based medicine in textbooks and elsewhere may find our division of topics surprising. For example, while we discuss the applicability of the results of studies in Part I, the critical appraisal of these studies is in Part II. The hyperlinks and cross-referencing throughout the book are also present to avoid any confusion caused by this deviation from the conventional ordering of these topics in standard EBM texts.

We also stress that you do not have to master Part I before moving on to Parts II and III. We hope you will read the book through and then, as you gain experience, return to those areas for which you require reinforcement.

Finally, we do not intend this text to teach every intricacy of evidence-based medicine. We have chosen to focus only on the intersection of EBM with clinical reasoning. In the additional reading section, we have listed a number of books, which uniquely elaborate the full skill set and teach evidence-based medicine in a rigorous and exhaustive fashion.

Well, enough of this introductory stage setting; let us begin the show . . .

MAKING DECISIONS: INCORPORATING EVIDENCE AND AVOIDING ERROR

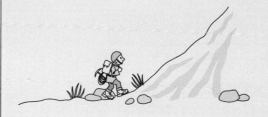

CHAPTER 1

GOOD DECISIONS

Emergency medicine is not a field for the indecisive; we need to make choices quickly and correctly. What we hope to teach in this portion of the book is decision-making by means of *critical thinking*. We can represent this process as shown in Fig. 1-1.

WHERE DOES THE EVIDENCE COME FROM?

We have just stated that making good decisions in the Emergency Department requires the consideration of the *best available evidence*. While searching for evidence and then evaluating its value during a clinical shift is occasionally possible, in most circumstances this is not an option. For a majority of our decisions, the evidence we use will have been *gathered* and *evaluated* before the patient presents. When we are making decisions at the bedside in the Emergency Department, the evidence can come from four places:

Evidence Given to us by an Attending or Colleague This is evidence that has already been assessed by someone we trust and who understands and has applied evidence-based evaluation. If our attendings can supply us with appropriately synthesized evidence, we can use it to make our own decisions (under their guidance) as opposed to just emulating practice.

Evidence we have Evaluated Ourselves This is evidence that we have previously examined and deemed to be good. In Part II, we discuss the methods of this evaluation. If we decide a piece of evidence adequately represents the truth, we can use it for future decisions.

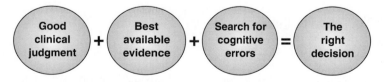

Good clinical judgment + Best available evidence + Search for cognitive errors = The right decision

— FIGURE 1-1

Evidence from Pre-Appraised Literature Sources   A number of resources are available that carefully evaluate studies for methodology and publish the results. If one of these sources has deemed a piece of evidence to represent the truth, we can use this evidence to make decisions. We discuss these sources of pre-appraised evidence in Part III.

Evidence from Consultants   Consultants may have access to and knowledge of important clinical evidence in their respective fields. If they can summarize it or direct us to it, we can use it to inform our decision-making. We are referring here to *evidence* from clinical research; this is different from the personal experience and knowledge of disease process that contribute, not inappropriately, to the opinions of our consultants. We may at times be forced to make decisions based largely on the opinions of others, but this is not the most desirable option.

THE PROGRESSION OF USE OF EVIDENTIARY SOURCES

At the beginning of our training, most of the evidence we use to make decisions will likely come from our attendings and colleagues. As we gain experience, we should turn to pre-appraised sources to fuel our need for evidentiary needs.

Link to Page 287

Throughout the rest of our careers, as we read journals and literature, we can use the skills of Part II to evaluate the quality and usefulness of this evidence. New patient presentations may spur us to search for evidence, both pre-appraised and primarily reported (usually after a good night's sleep). Part III teaches how to perform such a search and then the lessons of Part II will again allow us to evaluate the evidence to see if we can use it for future decisions. Since we cannot be experts on every rare presentation, even after years of practice, some of the decisions we make will be based on evidence from other authorities and consultants.

HOW MUCH INFORMATION FROM A STUDY DO WE ACTIVELY USE?

When we talk about using evidence for bedside decisions, we do not mean carrying a satchel full of photocopied studies around with us during a shift. The time it would take to reread an entire article each time we wanted to use evidence for decision-making would quickly destroy our patient flow.

The abstract of a study would certainly be quicker to read, but it may not contain the exact data we need in order to use the evidence and apply it to our individual patient. Besides, even the abstract is too long to read each time we need to make a decision.

The amount of information we actively use from a study is small, but incredibly important. We need to conceptually distill a study to the barest essentials needed for bedside decision-making. To describe this concept, we use the term NEEDLE.*

- **N**ecessary
- **E**vidence for
- **E**mergency
- **D**ecisions:
- **L**isted and
- **E**valuated

A NEEDLE is an extraction of just the data we need to make decisions. In the journalistic vein, we can describe NEEDLEs as the Why, What, Who, Where, How, and When of a piece of evidence.

- **Why** is why we should bother to perform a test, use a treatment, or utilize prognostic evidence. Why is expressed in quantitative terms.
- **What** describes what downsides are associated with the intervention; in other words, the risks of a treatment or the side-effects of a test.
- **Who** is which patients were actually studied; it is a brief description of the study population.
- **Where** is where the study took place. It includes description of the level and type of hospital as well as whether the study was performed in the Emergency Department or another patient area.
- **How** describes the manner in which the interventions or diagnostic testing was performed.
- **When** is when the evidence was published; it is just a citation of the study reference.

We can reduce these six questions into the following necessities:

1. The risks and benefits (the why and what)
2. Applicability information (the who, where, and how)
3. Citation (the when).

---

*NEEDLE is a new term created by one of the authors (SW). It is just as useful for non-emergency medicine decisions in clinical settings. In that case, just substitute everyday for emergency in the acronym.

The term *applicability* refers to adapting a piece of evidence to our individual patient. It is easy to see why the patient population, setting, and means of performing a test or treatment are essential to see if the evidence is applicable to our patient and clinical scenario.

A Modicum of Information on Study Quality or Precision

The essential parts of a NEEDLE for use in decision-making are listed above. We have stressed that the evidence used in a NEEDLE has already been evaluated; however, a savvy clinician should include a concise summary estimate of the study quality and precision of results as part and parcel of placing the evidence in the proper context. NEEDLE summaries therefore contain one to two sentences about the validity and precision of the results of a study, as in Fig. 1-2. We discuss these terms extensively in Part II; all that is essential to understand now is that these two concepts describe whether a study is good evidence.

If we have just the amount of evidence contained in a NEEDLE, we can use the knowledge from Part I of this book to immediately make decisions.

Diagnostic Evidence: Elisa d-dimer for Pulmonary Embolism

Benefits/Downsides

● LR + 1.73, LR – 0.11

● No risks, cost minimal

Applicability

● Adult patients in outpatient setting

● Performed in normal hospital laboratories; interpreted by laboratory staff

● Specificity lower in patients >70; sensitivity and specificity lower if symptoms >3 days

Brown MD et al. Annals Emerg Med 2002;40(2):133-144
-Valid meta-analysis. (Sens 95% CI 0.88-0.97) (Spec 95% CI 0.36-0.55)

— FIGURE 1-2 — *An example of a diagnostic NEEDLE. All of the terms included in the NEEDLE will be explained in the sections that follow.*

We can make decisions even before we become experts on *evaluating* or *finding* evidence; we simply need to understand what the results mean and how to apply them to our individual patient.

EXAMPLE

We are examining a patient we suspect of having a pulmonary embolism. Our attending relays to us all the information contained in the diagnostic NEEDLE example in Fig. 1-2. Since we have already finished reading Part I, we understand all of the terms and how to apply the evidence to our patient. We decide that if the d-dimer is negative, it will drive the probability of our patient having a PE to below a level where we would have to continue to entertain the diagnosis. We are able to use this evidence, even though we have not read the study from which it was derived.

FORMS OF NEEDLES

A NEEDLE can be merely a framework for us to relay and receive information about evidence. They can also take tangible form and be passed from one clinician to another. Some NEEDLEs we will commit to memory, because we use them so frequently. However, due to the large amount of varied decisions we make in emergency medicine, our memory is often not sufficient to retain all of the NEEDLEs we will need over the course of a shift. Attempting to memorize the essential parts of many studies may cause us to inevitably misquote or subconsciously alter the results and applicability information.

NEEDLEs can be easily written down on note cards or even on a matchbook cover. Perhaps the ideal form of NEEDLEs is electronic: placed on a personal digital assistant (PDA) or recorded online, they are immediately available for bedside decisions. NEEDLEs can also be part of, or be derived from, Critically Appraised Topics (CATs). CATs are a form of evidence summary, which is useful for saving a search, evaluation, and results from an evidentiary query. We extensively discuss the creation of NEEDLEs and CATs in Part III.

Link to Page 323

TYPES OF DECISIONS

This part of the book is divided into three further chapters: Diagnostic Decisions, Treatment Decisions, and Decisions about Prognosis. These deal with three of the four classic categories of evidence in evidence-based medicine (EBM):

- Diagnosis
- Treatment
- Prognosis

In emergency medicine, *harm*, the last classic category, is often inextricably entwined with treatment, so we discuss it in the treatment section.

SOURCES OF ERROR

Part I also delves extensively into cognitive errors and the mistake-prone environment of the emergency department. By discussing these potential errors, we hope to decrease their occurrence.

A METHOD TO OUR MADNESS

We can now expand our schematic representation for this book. The scheme in Fig. 1-3 offers a means of making decisions even before we learn all of the skills of evaluating and finding the evidence.

The subsequent pages describe the very heart of our practice. Our value as clinicians is our ability to make the right decision at the right time. We hope you enjoy and learn from what lies within.

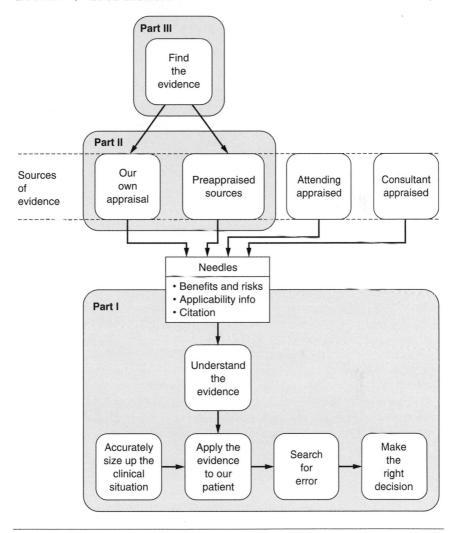

— FIGURE 1-3 — *The refined structure of this book.*

DIAGNOSTIC DECISIONS

CASE: THE CLOT THICKENS

It is a busy Monday at 3 p.m., and Dr Wayne is signing out his patients to you. You both walk over to bed #10 where a young woman looks up from the gurney. He tells you that he picked up the chart of this 25-year-old woman just 15 minutes ago, but the case is an easy one. She has just returned home after an eight-hour plane ride and is now complaining of a "little" shortness of breath and some reproducible chest pain. He goes on to tell you that he ordered a V/Q scan, which has not yet been done. He advises: "If it comes back normal or low probability, send her home. If it comes back intermediate or high, just put her on heparin and admit her as a confirmed PE." He finishes sign-out and leaves the department to you. You decide to start over with bed #10. *To be continued...*

MAKING THE DIAGNOSIS

In the emergency department, we are expected to diagnose potentially life-threatening illnesses based on scant information in limited amounts of time. Our patients are often unknown to us prior to their presentation and they are not at their best or most cooperative. Inundated with stimuli, distractions, and chaos, we practice in an environment far from the ideal for contemplation. Rarely do we have the luxury of devoting our full attention to any individual decision, but must instead juggle numerous cognitive processes at once.

To compound these difficulties, we often lack the assurance of certainty; we instead treat based on the "most likely." How we drive our decisions to this point of acceptable likelihood can be a combination of our clinical judgment and diagnostic testing.

Experienced clinicians make an enormous number of decisions in the course of a single shift in the emergency department. Given this density of decisions, we make surprisingly few errors. However, a large number of the errors that lead to poor patient outcome and malpractice suits are cognitive errors of diagnostic decision-making.[1]

Ill-structured Domain

From the perspective of decision-making, medicine is considered an ill-structured domain; this is in contrast to well-structured fields such as mathematics and the hard sciences. Well-structured domains are defined by rules that translate from one decision to the next.[2] The problems of medical decisions in general are only compounded in emergency medicine.

Components of the Ill-structured Domain of Emergency Medicine Decisions

- Complete information is often not available at the onset of the decision-making process. At times, complete information will never become available.
- Problems are dynamic; changes occur even in the midst of the diagnostic process.
- Approaches to problem-solving are often not generalizable to future patients.
- We lack the feedback to know if our decisions were correct; often the final diagnosis is decided only after the patient has left our care.

For all of these reasons, our decisions are more difficult and we require increased vigilance against cognitive pitfalls. By utilizing an approach to diagnostic decisions embracing critical thinking, we can minimize our potential to fall prey to the above errors. In the subsequent sections, we discuss each step of the process of diagnostic decision-making. We will then discuss the potential sources of error inherent in the process (Fig. 2-1).

DIFFERENTIAL DIAGNOSIS

The creation of a differential diagnosis is directly dependent on a clinician's skills and depth of experience. If we do not consider a disease as a possibility, even a full armamentarium of evidence-based medicine may not prevent us from missing the diagnosis.

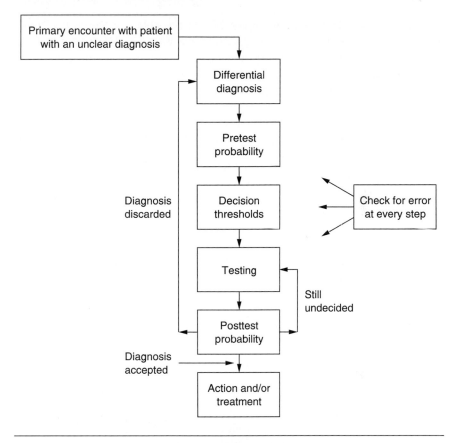

— FIGURE 2-1 — *The steps of diagnostic decision-making.*

A differential diagnosis is formed based on a history, a focused physical exam, and possibly a limited array of bedside tests, such as fingerstick glucose, 12-lead electrocardiograms, etc. We must critically analyze the data from these assessments and measurements and utilize them carefully to avoid error and bias.

Strategies for Forming a Differential

Exhaustive Method

As medical students, we arrived at our differentials via a laborious history, an all-inclusive review of systems, and an extensive physical exam. We then proceeded to list every possible cause of each stated symptom and discovered sign. This might have required a search through a backbreaking general medicine text looking for all of the possible disease entities consistent with each and every finding. Often we would follow this extensive differential with a suggestion for the scores of tests we should order to narrow down the compendium of possibilities.

We also refer to this strategy as "shotgunning" or the "blunderbuss method."[3] This exhaustive process is *inductive*; i.e. we gather information and then use it to formulate a hypothesis.[4,5]

Unfortunately, even experienced clinicians, under the rubric of defensive medicine, sometimes utilize the exhaustive method. This tendency may be reinforced during residency training; residents on medical wards frequently order tests only because they know they will be asked about the results on rounds. They may perceive it to be more expedient to simply order the test than to have to argue that they considered that the likelihood of the relevant target disorder was too low to justify testing for it. This leads to costly, unnecessary testing of no benefit to our patients. It also blunts our ability to think analytically about the use of diagnostic testing.

While it may seem counterintuitive, the history and physicals of expert clinicians are actually shorter than those of novices.[6] This brevity is not the result of carelessness, but instead reflects the ability of the seasoned physician to focus the interview while in the midst of it. The following diagnostic method explains this process.

Hypothetico-deductive Method

As we gather experience, the exhaustive strategy is replaced by a hypothetico-deductive method.[4,7] The patient's chief complaint guides our history-taking and systems review, which we then use to focus our physical exam. We are constantly considering and discarding diagnoses even as we are gathering further information to formulate a differential. As the name would indicate, this is a *deductive process*; we form a hypothesis and then we gather data to support or refute it.[5] In this way, we can create a list of differential diagnoses with a minimum of information. Kassirer termed this strategy the "method of steepest ascent"; a skilled emergency physician can come to the correct diagnosis with an extremely limited data set.[8]

Illness Scripts

The means by which we decide if a diagnosis is plausible is by comparing the current patient's presentation with our stored illness scripts.[9] Illness scripts are chunks of information about the presentation of a disease, including symptoms, signs, and the mental picture of patients previously encountered with that disease.[6] The illness script is a culmination of all of the patients we have seen with the disorder as well as any virtual exposures we have garnered through readings and case presentations. As our experience grows, we assimilate atypical presentations into the illness scripts. The scripts are stored in our long-term memory; when a patient presents, we move them into our short-term memory. Due to the limits of short-term memory, we generally can consider only three to five scripts at a time to see if they match our current patient's presentation.[3] We eliminate the scripts that do not match to allow others into consideration.

The hypothetico-deductive method is much quicker than the exhaustive strategy. We begin forming hypotheses as soon as we pick up the chart. Most presentations can be matched against one or a few illness scripts within one to seven minutes.[11] The rapidity with which we form our differential is indicative of our assurance. In other words, when we can form a differential diagnosis quickly, we are more likely to be correct.[2,6,12–13]

Backwards versus Forward Reasoning

The hypothetico-deductive method is an example of *backward reasoning*. This is something of a misnomer, because backward thinking is not outdated or inferior as the name may suggest, but instead is the quicker and more accurate means of clinical diagnosis.[14] The "backwards" refers to the fact that the situation immediately suggests diagnoses; we then work backwards to see if they fit. The inferior mode of forward reasoning is demonstrated by the exhaustive methods of novices.

Some diagnoses are made within moments of seeing a patient, an EKG, or a radiograph; the method that allows for this instantaneous provisional diagnosis is *pattern matching*.

Pattern Matching

When we see ST-elevations on an EKG, or an ashen, diaphoretic patient clutching his or her chest, we do not engage in extensive cognitive processing. Striking patient appearance or pathognomonic presentations can immediately suggest a diagnosis. However, clinicians experienced with a particular disease may effectively rely on pattern recognition even for atypical presentations. Diagnoses formed by pattern matching occur within seconds of exposure and require little conscious thought.[2,6]

Pattern matching is operative mostly for visual diagnoses such as rashes, radiographs, and patient appearance. It is also used for haptic pathology such as the pulsating mass in the abdomen of a patient with an abdominal aortic aneurysm. Illness scripts may still play a role as the source of the pattern to which we match the patient presentation. In fact, if we are already considering a diagnosis, we are more likely to be able to appreciate the stimulus which cues the pattern matching.[15,16]

EXAMPLE

If a patient's triage sheet documents a history of renal failure and five days of missed dialysis, our ability to immediately pattern match the electrocardiogram to the diagnosis of hyperkalemia is augmented.

Recognition-primed Decision Model

Klein first described this model, which emerged from studies of the critical decisions made by firefighters and military personnel.[17] The process allows the clinician to rapidly set diagnostic priorities, recognize and filter diagnostic cues, project what is expected on further examination, and mentally test numerous diagnoses to see if they fit with the patient presentation. It is essentially a distillation of clinical judgment to rapid decision-making. Psychologists describe similar processes as *gestalt*. The recognition-primed decision model integrates the previous three methods we have just discussed. As can be seen in Fig. 2-2, depending on the complexity of the presentation, we shift between the various decision-making strategies.

Literature Support

Reports of Clinical Manifestations of Disease   This type of study assesses the frequency of various signs and symptoms among series of patients independently identified as having a target disease.[18] By using the data from this research, we can decide whether a disease we are considering accounts for all of the important elements of a patient's presentation. If it does not, an alternative or additional diagnosis may need to be entertained.

Differential Diagnosis Lists   There are whole textbooks and review articles, which provide a precompiled list of differentials for any given sign or symptom. This form of literature can also be helpful to suggest possibilities that we might not have considered or remembered.[19,20]

Summary

The differential diagnosis provides a list of diagnostic hypotheses. After generating this list, we must systematically evaluate each possibility to determine whether it merits active consideration. We may be confident in quickly dismissing many of the possibilities on the basis of our illness scripts or pattern matching. If we feel obligated to actively consider more

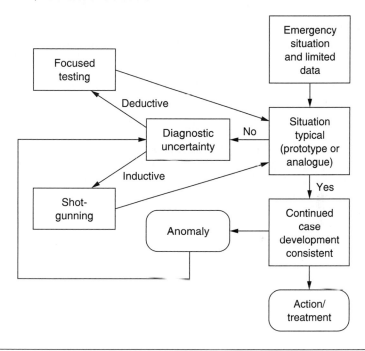

— FIGURE 2-2 — *Recognition primed decision-making.*

than one diagnosis, we need to use validated clinical criteria, laboratory testing or imaging to further narrow the possibilities. The next sections provide a pathway to critically evaluating the possible diagnoses to come to the truth and avoid error.

THE STATISTICS OF LIKELIHOOD

Before we delve into further discussion of the art of diagnostic decision-making, we must digress for a quick review of the mathematics of likelihood.

Likelihood

Likelihood is the soul of diagnostic decision-making. It is traditionally expressed in two ways: probability and odds. Each has its uses, so we must be proficient with both.

Probability

Probability is the measurement of likelihood most familiar to us. It is the ratio of one outcome to all outcomes.

$$\text{Probability} = \frac{\text{Particular outcome}}{\text{All outcomes including that particular outcome}}$$

It is usually expressed as a percentage from 0 to 100%. To change the equation above to a percentage, simply multiply by 100. If doing calculations with probability, it should remain as a decimal ranging from 0 to 1.

EXAMPLE

You want to see how many times heads comes up when you flip a coin 100 times. If it comes up 50 times, then you can calculate the probability as:

$$\frac{50\,\text{heads}}{100\,\text{flips}} = 0.5 = 50\%$$

The probability would be 0.5 or 50%.

Odds

Odds are less familiar to physicians, but aficionados of horseracing and Las Vegas excursions are quite used to the terminology. Odds describe the possibility of an event as a *ratio* of one outcome and all of the outcomes that are not that outcome.

$$\text{Odds} = \frac{\text{One outcome}}{\text{All other outcomes except that outcome}}$$

In Las Vegas, the casinos express odds as a number to one. For example, the odds against a ball stopping on the number 19 on the roulette wheel are 35 to 1.* In medicine, we just eliminate the one; we would call those same roulette wheel odds 35.

---

*The roulette wheel odds are a bit misleading, as the wheel contains the numbers 0 through 36. This would make the actual odds against the number nineteen 36 to 1, but the odds (and therefore the payoff for a winning bet) are listed as 35 to 1 to keep the casino's coffers full. Hence, no one familiar with likelihood plays roulette.

EXAMPLE

If the same coin flip experiment as above is expressed in odds, it would look like:

$$\text{Odds of heads} = \frac{50\,\text{heads}}{50\,\text{not heads (tails)}} = 1.$$

Odds of 1, otherwise known as *even odds*, are the same as a probability of 50%. Any probability less than 50% will be represented by odds between 0 and 1. Probabilities greater than 50% are represented by odds greater than 1. As probabilities get smaller and smaller, they begin to match the odds. For instance, a probability of 10% (0.1) is the same as odds of 0.11. Odds of 20 are the same as a probability of 95%; odds of 100 are equivalent to a probability of 99%. Since odds can go up to infinity, for most decisions we consider odds greater than 100 to be 100% probability.

Converting between odds and probability is quite simple, using these equations:

$$\text{Odds} = \frac{\text{Probability}}{1 - \text{Probability}} \qquad \text{Probability} = \frac{\text{Odds}}{1 + \text{Odds}}$$

At this point, you might be questioning why we ever need to think in terms of odds, since probability is more familiar, and often more intuitive. As we will be discussing in subsequent sections, many types of association can only be measured using odds.

PRE-TEST PROBABILITY

Pre-test probability takes the comprehensive list of the differential diagnoses and assigns likelihood to each.

Probabilistic Thinking

In the previous section, we discussed the generation of a differential diagnosis; we now must decide the likelihood of each disease on the list. This method of probabilistic thinking will guide the further diagnostic process. We call this likelihood the *pre-test probability*. As the name would indicate, it requires the assignment of probability *before* we perform further diagnostic testing.

It may seem counterintuitive to assign a value to likelihood prior to testing. It evokes the clamoring of "Is that not why we are doing the test in the first place?" Given the presence of perfect diagnostic tests, it would be a valid complaint. The problem is that very few, if any, of our diagnostic tests are perfect, so we must interpret all of them in light of our pre-test probability. This is an adaptation of the principles of *Bayesian analysis*.

Bayesian Analysis

The reverend Thomas Bayes was an English mathematician in the 1700s. His theorem discussed the alteration of prior probability by new events. After these events, a new post-event probability is created. All of our diagnostic decisions are an adaptation of this theorem. An "event," in the context of clinical diagnostic reasoning, may be a patient's answer to a question we ask, information from our physical examination, or the result of a diagnostic test we perform on the patient. We can express the use of Bayes' theorem in this context with the equation:

Pretest probability × Effects of diagnostic test result = Post-test probability.

The application of this theorem takes what is often an informal process:

> I think he may have appendicitis...
> ... so I'll get a CT scan.
> CT shows appendicitis ...
> ... so I'll call the surgeon.

and adds structure, a pathway for critical examination of our thought processes. Mainly, the theorem makes clear that our interpretation of assessments and tests must depend not only on the results, but also on a factor that is entirely independent of the result. We call this the "pre-test" or "pre-assessment" probability of the condition we are considering. This formal decision-making process can appear onerous to perform in our frantic environment, yet we are already performing each step, but perhaps not with the necessary awareness and rigor.

EXAMPLE

You have a patient complaining of acute pain to his right ankle which you note on exam is swollen and painful. Before you had a chance to evaluate the patient, the triage nurse sent a white blood cell (WBC) count. You notice the result of the WBC count is $14 \times 10^3/\text{mL}$. If the patient was asymptomatic until twisting his ankle at a soccer game 30 minutes prior to arrival, your pre-test probability for infection would be extremely low. If, instead, the patient was complaining of a fever, your pre-test probability for an infectious cause would be much higher. How we interpret the WBC count, an imperfect test for infection, is directly dependent on pre-test probability. If, however, the WBC count was a perfect test for infection,* then pretest probability would be irrelevant and a reevaluation of your soccer player for an infectious source would have to be undertaken. This also illustrates the dangers of sending tests before determining their need and utility.

To use Bayesian analysis to its fullest advantage, we need to estimate our pre-test probability. It is often easier to say that a diagnosis is "unlikely, but possible" than to say your pre-test probability is 10%. The risk stratification of low, moderate, or high probability is often familiar to emergency physicians. This level of pre-test stratification will suffice for most diagnostic decisions. To use these qualitative descriptions requires us to already have familiarity with the situation and the abilities of our diagnostic tests.

Committing to an estimate of pre-test probability allows us to explore the power of new tests and deal with situations we have not thought through in the past. The formal decision-making process we will discuss in subsequent chapters requires a quantitative assessment of pre-test probability. Defining an estimate of pre-test probability also permits subsequent interpretation by other clinicians.

A written notation of moderate pre-test probability is far easier for the physicians on the floor to utilize than jotting down "I sort of suspect he has a dissection." Even more useful is the commitment to a 35% pre-test probability in the chart.[21]

A study by Bryant illustrates the difficulties of using qualitative words in lieu of numeric probability. In this study, physicians were asked to express numeric equivalents of the words we often use to express pre-test probability.[22] The wide ranges in Fig. 2-3 show that the words led to very different assignments of probability amongst the study participants.

The study provides an estimate of the probability ranges to which clinicians frequently assign qualitative estimates of the various descriptive terms:

- Low probability ~10%
- Unlikely ~20%
- Possible ~40%
- Suggestive/moderate ~50%
- Likely/probable ~80%
- Pathognomonic/classic ~90%.

*In this context, a perfect test refers to one that will always be negative in the absence of disease and will always be positive when the patient has the disease. Perfect tests and assessments are exceedingly rare, as we discuss in subsequent sections.

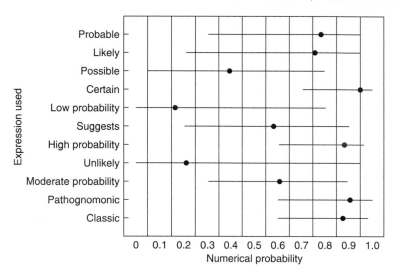

— FIGURE 2-3 — *Ranges of probability associated with qualitative descriptions. The points are the means and the lines are ranges of the physician responses.*

It is not important if the estimate of pre-test probability is off by a small amount, it is only a problem when it is off by orders of magnitude. There will be very little difference if a pre-test probability is estimated at 70% rather than 60%.

EXAMPLE

One of your colleagues from the medicine service stops by the department to give you follow-up on a patient admitted last week with abdominal pain. It turns out the patient had acute intermittent porphyria. In an attempt to avoid missing this diagnosis with future patients, you vow to consider this in the differential of every patient presenting with abdominal pain. Since it is in the differential, you decide to assign a pre-test probability of 10% to the diagnosis in the next patient you see with abdominal pain, despite the absence of any suggestive symptoms or signs. A true estimate of the pre-test probability of this disease in undifferentiated abdominal pain is closer to 0.001%.[23]

It is fine to consider rare diagnoses, but this consideration should be tempered with accurate estimations of pre-test likelihood. The evidence for their consideration (from our history, physical, and bedside testing) should be compelling and they require the use of the threshold approach to decision-making, which we discuss shortly.

If we are considering more than one diagnosis, the combination of pre-test probabilities should total 100%. Assigning a patient a 50% pre-test probability of appendicitis, 50% for gas pain, and 45% for diverticulitis offends the tenets of mathematics and evidence-based medicine alike.

Aids to the Estimation of Pre-test Probability

Literature Support

The literature can guide us in the estimation of pre-test probability, thereby removing some of the difficulties of quantitative assignment. Ninety percent of patients in a survey done by Richardson had conditions in which evidence existed in the literature to guide the estimation of pre-test probability.[24] Published studies can serve as an aid to the estimation of pre-test probability in three ways.

Published Prevalence

If we can find diagnostic studies with patient populations similar to the patient we are evaluating, we then have a powerful tool for determining pre-test likelihood. By looking at the final number of patients who had gold-standard evidence of a disease, we can obtain a point of departure for estimating the pre-test probability of our individual patient.

EXAMPLE

You have a young patient who presents with the worst headache of her life. You remember reading an article on the use of CT scans to diagnose subarachnoid hemorrhage (SAH). The article had 17% of its patients with the worst headache of their life diagnosed with SAH with lumbar puncture evidence or angiographic evidence.[25] Starting with 17% as the average likelihood of these patients, you can consider whether your own patient may have a somewhat greater or smaller individual pre-test probability.

Studies of Differential Diagnosis

This form of literature examines a particular presentation and reports the diseases, which the study patients were eventually proven to have. These studies can give us a rough estimate of pre-test probability.

EXAMPLE

A study is performed to discover the eventual diagnosis of 200 patients presenting with syncope.[26] Fifty are found to have a cardiovascular cause, 50 are found to have a neurogenic cause, and the remainder have no etiology found for their loss of consciousness. Based on this study, we can set our pre-test probability for a cardiac cause at approximately 25% if a patient presents with syncope.

Clinical Prediction Rules

The second way the literature can aid pre-test probability assignment is by establishing clinical prediction rules (CPRs) that yield pre-test probability stratification. This form of literature identifies independent signs and symptoms that would indicate the presence of the disease. These signs and symptoms are then validated through additional studies to assure that the components of the CPR accurately predict disease probability. By assigning points to these components, an estimation of pre-test probability is generated.[27,28] When this form of evidence is available, it provides the highest level of literature support. Clinical prediction rules are discussed more extensively in Part II.

Link to bottom Page 228

EXAMPLE

You have a patient with unilateral leg swelling and recent surgery. An article by Wells allows points assigned to these characteristics to place the patient in a moderate pre-test probability group with a range of 40–50%.[29]

Using literature aids increases the precision of our pre-test probabilities. Studies show a lack of reproducibility when physicians are asked to evaluate pre-test probabilities using gestalt.[30] However, the accuracy of the estimates of *experienced clinicians* in disorders such as pulmonary embolism and acute coronary syndromes is quite good.[31] The problem with relying on gestalt is that we may not be as experienced with a disorder as we may think, unless we have done a self-comparison of our estimates and a decision rule. For this reason, if a prediction rule or other literature support is available, then it is beneficial to consider the pre-test probability it generates.

We do not need to disregard our gestalt estimate to use these literature-based aids, but instead the two should work in tandem to arrive at the most accurate pre-test probability for the unique patient presentation.

Computer-aided Pre-test Probability

Work is being done on complex Bayesian networks, as well as artificial intelligence to aid diagnostic decision-making. While these technologies are in their early stages, computer aid is currently available for the estimation of pre-test, probably in the form of large patient databases. If the patient's demographic data and symptomatology are cross-referenced with a large database of patients with known disease status, a pre-test probability can be derived.

Deciding upon the Pre-test Probability

At first, it may seem daunting to choose an exact number for our estimate of pre-test probability. Often, emergency physicians choose to use only pre-test risk categories. If pre-test probability can be qualitatively split into low, moderate, and high probability, the diagnostic process can still go forward.

EXAMPLE

A reliable practice guideline informs us that we may use an ELISA d-dimer assay in patients we suspect have pulmonary embolism, if we estimate them to be in the low pre-test probability group.[32]

If validated clinical guidelines are available, then this strategy is even more viable.

EXAMPLE

A validated strategy for the evaluation of pulmonary embolism offers a path for the work-up of patients placed into low, moderate, or high risk groups.[33] Numeric estimations are unnecessary, because each of the qualitative categories has an associated diagnostic pathway.

For some diseases, no clear literature exists to provide us with *diagnostic strategies* based on qualitative risk stratification. In these situations, we *need* to use numeric estimates. If we master the skills necessary to make these quantitative estimations, we then have the ability to evaluate *any* diagnostic test or process on our own. The methods we use to make this evaluation are the subject of the next section.

DECISION THRESHOLDS

Just as important as the assignment of accurate pre-test probabilities is choosing the probabilities at which we will discard a diagnosis or accept it. We will refer to these probabilities as "decision thresholds." Pauker and Kassirer first described the use of the threshold approach in diagnostic decision-making.[34]

In an ideal world, we would accept a diagnosis only with a probability of 100% and would reject it only with a probability of 0%. And we would have cheap, quick, non-invasive tests that could easily achieve this level of certainty in all situations. Such a high level of assurance is rarely achievable in medicine and even less so in the tumultuous environment of the emergency department. In the rare circumstances when it is possible to achieve this degree of certainty, the costs are often prohibitive.

We can often decrease, but rarely completely eliminate, uncertainty regarding whether a particular diagnosis is present or absent. Therefore, for every diagnosis we must factor in the risks of underdiagnosis and over-diagnosis. We must consider the costs, risks, and time expenditures of testing as well.

The concept of decision thresholds is that instead of an absolute assurance, we necessarily seek to drive the likelihood of a diagnosis past a point where we are comfortable either accepting or discarding it. This level will be affected by patient values and concerns; the severity of the potential outcomes; the availability, costs, and invasiveness of relevant diagnostic technology; and many other situational factors.

The best way of representing decision thresholds is graphically. First, we will make a bar showing probabilities from 0 through 100% (Fig. 2-4).

Discard Threshold

We can next add a line representing the probability below which we will discard the diagnosis in question. We will call this probability the "discard threshold" (Fig. 2-5A).

In life-threatening diseases or ones associated with significant morbidity, we might place this threshold at 1% or even lower (Fig. 2-5B). For instance, the diagnoses of myocardial infarction, aortic dissection, pulmonary

0% [   ] 100%

— FIGURE 2-4 —   *Probability bar.*

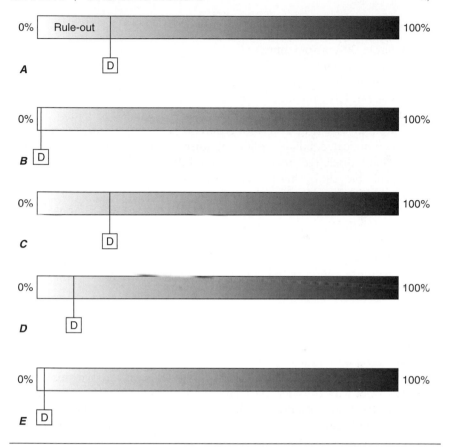

— FIGURE 2-5 — **A** *Discard threshold: probabilities below this level will cause us to discard the diagnosis.* **B** *Discard threshold of 1% in life-threatening conditions.* **C** *Discard threshold of 20% for strep pharyngitis in adults.* **D** *Discard threshold for cholecystitis in a healthy, young patient with suspected cholelithiasis.* **E** *Discard threshold for the same scenario, but in a less reliable patient.*

embolism, and all other life threats, would certainly have a discard threshold of approximately 1%.

In relatively benign diseases in which an underdiagnosis would represent very little damage to the patient, the discard point can be set higher (Fig. 2-5C). For instance, the discard threshold for strep pharyngitis in healthy adults may be as high as 20%, as the risks of missing the diagnosis are extremely small and the disease will usually resolve on its own, even without treatment.

Even given the same disease state, patient characteristics can dictate the set point for the discard threshold.

EXAMPLE

A reliable 30-year-old presents with mild epigastric and right upper-quadrant abdominal pain. Your ultrasound exam indicates the presence of gallstones. You observe the patient for four hours in the emergency department. His pain gets better and he is able to eat one of the mystery meat sandwiches from the refrigerator. We might set the discard threshold at 10% (Fig. 2-5D) for a diagnosis of cholecystitis (as opposed to uncomplicated biliary colic), because if this patient is sent home with good discharge instructions and follow-up at the surgery clinic for probable cholelithiasis, we can expect him to return if he has intractable pain or he develops a fever.

However, if a homeless patient with known substance abuse issues presents with the same scenario, the discard threshold point may have to be lowered (Fig. 2-5E). This patient is less likely to return if his condition declines. Setting his discard threshold at 2% for cholecystitis may be more appropriate because of these factors.

Accept Threshold

Next, we need to add a point on the bar above which we will "rule-in" the disease in question (Fig. 2-6A). At any probability above this accept threshold, we will consider the patient to have the diagnosis and, if necessary, treat accordingly (in this discussion, treatment may run the gamut from medications to consultation to admission to simply considering the diagnostic process complete).

The accept threshold is modified by the risks of treatment as well as the risks of overdiagnosis. A patient falsely diagnosed with a pulmonary embolism will suffer both the risks of anticoagulation as well as problems with obtaining health and life insurance. A patient falsely branded with this diagnosis in a medical history will also be potentially misdiagnosed any time he or she presents to a medical professional subsequently with a complaint of chest pain or shortness of breath. Therefore the accept point should be set relatively high in this patient, perhaps at 85% (Fig. 2-6B).

In a patient with epigastric burning, the accept point for peptic ulcer disease can be set much lower, as there is very little risk to falsely over-diagnosing this disease in the emergency department, as long as the patient is given appropriate follow-up (and we are not missing a more serious diagnosis such as MI). The risk of treatment with proton pump inhibitors is quite small and there are no stigmata from this diagnosis. We can therefore pick an accept level of around 60% (Fig. 2-6C).

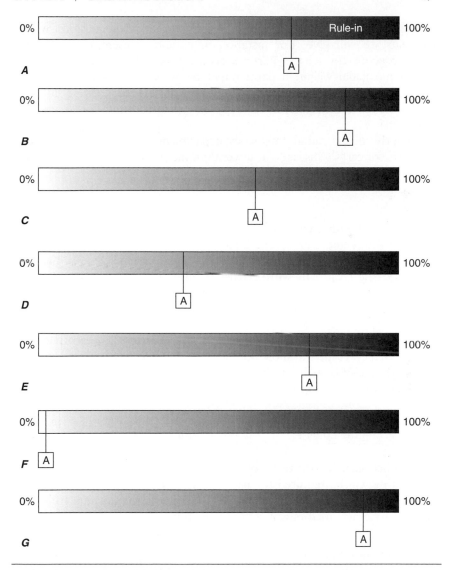

— FIGURE 2-6 — *A The accept threshold: above this probability, we will "rule-in" the diagnosis. B Accept threshold is set high in diseases in which overdiagnosis or treatment is risky. C In diseases in which overdiagnosis or treatment is not dangerous, the accept threshold can be lowered. D An accept threshold of 40% for acute coronary syndrome may be established to give heparin. E An accept threshold of 75% may be established to more aggressively treat acute coronary syndrome in the emergency department. F A low accept threshold for the diagnosis of partial extensor tendon laceration in the emergency department. G The surgeon providing follow-up the next day will set the accept threshold for the same diagnosis much higher.*

Sometimes, the level of accept threshold will vary depending on which treatments we will give. For instance, in patients presenting with chest pain, the acute coronary syndrome accept threshold for giving aspirin and low-molecular-weight heparin might be 40% (Fig. 2-6D). However, to give that same patient IIb/IIIa inhibitors, our accept threshold may be 75% (Fig. 2-6E), as this therapy is expensive and has increased side-effects.

Similarly, in the initial emergency department visit, we will set accept thresholds for certain diseases far lower than the physician who will provide follow-up.

EXAMPLE

In a patient with a cut from a knife to the dorsum of the first phalanx of the forefinger, our accept threshold for the diagnosis of a partial tendon laceration should be set quite low, perhaps 2%, if there is any question of pain with extension, even in the presence of good strength testing (Fig. 2-6F). If we accept this diagnosis in the emergency department, we will splint the patient and give follow-up with a hand surgeon.

When the hand surgeon reexamines the tendon in her office, she will set the accept threshold for the same diagnosis at a much higher level (Fig. 2-6G), as it will be the difference between weeks of splinting or a simple laceration repair.

Indeterminate Zone

The area between the two thresholds is the indeterminate zone (Fig. 2-7A); more testing will be required for us to make a decision if a probability is in this area. Sometimes we elect to admit patients to the hospital from this zone and let other doctors worry about the final decision.

Pre-test Probability

After plotting the two decision thresholds, we can add our pre-test probability to the bar (Fig. 2-7B).

If the pre-test probability lies below the discard threshold we have chosen (Fig. 2-7C), then further testing for this diagnosis is unnecessary and we should seek another explanation for the patient's complaints. If it lies above the accept threshold (Fig. 2-7D), then further testing may not be necessary and the diagnosis has been made. If it lies between the two thresholds (Fig. 2-7E), then further testing is needed.

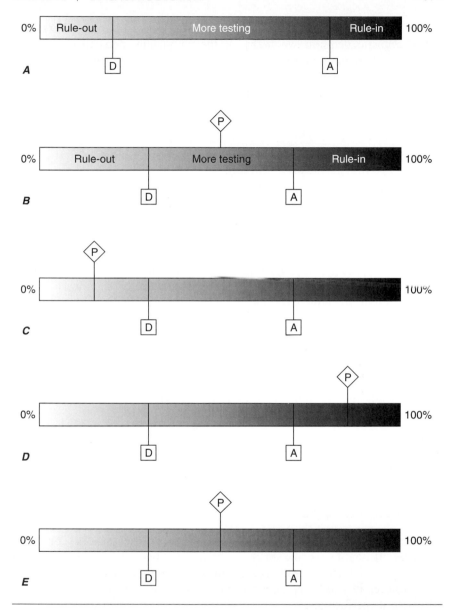

— FIGURE 2-7 — **A** *The probability bar with both accept and discard thresholds.* **B** *Pre-test probability can be placed on the bar.* **C** *Pre-test probability below the discard threshold: no testing needed.* **D** *Pre-test probability above the accept threshold: no testing needed.* **E** *Pre-test probability is between the thresholds: additional diagnostic tests are necessary.*

We do not advocate the routine drawing of probability bars for each diagnostic decision we make in the emergency department. Often we perform these manipulations mentally, without the need for a sketchpad. We have found that actually drawing the probability bars is an extremely effective technique for teaching house staff and medical students during a shift.

Estimation of Thresholds

Often the discard threshold is simple to estimate, being very low in dangerous conditions and higher in diseases without sequelae. The accept threshold is often more difficult to pin down precisely. The key point is that the accept threshold is rarely as critical an issue as the discard threshold. If short-term treatment does not carry risk, then a lower accept threshold will not be a problem. A higher accept threshold may result in unnecessary testing, but most tests are without significant side-effects, though they increase the cost of care. In contrast, setting the discard threshold too high can result in the serious consequences of missed diagnoses.

There are complex formulas that we can use to quantitate the thresholds, but they are unwieldy.[44] Instead, just as in pre-test probability, we should choose a number that best represents the combination of our clinical estimation and the available evidence and not worry about a few percentage points in either direction.

CHARACTERISTICS OF DIAGNOSTIC TESTS

Perfect Diagnostic Test Performance

A perfectly performing test would not have any false positives or false negatives. If the test came back positive, the patient would have the disease and a negative result would only be present in a healthy patient. Furthermore, it would be inexpensive, rapid, and bring no associated risks with its performance.

If such tests existed, we would not need to invest time and effort in the calculation of pre-test probability, the assignment of decision thresholds, or even agonize over a complete differential diagnosis. We could just order the ER Screen[TM], a panel of assays for life threats; our job would be to treat whichever tests returned positive.

We do not have access to many tests even approaching this level of perfection. The ones that are available often exact a high cost to provide us with a high degree of certainty. Therefore, when we order an imperfectly performing diagnostic test, we can only interpret its results based on its characteristics.

Testing Vocabulary

Gold Standards

The government used to back all paper money by its value in precious metal; hence the term "gold standard." Medicine adopted the term to refer to the most accurate means of diagnosing a disease. Often these tests are expensive, time-consuming, invasive, or unsuitable for the clinical environment. When the gold standard is a 6-month follow-up or autopsy, the standard is obviously not feasible in the emergency department.

Even the gold standard test is not necessarily diagnostically perfect, as sometimes these tests have false positives and negatives. It would be better if we could evaluate new diagnostic tests against the Clinical Truth. However, just as in all of life, the truth in medicine is a concept that is wily and difficult to locate. We must instead make do with the best standard available. Hence, a better descriptive term for the gold standard is the *criterion* or *reference standard*, as this does not imply perfection; it just implies that this is the best means of diagnosing a disease currently available to us.

Often the tests we actually perform in the emergency department are surrogates for the criterion standard. Their value was established in well-done (hopefully) comparisons to a *criterion standard*.

The comparison of these surrogate tests to the criterion standard is often plotted on a 2 × 2 table (Fig. 2-8). The table is traditionally drawn with the known disease status or criterion standard testing on the horizontal and the results of the new test on the vertical. Each of the four boxes on this table will represent one of the following:

- *True positive:* a patient with the disease who tests positive on the new diagnostic test
- *False negative:* a patient with the disease who tests negative on the new diagnostic test
- *True negative:* a patient without the disease who tests negative on the new diagnostic test
- *False positive:* a patient without the disease who tests positive on the new diagnostic test

Disease

Present   Absent

— FIGURE 2-8 —   *The 2 × 2 table you learned to hate in medical school.*

Accuracy

An accurate test will give results that mirror the truth. We can represent the accuracy of a diagnostic test quantitatively by the equation:

$$\text{Accuracy} = \frac{\text{True positives} + \text{True negatives}}{\text{All patients in the study}}.$$

Accuracy attempts to represent the utility of a test using just a single number. This is an oversimplification, because a test is frequently good at ruling-in or ruling-out a disease, but rarely both. The accuracy equation gives little indication of this fact.

Precision

A precise test will have reproducible results time after time. These results do not necessarily represent the truth; they just need to be consistent (Fig. 2-9). A rifle, which shoots 10 inches to the right of the target every time it is fired is very precise, though not much use for hunting.

▦ Interpreting Test Results

When we scan a journal article on diagnostic testing, we may see many different parameters used to evaluate a test.* The problem with the common, traditional test evaluation parameters is that they do not address the meaning of a test result. In the emergency department, we need to know

*The classic parameters are sensitivity and specificity, which we define later.

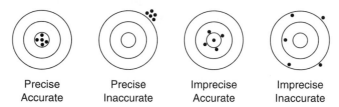

| Precise | Precise | Imprecise | Imprecise |
| Accurate | Inaccurate | Accurate | Inaccurate |

— FIGURE 2-9 — *Precision and accuracy.*

what to do with the results of the tests we perform on the individual patient we are treating. The ideal test parameter would not only indicate the meaning of a test result, but would also allow us to use it directly in the Bayesian equation we have discussed in the previous section:

Pretest probability × Effects of diagnostic test result = Post-test probability

Furthermore, we should be able to predict whether any of the test results will allow us to make a change in our clinical suspicion before we even perform the test. If we realize, prior to its performance, that a test will not affect our actions, regardless of whether it is positive or negative, then we can save much time and expense by not using it.

Luckily, we have a way of evaluating test results that fulfills all of these criteria: *likelihood ratios*. Though it is a departure from the typical didactic order, we will discuss likelihood ratios, then segue into the older parameters of sensitivity, specificity, and predictive values.

Likelihood Ratios

Likelihood ratios (LRs) allow us to understand the meaning of a test result and use this to alter our pre-test probability. They are the best representation of the accuracy of a test result.

We can define LRs as the ratio of the probability of a test result in patients with disease to the probability of the same test result in patients without disease:

$$\text{LR result} = \frac{\dfrac{\text{Patients with disease and with result}}{\text{All patients with disease}}}{\dfrac{\text{Patients without disease and with result}}{\text{All patients without disease}}}.$$

The mnemonic for this formula is WOWO, referring to With disease Over WithOut disease.[35]

- Tests results with likelihood ratios greater than 1 are more likely to occur in patients with the disease than in patients without the disease. LRs above 1 increase our post-test probability of a disease.
- Tests results with likelihood ratios less than 1 are more likely to occur in patients without the disease than in patients with the disease. LRs below 1 decrease our post-test probability of a disease.
- If the likelihood ratio of a test result equals 1, then it is just as likely to occur in a patient with the disease as in a patient without the disease. These test results have no effect on post-test probability and therefore do not help us make a diagnosis.

To reinforce these concepts, consider a likelihood ratio of 10. This means that the result is ten times *more likely* to occur in a patient with the disease than a patient without the disease. This is not bad for a test result, which we would consider "positive"; however, we would certainly prefer an LR of 100 for this purpose.

By the same token, a test result with a likelihood ratio of 0.1 is ten times *less likely* to occur in a patient with the disease than in a patient without the disease. We can consider this result negative, though a likelihood ratio of 0.01 would be even better.

Another way of contemplating likelihood ratios is by their effect on *pre-test odds*. A test result with a likelihood ratio of 20 will yield *posttest odds*, which are twenty times greater than pre-test odds.

EXAMPLE

If our pre-test odds were 4, then a test result with a likelihood ratio of 20 will yield post-test odds of 80.

You may be questioning why we have suddenly gone from the pre-test probabilities of the previous chapter to the irksome pre- and post-test odds. Likelihood ratios can only be directly multiplied with odds, but we will shortly describe how to easily shift back and forth between probabilities and odds. Through these methods, likelihood ratios will allow us to directly modify our pre-test probabilities to yield accurate post-test probabilities.

At first, it may be easier to approach likelihood ratios as they apply to dichotomous test results.

Likelihood Ratio Positive

This value represents the change in pre-test probability caused by a positive test result. It ranges from 1 to infinity and can be represented mathematically as:

$$\text{LR positive} = \frac{\dfrac{\text{Patients with disease who tested positive}}{\text{All patients with disease}}}{\dfrac{\text{Patients without disease who tested positive}}{\text{All patients without disease}}}$$

or

$$\text{LR positive} = \frac{\dfrac{\text{True positives}}{\text{True positives} + \text{False negatives}}}{\dfrac{\text{False positives}}{\text{False positives} + \text{True negatives}}}.$$

Test results having values greater than 5 are moderately useful and those with values greater than 10 have the power to truly alter decision-making. Test results with values from 1 to 5 do very little to alter pre-test probability.

Likelihood Ratio Negative

This value represents the change in pre-test probability caused by a negative test result. It ranges from 0 to 1 and can be expressed mathematically as:

$$\text{LR negative} = \frac{\dfrac{\text{Patients with disease who tested negative}}{\text{All patients with disease}}}{\dfrac{\text{Patients without disease who tested negative}}{\text{All patients without disease}}}$$

or

$$\text{LR positive} = \frac{\dfrac{\text{False negatives}}{\text{True positives} + \text{False negatives}}}{\dfrac{\text{True negatives}}{\text{False positives} + \text{True negatives}}}$$

Test results with values of less than 0.5 are moderately useful and values less than 0.1 are truly significant and can alter decision-making. Values from 0.5 to 1 do very little to alter the original pre-test probability.

Non-dichotomous Likelihood Ratios

One of the many advantages of likelihood ratios is that they can also easily represent the effects of non-dichotomous test results.

To calculate the likelihood ratio of each test result, we return to our original formula:

$$LR\ result = \frac{\dfrac{\text{Patients with disease and with result}}{\text{All patients with disease}}}{\dfrac{\text{Patients without disease and with result}}{\text{All patients without disease}}}.$$

EXAMPLE

The former study of choice for the initial evaluation of pulmonary embolism was a nucleotide ventilation/perfusion scan (V/Q). Instead of being reported in dichotomous positive/negative values, scans are reported as four results: normal, low probability, intermediate probability, and high probability. We can calculate likelihood ratios for each of these results by using the values provided in the PIOPED study:[36]

SCAN RESULT	PE	NO PE
Normal	5	126
Low probability	39	273
Intermediate probability	105	217
High probability	102	14
Total	251	630

We now have enough information to calculate likelihood ratios for each value:

$$LR\ normal = \frac{\dfrac{5\,(\text{with disease and result})}{251\,(\text{with disease})}}{\dfrac{126\,(\text{without disease and with result})}{630\,(\text{without disease})}} = 0.1.$$

In the same way, we can calculate the likelihood ratios for each of the other results:

- LR low probability = 0.4
- LR intermediate probability = 1.2
- LR high probability = 18.3

Based on these likelihood ratios, it is apparent that a high or normal scan can significantly alter our pre-test probability. On the other hand, the low and intermediate values will not greatly change our pre-test probability. This has led to the reporting of a low or intermediate scan as non-diagnostic. From the perspective of diagnostic decision-making, we gain very little information from either of these two results.

Scalar Likelihood Ratios

Even intervals of scalar values can be reported using likelihood ratios. This avoids the problems created by having just one dichotomous cutoff when interpreting scalar tests.

EXAMPLE

It is a common situation for consultants to ask for a white blood cell (WBC) count when being called to evaluate a patient for appendicitis. The problem with this strategy is that rarely are realistic cutoffs for the results established before ordering the test. Using data from a prior study,[37,38] Brown and Reeves reported likelihoods for various intervals of the WBC count for patients suspected of appendicitis:[39]

WBC COUNT ($\times 10^3/\text{mL}$)	LIKELIHOOD RATIO
4–7	0.1
7–9	0.52
9–11	2.8
13–15	1.7
15–17	2.8
17–19	3.5

It can be seen that the WBC count has very little diagnostic effect unless it is below 7 or above 17. This makes the WBC a less than optimal test for appendicitis. If we use an arbitrary cutoff such as >11 instead of interval likelihoods, the test is even less functional.

The power of likelihood ratios is that they simultaneously embrace both the true and false rate for any test result. For instance, the likelihood ratio positive encompasses both the true positive and false positive rate of a test. As we will see shortly, other testing parameters are not capable of this necessary duality.

Ideally, all journals would report likelihood ratios for all studies of diagnostic tests. The literature is unfortunately not yet at this point of sophistication, so we must be familiar with some of the less useful, but more prevalent, test parameters.

Sensitivity and Specificity

Sensitivity and specificity were originally developed for use in chemistry research to rate the ability of assays to detect substances.[35] Medicine adopted the terms for use in the description of diagnostic tests; like many makeshift measures, they are not ideal for their intended use. The problem is that they measure the likelihood of a test result in patients with the disease status *already known*.[35] In the emergency department we need just the opposite; we want to know the likelihood of the patient having the disease once we have the test result. This can only be tangentially answered by sensitivity or specificity.

Sensitivity

A test with perfect sensitivity would be *positive* in every patient *with the disease*.* The classic mnemonic is PID, reminding us that the test is Positive In Disease (Fig. 2-10). Another way of thinking about sensitivity is that a patient with disease will never have a negative result on a perfectly sensitive test.

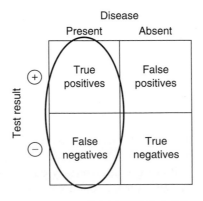

— FIGURE 2-10 — *Sensitivity represents true positives divided by all patients with disease.*

*In this sense, perfect refers to a sensitivity of 1, or 100%.

We can express sensitivity mathematically as:

$$\text{Sensitivity} = \frac{\text{True positives}}{\text{True positives} + \text{False negative}}.$$

Since tests rarely have perfect sensitivity, there will be a number of false negatives; i.e., patients who have the disease but still test negative. The more sensitive the test, the less false negatives there will be. The false negative rate can be expressed as:

$$\text{False negatives} = 1 - \text{Sensitivity}.$$

Negative results on a highly sensitive test are powerful. Sensitive tests are important because they have the ability to aid in ruling-out a disease. Conceptually, a negative result on a sensitive test will sharply decrease the post-test probability.*

This has lead to the superior mnemonic of SNOUT to represent that a SeNsitive test helps to rule OUT disease.[40]

Specificity

A test with perfect specificity would be *negative* in every patient *without the disease*. The classic mnemonic is NIH, reminding us that the test is Negative In Health (Fig. 2-11). Another way to think about specificity is that a patient without the disease will never have a positive result with a perfectly specific test. To express specificity mathematically.

$$\text{Specificity} = \frac{\text{True negatives}}{\text{True negative} + \text{False positives}}.$$

Since tests rarely have a perfect specificity, there will be a number of false positives; i.e., patients who are healthy but test positive. The more specific the test, the less false positives there will be. The false positive rate can be expressed as:

$$\text{False positives} = 1 - \text{Specificity}.$$

Positive results on highly specific tests are important, because they have the ability to aid in ruling-in a disease. Conceptually, a positive result on a

---

*We say conceptually, because sensitivity is the likelihood of a positive result in the presence of disease, not the likelihood of the absence of disease with a negative result. The latter concept is the definition of the negative predictive value. However, since sensitivity is proportional to the negative predictive value, a negative result on a perfectly sensitive test should rule out the disease. This entire quagmire can be avoided by using likelihood ratios.

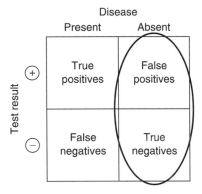

— FIGURE 2-11 —   *Specificity represents true negatives divided by all patients without the disease.*

specific test will sharply increase the post-test probability. This concept is represented with the mnemonic SPIN to represent SPecific tests help to rule IN disease.[40]

Often, to increase sensitivity requires a loss of specificity and vice versa. This is because many seemingly dichotomous tests actually generate a wide range of values. The researchers convert these scalar values to a dichotomous result by picking a cutoff for positive and negative. The cutoff for many dichotomous tests is picked from a range of possible points each with a sensitivity/specificity tradeoff.

EXAMPLE

You decide to create a new machine to test for hypoglycemia in diabetics, but instead of reporting the numeric value of the finger-stick sugar, it reports two results: either hypoglycemic or normal. If the machine is set to report hypoglycemia with any sugar level below 100 mg/dL, then it is unlikely that any cases of hypoglycemia will be missed, making the test extremely sensitive. However, at that cutoff point, many patients with normal glucoses will be labeled hypoglycemic; therefore, the test will have low specificity. If the machine was reset to report hypoglycemia below 40 mg/dL, the specificity would increase at the expense of sensitivity.

The sensitivity and specificity will change for any individual value chosen as the cutoff point, as was shown in the preceding example. We rarely have access to any of these sensitivities or specificities other than the one point chosen by study researchers. We can partially overcome

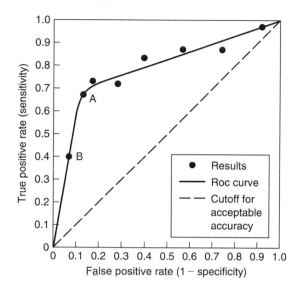

— FIGURE 2-12 — *Receiver operator characteristics curve.*

this problem by obtaining the receiver operator characteristics curve for a test.

Receiver Operator Characteristics (ROC) Curves

These are a graphical representation of true positive rate (sensitivity) on the vertical axis and false positive rate (1 − specificity) on the horizontal. Using these graphs, we can see an estimation of the sensitivity and specificity for the individual values of a scalar test (Fig. 2-12).[41,42]

Area Under the Curve If we examine the ROC curve, we can appreciate that the greater the area under the curve (AUC), the more accurate the test. If the AUC is 0.5 (represented by the diagonal line in the diagram), then the test is no better than chance alone. If the AUC is 1.0, then the test has perfect accuracy.

Cutoff Values When researchers pick a cutoff value for the positive/ negative level of a test, they must first decide whether they wish to maximize sensitivity or specificity. They can then pick a point on the curve, which makes that characteristic highest with minimal false results. Point A on the curve in Fig. 2-12 will maximize sensitivity with the minimal loss of specificity. Point B will give the highest specificity with a minimum of false negatives (sensitivity).

We can also use the ROC curve to observe the likelihood ratios of both individual points on the curve as well as scalar ranges. An article by Choi describes using the slope of various points of the ROC curve to arrive at the appropriate LRs.[42]

The Dangers of Being Alone

Another serious shortcoming of these sensitivity and specificity tests is that they are often viewed in isolation of each other. The most sensitive test available is useless if it is non-specific. It will help to rule-out a disease if it is negative, but it will be negative so infrequently as to make it clinically useless.

EXAMPLE

A new laboratory test for septic arthritis has a sensitivity of 99.5% and a specificity of 1.8%. You are excited to try the test in the pediatric emergency department, because you have had difficulty easily making this diagnosis in children. You surmise that if the test is negative, you have virtually ruled-out the diagnosis of septic arthritis in your patients. You are frustrated to find that the first twenty patients you send the assay on have positive results. You finally stop using the new assay, because it never helps you make a clinical decision.

A converse of this problem is seen with specific, but insensitive, tests. They may be helpful if they are positive, but they will be negative most of the time.

- If sensitivity + specificity ≤ 100, then test = useless!

If we find that the sum of the sensitivity and specificity is less than or equal to 100%, the test is absolutely clinically useless. If we calculate the likelihood ratios of this type of test, by the method we are about to describe, we can prove this to ourselves.

Making Better Use of Sensitivity and Specificity

For the reasons we have mentioned, sensitivity and specificity are not ideal parameters for emergency medicine decision-making. Luckily, we can easily convert these parameters to the far more powerful *likelihood ratios* (positive and negative). Likelihood ratios avoid all of the above problems.

$$\text{LR positive} = \frac{\text{Sensitivity}}{1 - \text{Specificity}};$$

$$\text{LR negative} = \frac{1 - \text{Sensitivity}}{\text{Specificity}}.$$

An astute reader will quickly realize that these formulas are merely a different way of expressing the WOWO formula for likelihood ratios, as mentioned above.

Predictive Values

There is another set of parameters which attempt to reconcile the problems of sensitivity and specificity. Predictive values do address the necessity of evaluating a *test result* (like likelihood ratios) as opposed to evaluating a *test* (like sensitivity/specificity). However, predictive values bring problems of their own; they are fixed values that reflect the population included in a particular study and rarely provide the information you need about your own individual patients.

Predictive Value Negative

Given a negative test result, the predictive value negative provides the probability of the patient being healthy. The value is linked to the prevalence of the study population; the predictive value negative *increases* as the prevalence of the disease *decreases*. Mathematically, it can be expressed as:

$$\text{Predictive value negative} = \frac{\text{True negatives}}{\text{True negatives} + \text{False negatives}}.$$

and on the 2 × 2 table as shown in Fig. 2-13.

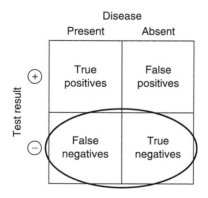

— FIGURE 2-13 — *Predictive value negative represents true negatives divided by all negatives.*

Predictive Value Positive

Given a positive test result, the predictive value positive provides the probability of the patient having the disease. The value is inextricably linked to the prevalence of the disease in the study; the predictive value positive *increases* as the prevalence *increases*. It can be expressed in the equation:

$$\text{Predictive value positive} = \frac{\text{True positives}}{\text{True positives} + \text{False positives}}.$$

and on the 2×2 table as shown in Fig. 2-14.

Problems with Predictive Values

Predictive values are linked to the prevalence of the disease in the study from which they were derived; this is problematic. If that study's prevalence matches or approximates the pre-test probability of disease in our patient, then we are able to use these characteristics. If not, then the predictive values may not be accurate to predict disease in our patient. A new pregnancy test that one of the authors is developing demonstrates the extremes to which prevalence can alter predictive values.

EXAMPLE

A new pregnancy test is developed consisting of a piece of loose-leaf paper with the phrase "You are pregnant" written on it in ballpoint pen. You tape this piece of paper to any patient and if it still reads "You are

— FIGURE 2-14 — *Predictive value positive represents true positives divided by all positives.*

pregnant," then the test is positive. Obviously, this test has perfect sensitivity (100%), as it will always be positive if taped to a pregnant patient. The specificity will be 0% as the test will never be negative when placed on a non-pregnant patient.

If we performed this test on an Ob/Gyn ward where 95 of the 100 patients on the floor are pregnant, the predictive value positive will be 95% despite the specificity of 0% (Fig. 2-15A). If we took the test to a general medical ward where 95 of the patients are not pregnant and 5 patients are pregnant, the predictive value positive will be 5% despite having an unchanged specificity of 0% (Fig. 2-15B).

Reported predictive values are a less than ideal solution to the problem of appropriately representing the value of a test result. They are inextricably linked to the disease prevalence in the study that reports them and they

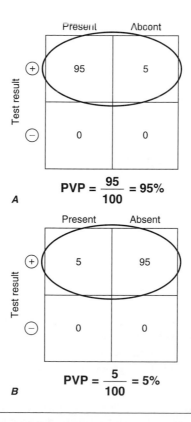

— FIGURE 2-15 — *A A new pregnancy test applied on an Ob/Gyn floor. B The same test applied to a general medical ward.*

cannot be directly applied to our patients, unless their pre-test probability exactly matches this prevalence.*

Likelihood ratios give us the information about the test result that really matters; they apply to *any* level of pre-test probability and can be directly inserted into the Bayesian equation.

Screening Tests

We do not routinely perform screening tests in the emergency department, though they are an essential part of our public health system. The difference between screening tests and diagnostic tests is that the individuals undergoing screening tests are asymptomatic for the diagnosis and we have no reason to suspect they have a greater risk of disease than the general population. The ideal screening test would be both sensitive and specific, but since most tests cannot be both, screening tests are often quite sensitive with a lower specificity. These less than optimal tests, when positive, would then require a second confirmatory test, which possesses high specificity. An example of this is HIV screening, which starts with a sensitive test, the ELISA. If the ELISA is positive, the extremely specific Western Blot is ordered to confirm the results.

One screening test, which we use routinely and appropriately in the emergency department prior to the administration of medication or radiography, is the urine pregnancy test for women of childbearing age. The urine pregnancy test is an example of an excellent screening exam as it has the power to take a pre-test probability of near zero:

> "Doctor, there is no way I can be pregnant. I haven't been with anyone for two years."

to a post-test probability of 100%. With a specificity of 100%, a sensitivity of over 98%, a likelihood ratio positive of infinite, and a likelihood ratio negative of 0.02 (it will miss a very early pregnancy which has not produced adequate b-HCG,) it is one of the most powerful tests in emergency medicine.

Unfortunately, we use many inappropriate diagnostic tests as if they were screening tests. To get a white blood cell count as a screen for infection is to guarantee uninterpretable results. The routine coagulation panel for all emergency patients is a gross waste of resources; it screens for

---

*Even worse, they are misleading even with respect to the original study population. They apply only to the patient whose individual probability of disease is exactly identical to the prevalence within the average of the study population. This may not be true for any individual patient in the entire study!

conditions that we have no reason to suspect. If a patient is receiving anticoagulation or is actively bleeding, then we order a coagulation panel (or better yet, we can break the panel strategy and just order the INR on our patients taking warfarin). Otherwise, there is no reason to support needless and costly standard emergency lab panels.

Playing Testing Jeopardy A practice, which is particularly frustrating, is the ordering of tests without considering their necessity or utility and then trying to determine their value after the results have arrived. This is akin to the American game show Jeopardy, in which an answer is provided and contestants must determine the question. Trying to figure out the meaning of test results that were ordered without indication is not a proper diagnostic strategy.

History and Physical Exam

Under the differential diagnosis section, we discussed how a patient's signs and symptoms can suggest diagnoses that we must consider and decide whether or not to evaluate. Our history and physical exam also have the ability to alter the pre-test probability; in this sense they are *diagnostic tests*. In order to make this process objective, we need test characteristics.

While many studies evaluate the test parameters of the components of our history and physical, perhaps the best source for this information is in an ongoing series published in the *Journal of the American Medical Association* (JAMA). The series, entitled The Rational Clinical Exam, takes different diseases and disorders and summarizes the performance of the signs and symptoms conventionally associated with the diagnosis. Particularly relevant to emergency physicians, the *Annals of Emergency Medicine* has begun to publish abstracts and commentaries summarizing the important information from the JAMA series that are relevant to emergency medicine.

The incredible value of this form of evidence is that, in addition to helping us make diagnoses in individual patients, it can allow us to retrain our clinical judgment and *illness scripts*.

EXAMPLE

When diagnosing appendicitis in the emergency department, we have always considered anorexia to be one of the hallmarks of the disorder. When one of our colleagues hands us a copy of the Rational Clinical Exam article on diagnosing appendicitis, we are surprised to see that the likelihood ratios positive and negative (respectively, 1.27 and 0.64) for this symptom are close to one.[43] In the future, we stop using anorexia to change our pre-test probability of appendicitis.

▨ What are we actually testing?

In order to derive the maximum benefit from the use of a diagnostic test, we must understand what is actually being tested. A pregnancy test does not test for pregnancy, it tests for bHCG; this is why it may test negative during the first two weeks after conception when bHCG levels are too low to detect. If we do not properly understand what a test result means, then we may be led astray from the true diagnosis.

EXAMPLE

We often use the FAST (focused assessment using sonography in trauma) exam to evaluate the abdomen of trauma patients. When we perform this study, we may think we are assessing for intra-abdominal injury. However, the FAST exam does not assess for intra-abdominal injury, it assesses for free intraperitineal fluid. Furthermore, it cannot detect small amounts of fluid, it requires at the very least a few hundred milliliters of fluid before the test will be positive. If we perform a negative FAST exam on a trauma patient who subsequently has a positive laparotomy, then the study may be branded a false negative. If the intra-abdominal injury was a bowel wall injury with mesenteric hematoma and only 20–30 mL of blood in the abdomen, then the ultrasound was not really a false negative. If, however, the injury was a splenic hematoma with a liter of blood, then the FAST exam was indeed falsely negative.

By the same token, if a FAST exam reveals large amounts of free fluid in a patient with cirrhosis, some would call this a false positive FAST exam. However, it is not really falsely positive, because there was fluid in the belly, it just was not blood.

As we can see, understanding what the test actually examines is vitally important, both to use the results and also to understand the testing characteristics derived from a diagnostic study. If one study uses the presence of fluid while another uses intra-abdominal injury as the test criteria, then the sensitivity and specificity of the FAST exam may be very different in the two studies.

If we understand what a test examines, then we can extrapolate the results to the clinical situation. Free fluid on the FAST exam in a normotensive patient with a grossly enlarged liver and caput medusa may be interpreted as a positive FAST exam that does not necessarily signify an abdominal injury.

APPLICABILITY OF DIAGNOSTIC TESTS

In the previous section, we discussed the process of understanding and using the characteristics of diagnostic tests. The next step is to evaluate whether these characteristics must be altered to account for our individual patient and unique clinical scenario. We call this process of evaluation, and possible adjustment, the *applicability* of evidence.

The evidence we need to determine applicability includes the setting, population, and interpretation of the original study. NEEDLEs can provide these facts in a readily usable form (Fig. 2-16). Using this information, we can decide if the evidence is appropriate to use for diagnostic decision-making in our patient.

Diagnostic Evidence: Elisa d-dimer for Pulmonary Embolism

Benefits/Downsides

- LR + 1.73, LR − 0.11

- No risks, cost minimal

Applicability

- Adult patients in outpatient setting

- Performed in normal hospital laboratories; interpreted by laboratory staff

- Specificity lower in patients >70; sensitivity and specificity lower if symptoms >3 days

Brown MD et al. Annals Emerg Med 2002;40(2):133-144
-Valid meta-analysis. (Sens 95% CI 0.88-0.97) (Spec 95% CI 0.36-0.55)

— FIGURE 2-16 — *NEEDLE: Necessary Evidence for Emergency Decisions, Listed and Evaluated.*

Applicability

Applicability directly relates to the question "Are our patient and practice setting sufficiently similar to those in the diagnostic study to directly use the study's test characteristics?" Factors that might cause us to change our interpretation of a test and its applicability are considered below.

Patients

A study of performance of a test in relationship to a disease may not apply to our patient and we therefore may not be able to use the information from such a study to assist in our diagnosis. Factors that may cause a test to be more or less accurate in a given patient include severity of disease, comorbidities, or age.

EXAMPLE

If a patient is pancytopenic, because of myelodysplastic syndrome, we would not think to use his or her white blood cell count to determine the likelihood for appendicitis, even though, ordinarily, a value of less than $7 \times 10^3/\text{mL}$ would have a useful likelihood ratio negative. In the absence of a study that reported WBC counts in pancytopenic patients being considered for appendicitis, a low WBC in this patient should not change our pre-test probability

Evidence for diagnostic tests may not be applicable to whole groups of patients. In this case, we may not even bother to order the test when we are practicing in this setting.

EXAMPLE

During one of your rotations through the surgical intensive care unit (SICU), you have a postoperative patient with sudden-onset shortness of breath. You consider pulmonary embolism in your differential and tell your attending that you want to order a d-dimer. Your attending explains that, while this test is useful in emergency department patients, its applicability is severely diminished in SICU patients. Postoperative patients almost uniformly will test positive regardless of the presence of embolism, therefore this test has very little utility in this setting.

Interpreters

When using a test, we must ask ourselves if its interpretation will be as accurate as in the original study.

EXAMPLE

CT angiogram was found to have very high accuracy for the early diagnosis of ischemic stroke in a well-done study. Fellowship-trained neuroradiologists interpreted the CT scans. At our institution, there are only general radiology residents with little familiarity with CT angiograms of the brain; we would not expect the sensitivities or specificities at our institution to be as high as in the study.

Equipment and Resources

Another part of the applicability of a diagnostic test hinges on the use of the same quality of equipment as in the original study. The accuracy of the test will be less if our diagnostic equipment is inferior.

EXAMPLE

Emergency department ultrasonographers perform an imaginary study demonstrating a likelihood ratio negative of 0.01 for the signs of pericardial tamponade in patients with pericardial fluid. The study was performed using a $150,000 echocardiography machine with a phased array transducer. It is doubtful that the quality of images using your cut-rate ultrasound machine from the early 1990s will allow the same test characteristics.

Clinical Scenario

Certain clinical scenarios will also allow and necessitate the adjustment of diagnostic test parameters. We can use this variance of testing characteristics in different clinical scenarios to our advantage. Tests that have only middling discriminatory ability can shine in certain circumstances.

EXAMPLE

We know that the FAST exam does not have 100% sensitivity for intra-abdominal injuries or even for the presence of free fluid. However, there are some situations in which we can use the test as if it has a near perfect sensitivity.[44]

If a patient comes to our trauma after *isolated* severe blunt trauma to the abdomen and pelvis, we are placed at a diagnostic nodal point. Should we go to the operating theatre for an exploratory laparotomy or send the patient to angiography for pelvic embolization? To aid our decision, we can perform a FAST exam. If it is negative, then we can conclude that the hypotension is a result of the pelvic fracture and send the patient to the angiography suite. Because the patient is hypotensive, we would expect any intra-abdominal injury significant enough to cause hypotension to have a large amount of free fluid. If we are able to get good windows with our FAST exam and we do not see free fluid, then we can presume that the bleeding is in the pelvis, even though there may be some free fluid in the belly missed by the ultrasound. We adjust the sensitivity of the FAST exam based on the spectrum of disease of our patient.

We can describe the complex thinking involved in this example:

- We have a hypotensive blunt-trauma patient.
- After a quick primary survey, a negative chest radiograph and subxiphoid transthoracic echocardiogram, we conclude that the patient has isolated trauma to the abdomen and pelvis.
- Therefore, we attribute the hypotension to active bleeding, not to spinal injury, cardiac tamponade, pneumothorax, or other medical causes.
- We deduce that there is no cause for the bleeding that may exist other than pelvic or abdominal after ruling out major extremity bleeding on clinical grounds.
- We decide that if there is not enough blood in the belly to account for the hypotension, then we are going to angiography to stop the pelvic bleeding.
- We consider that an ultrasound of the abdomen, if negative, will have a very low LR for the amount of bleeding that we have decided must exist in order to cause the hypotension. In other words, even though the LR negative for the FAST exam may not be significant enough to rule-out any abdominal bleeding in this patient, we are confident that the sensitivity of US for detecting the amount of blood required to make our patient this hypotensive would be much higher than for the usual minimum threshold for detection, and that the LR for a negative US would therefore be low enough to rule-out the diagnosis of *significant* intra-abdominal bleeding.[44]
- As a result of the negative FAST exam, we conclude that the immediately important bleeding must be retroperitoneal from a severe pelvic fracture and we send the patient to the angiography suite.

This adjustment of test result interpretation to fit the clinical scenario is the hallmark of an adept clinician.

Sensitivity Analysis

The adjustment of a test to make it applicable to our patient and clinical scenario is often more of an art than a science. In some circumstances (e.g., the WBC in the myelodysplastic patient), we will simply decide we cannot use the test.

In other circumstances, semi-quantitative adjustment is possible through a process called *sensitivity analysis*.[40] This process involves deciding how much loss of accuracy we can accept and still be able to use the test to make a decision. If the test result would normally allow us to make a decision with a wide margin of certainty, but our applicability assessment causes us to downgrade the accuracy, we may still use the test. If, however, a test result barely would allow us to cross a decision threshold, we may no longer be sure that a test with diminished applicability will allow us to make the decision. The next section will deal with the determination of this margin of error for our decision-making.

POST-TEST PROBABILITY

With an understanding of the power and pitfalls of diagnostic tests, we can see how they alter our pre-test probability of disease. The most efficient method utilizes likelihood ratios, as they allow direct calculations of post-test probability.

Obtaining Post-test Probabilities

We started with the equation:

Pretest probability × Effects of diagnostic test = Post-test probability.

We can now alter the equation to include the use of likelihood ratios:

Pretest odds × Likelihood ratio = Post-test odds.

Unfortunately, likelihood ratios can only be directly multiplied with pre-test odds and not pre-test probability.

To convert pre-test probability to odds, use the formula:

$$\text{Odds} = \frac{\text{Probability}}{1 - \text{Probability}}.$$

To convert post-test odds back to post-test probability, use the formula:

$$\text{Probability} = \frac{\text{Odds}}{1 + \text{Odds}}.$$

If this seems like a lot of calculating, there is a much easier solution; a nomogram exists that takes pre-test probability and LR and gives the post-test probability (Fig. 2-17A).[45] Using the nomogram involves simply

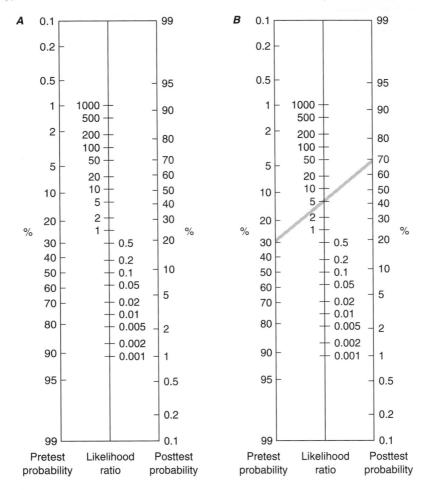

— FIGURE 2-17 — **A,B** *Nomograms for calculating post-test probability. (Adapted from Fagan, 1975[45])*

drawing a line through the pre-test probability and likelihood ratio of the test result to yield the post-test probability.

EXAMPLE

If our pre-test probability is 30% and the LR for our positive result is 5, then our post-test probability is 70% (Fig. 2-17B).

In addition to the nomogram, there is software available for PDAs (personal digital assistants) that will calculate post-test probability as well as convert sensitivity/specificity to likelihood ratios. A free version can be found at www.cebm.utoronto.ca. There are also online calculators for post-test probability, which allow us to avoid calculating odds: http://araw.mede.uic.edu/cgi-bin/testcalc.pl.

Plot the Post-test Probabilities *before* Performing the Test

Before even performing a test, we can plot the post-test probabilities of its results on our decision bar, using the likelihood ratios of each result. In Fig. 2-18A, the post-test probabilities of each test result cross the decision thresholds. If we perform this test, it will allow us to make a decision no matter what its results. If this is the case, it is a fortuitous situation; however, a test will often only allow the crossing of one decision threshold (Fig. 2-18B). If you plot the post-test probabilities and realize that neither result will cause a crossing of a decision threshold, do not perform the test.

If a test has a result that will allow the crossing of at least one decision threshold, then it can help make the diagnosis.

Perform Testing

After the results return, we can see where on the decision bar the post-test probability lies. If we are below the discard threshold (Fig. 2-19A), then we must seek another diagnosis. If we are above the accept threshold (Fig. 2-19B), then we have "ruled-in" the diagnosis and should take action.

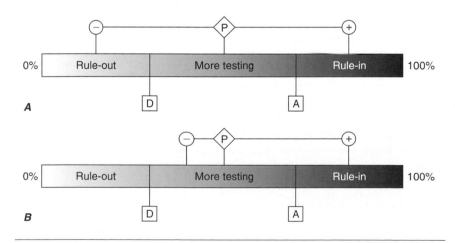

— FIGURE 2-18 — *A Post-test probabilities plotted before testing.* *B Only one of the test results crosses a decision threshold.*

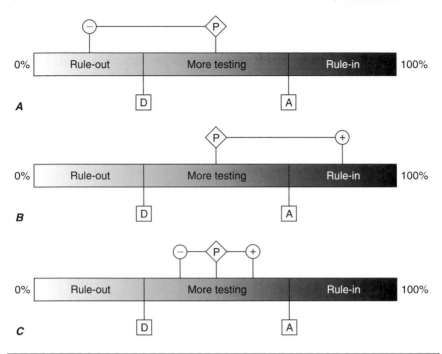

— FIGURE 2-19 —   *A The post-test probability is below the discard threshold. **B** The post-test probability crosses the accept threshold. **C** The post-test probability is still in the indeterminate zone.*

This action may be to administer a medication, admit the patient, call a consultant, or simply give the patient appropriate discharge instructions and a follow-up appointment.

If the post-test probability still lies within the indeterminate zone (Fig. 2-19C), then we still have not made or eliminated the diagnosis and further testing is needed. The venue for this continued testing depends on the clinical situation. It can take place in the emergency department, in the hospital, or as an outpatient.

The diagnostic testing we have already performed may not have been a waste of time. The post-test probability after the first round of testing becomes the new pre-test probability for any further tests we order (Fig. 2-20).

SOURCES OF ERROR

In emergency medicine, we need to make rapid, accurate diagnoses. A good deal of emergency medical cognition is performed subconsciously, almost automatically. The impetus for many of our diagnostic decisions

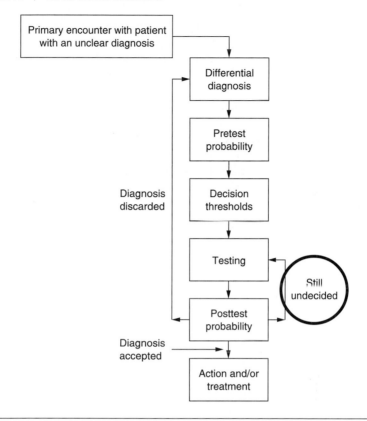

— FIGURE 2-20 — *If our post-test probability has not allowed us to discard or accept the diagnosis, then we must perform further testing. We then use the generated post-test probability as our new pre-test probability for this additional testing.*

comes from behind the scenes. If we have integrated flawed reasoning into our diagnostic methodology, we are prone to make errors. By recognizing this potential and systematically eliminating sources of error, we can free our decision-making process from the potential pitfalls.

Diagnostic Errors

Error in medicine has received an enormous amount of attention in recent years. Kassirer has delineated the types of error that occur during the process of diagnostic decision-making:[46,47]

- *Faulty triggering:* The signs and symptoms do not lead us to a consideration of the diagnosis.

- *Faulty context formulation:* We assign an improper diagnosis because of the setting or other external factors.
- *Errors in gathering or processing information:* We make an error because we have performed a poor history, conducted a flawed exam, or ordered the wrong test.
- *Faulty interpretation of clinical testing:* We draw improper conclusions from test results, leading to misdiagnosis.
- *Errors in verification:* We prematurely discard or accept a diagnosis before a sufficiently thorough evaluation
- *No-fault errors:* We miss the proper diagnosis, but in retrospect, no clear cognitive missteps can be found.

We can simplify this schema even further by dividing the cognitive missteps of diagnostic decision-making into errors of information gathering and errors of information integration.[48]

Errors pertaining to the gathering and acquisition of information are known as *slips* and *lapses.*

Slips and Lapses

These forms of error involve the gathering of false data; by virtue of this erroneous information, our diagnostic pathways are compromised. Many slips and lapses are caused by the frequent interruptions and multiple simultaneous stimuli characteristic of the environment of a typical emergency department.

Slips

If we are distracted, our inattention can cause us to misread or falsely receive information. We may look at the number 1.1, but see 11; if this number is the white blood cell count in an oncology patient, the results of this error can be serious. When looking at a chest radiograph, if we are simultaneously signing an order sheet, a subtle pneumothorax can easily be missed.

Cognitive drift is the cause of many slip-type errors. Optimally, we process one task or thought pattern at a time. If we want to check labs, but the computerized information system takes 45 seconds to start-up, we naturally might use this time to think of other things than the values we wanted to check. When the computer system does eventually start, we may be distracted. Informatics experts therefore view sub-second computer information system response times as essential to avoid error due to cognitive drift.[49]

Lapses

Lapses are errors of memory. Just as in slips, distraction can play a role in causing us to forget information we normally can recall readily. Often these lapses deal with skills and tasks we normally would perform automatically. If in the course of the preparations for suturing an arm laceration, we look up at the full chart rack, we may forget to perform our standard search to diagnose foreign bodies. Ordinarily, we have a set order for our preparations: first we inject anesthetic, then we clean the wound, then the search for foreign bodies, and finally we suture. However, a distraction can cause us to deviate from this routine and forget our normal process, leading to a missed diagnosis.

It is also a lapse when we place drops of urine on a bedside pregnancy test and read the results as soon as the indicator lines appear. We are forgetting the necessity of waiting the proscribed period of time for the reagents to mix with the urine. This lapse can lead to a false diagnosis of a patient's pregnancy status.

Mistakes

Slips and lapses cause us to bring *false data* into our diagnostic decision-making process. If the data we assimilate is correct, but we process it erroneously, cognitive psychologists would refer to this error type as a *mistake*.

While slips and lapses were errors of information gathering, mistakes are errors of information processing and utilization. The difficulty of using information to make diagnoses in the emergency department is the rapidity with which we must make decisions. One factor which contributes to our ability to make decisions in the rapid manner necessary in our practice, is the use of heuristics.[50]

Heuristics

Croskerry provided a definition of heuristics as a

> "Cognitive process that simplifies clinical decision-making operations, describing the everyday intuitive decisions that emergency physicians make without resorting to formal decision analysis."[51]

While heuristics can aid in the urgent formulation of a diagnosis, these rules of thumb can also lead to error. Non-beneficial heuristics are often referred to as "biases," though the ambiguity of this term has lead Croskerry to call them a *cognitive disposition to respond* (CDR).[7,50]

Comprehensive lists of heuristics that may affect the thinking of emergency physicians can be found in the literature.[7,52]

Ultimately, the use of heuristics is unavoidable. McDonald advises physicians to become aware of the heuristics used in decision-making and to consider an ongoing process of pruning and re-examining such criteria.[53] Awareness of potentially flawed or failed heuristics can prevent them from negatively influencing our decisions. Relevant clinical evidence can be a powerful adjunct to rejecting or revising erroneous heuristics. What follows is a discussion of the potential errors inherent in each phase of diagnostic decision-making.

Errors in the Creation of a Differential Diagnosis

If our illness scripts are well-developed and extensive, we are able to accurately and quickly develop a differential. If inexperience or an anomalous patient presentation forces us to into a state of diagnostic uncertainty, we are more prone to error. It is in this state that we are most subject to biasing heuristics.

ROWS: Rule-out Worst Scenario

It is our nature as emergency physicians to assume the worst. Asking the question "What is going to kill this patient?" is one of the foundations of emergency medicine decision-making. We always search for the most serious or life-threatening explanation for a patient's presentation and then attempt to "rule-out" these dangerous diagnoses. In most circumstances, this heuristic is beneficial and essential given the unique nature of our practice. If taken too far, it can lead to needless work-ups for benign conditions.[7]

Availability Bias

Diseases that are easier to remember will spring to mind readily; diseases that are difficult to remember are often not considered. This heuristic can cause us to leave infrequently encountered disorders off the list of differential diagnoses.[50,54]

Confirmation Bias

This heuristic deals with the momentum that occurs when a clinician latches on to one diagnosis. Often, we will accept new evidence only if it confirms this working diagnosis and ignore the information if it does not. This is a form of "anchoring"; it is human nature to regard positive, confirmatory evidence more highly than negative information.[55] When we set our stakes on one diagnosis, other potential entities can be missed.

Occam's Razor

William of Occam, a medieval philosopher, postulated the principle of parsimony; i.e., "Plurality should not be posited without necessity." This principle demands the search for the simplest explanation for any course of events. When found, that simplest explanation will likely be the correct one. To state the theory another way, "One should not increase, beyond what is necessary, the number of entities required to explain anything."[56] While it is quite satisfying to postulate a unifying diagnosis for all aspects of a patient's presentation, we must keep in mind that two or more problems might have caused the patient to arrive in the emergency department. While beneficial as a general mindset, if only singular explanations are considered, we will miss diagnoses.[7,50]

Search Satisficing

Similar to confirmation bias above, this source of error stems from the lack of consideration of other diagnoses once we are positive about one diagnosis. A Nobel Prize winning economist, Herbert Simons, first described the concept; the term is a combination of satisfying and sufficing.[57] This heuristic causes us to abandon the search for further fractures on a radiograph once one fracture is found. In the same vein, if after exploration a foreign body is discovered in a laceration, there is a strong urge to cease the search for additional foreign bodies.[7,17] This bias is a form of premature closure, a cessation of the search prior to finding *all* of the correct diagnoses.

Prior Extensive Work-ups

When we deal with a patient with multiple presentations and/or an extensive work-up preceding the current visit, it can predispose us to error. This bias causes a narrowing of the differential in such patients as they have already been worked up the "yin-yang."[7] The danger lies in the possibility that such patients may have a new condition or a missed diagnosis despite their prior exhaustive work-up. "Frequent fliers" also fall into this category; this bias causes us to miss the intracranial bleed on the inebriated gentleman who has visited the emergency department every night for the past three years.

Errors in Assigning Pre-test Probability

The process of assigning pre-test probabilities is not free of cognitive pitfalls. Just as heuristics affected differential diagnosis, they can lead to errors in the estimation of pre-test probability. Though there are many forms of bias that can cause false estimation of pre-test probability, the following are common in emergency medicine.[7]

Sampling Bias

Limited or skewed exposure to the diseases that cause various presentations can lead to an over-representation of rare diseases or an under-representation of common ones. If this biased exposure is applied to a different population, then it can foil pre-test probability estimates.[50]

EXAMPLE

A medical student has worked on the wards at a referral center for pulmonary hypertension patients. Three of his first five patients with shortness of breath had this disease as the etiology of their dyspnea. When he rotates to the emergency department and presents his sixth patient with shortness of breath to his attending, he naturally places the pre-test probability of pulmonary hypertension at 60%. In the general emergency population with dyspnea, the prevalence of pulmonary hypertension is actually much lower than 60%.

This heuristic also pertains to diseases that receive extensive journal coverage. Some rare conditions receive literature coverage out of proportion to their prevalence; this can lead to faulty estimation of pre-test probability.[58]

Saliency Bias

When assigning pre-test probabilities, certain diseases come to mind more quickly than others do. For instance, we may have seen a striking example of the disease on our previous shift; this form of the bias is motivated by a recency effect. Novel clinical features of a disease may make it more striking than others with equal prevalence. If a previous misdiagnosis has led to legal action or embarrassment, a clinician will often vow consciously or subconsciously to never miss this diagnosis again. The *salience* of these diagnoses may lead us to assign a higher than accurate pre-test probability. This source of error is similar to the availability bias we discussed under differential diagnosis.[52]

Link to Page 62

EXAMPLE

A patient presenting with isolated substernal chest pain wound up dying in the department from a thoracic aortic dissection during one of your shifts. From that point on, you assign high pre-test probabilities to the diagnosis of dissection in all of your chest pain patients. This falsely elevated pre-test probability requires you to send all of these patients for CT angiograms. Without this bias, in a majority of these patients your history and physical would allow you to discard the diagnosis of dissection without testing.

Equal Weighting of Clinical Characteristics

This form of bias assigns equal value to clinical characteristics despite the varying significance of these characteristics. Examining articles on the clinical manifestations of disease can aid in the elimination of this negative heuristic.

EXAMPLE

A patient presents with fever and headache, but no Kernig's sign or Brudzinski's sign. If we give the same weight to the absence of the latter two signs as to the presence of the first two, we would calculate a falsely low pre-test probability for the diagnosis of meningitis. The presence of fever and headache are much more predictive of meningitis than the absence of the latter two signs.[59]

Avoidance of this form of bias relies on the integration of the frequency of the clinical manifestations of disease into our illness scripts.

Base Rate Neglect

This bias causes the assumption that all possibilities in the differential list have equal pre-test probability despite varying prevalence. This can be a byproduct of the ROWS heuristic causing us to assign the same probability to all life-threatening diagnoses as we would to less dangerous, but more common, diagnoses.[7]

Link to Page 62

EXAMPLE

A patient comes to the emergency department with crushing chest pain. You quickly make a differential consisting of acute coronary syndrome, pneumothorax, pericarditis, pulmonary embolism, and Booerhave's rupture of the esophagus. If you calculated a pre-test probability of 20% for each of the disorders, you would be ignoring the fact that Booerhave's is much less common than the other diagnoses.

Novices also commonly fall prey to this form of error, as it is often easier to create a differential than to accurately assign pre-test probabilities to each of its constituents. Assigning an equal value to each part of the differential is an easy but flawed way of dealing with this difficulty.

Gamblers' Fallacy

If an uninformed gambler sees the roulette wheel stop on red five times in a row, he assumes that the bet on black for the next spin is a "sure thing." In decision-making, this bias causes the erroneous assumption that if we diagnose a number of patients with a serious condition, it is less likely for the next patient to have this same serious condition.[2] This misconception of chance can result in a false decrease in our estimation of pre-test probability.[50]

EXAMPLE

During your shift, you have three patients in a row present with chest pain who then have enzyme evidence of myocardial infarction. If a fourth patient comes in with chest pain, this bias would cause the underestimation of pre-test probability of myocardial infarction as the etiology of his chest pain.

Prototypical Error

This bias causes the underestimation of pre-test probability when a presentation of a disease is not the one described in the textbooks. It is particularly dangerous when *atypical* presentation is far more common than the *classic* presentation. This failed heuristic is most prevalent during the nascent stages of our development of illness scripts. As we progress through our career, our illness scripts embrace a wide range of disease presentations. Inevitably, we begin to understand that the classic presentation is very infrequently the same as the *typical* presentation.

EXAMPLE

A 70-year-old diabetic woman presents with epigastric pain and shortness of breath. This patient's pre-test probability for ischemic heart disease should be quite high regardless of the fact that she does not have retrosternal chest pain.

Errors in the Decision to Perform Diagnostic Tests

As we discussed in the prior sections, testing without diagnostic uncertainty is not only unnecessary, but can lead to false results. Cognitive biases can lead to performing tests we do not need and can obscure the diagnostic process.

Commission Bias

In this context, commission bias refers to the performing of diagnostic testing even if the pre-test probability lies above the accept threshold or below the discard threshold. We often feel the need to *do something*. This bias is operative when we do not feel that our clinical reasoning is a tangible *something* or confidence in our decision-making is lacking. In other situations, it will be the patient directly requesting an objective test as opposed to the supposedly subjective judgment of the clinician. Most patients are quite satisfied with an explanation of the thought process that led us not to need a test, if we take the time to delineate our reasoning. If we still feel the need to order a test, instead of one that would simply confirm what we already have decided, the more worthwhile test would be one that has the potential to alter our diagnosis.

EXAMPLE

You have two 5-year-old patients complaining of a sore throat. The first has anterior cervical lymphadenopathy, exudate on his tonsils, and a low-grade fever. He is not complaining of a runny nose or a cough. You set your pre-test probability at 85% for strep pharyngitis. You set your discard threshold at 15% as missing this diagnosis is unlikely to result in harmful sequelae.[60] You set your accept threshold at 60% as the risks of over-treatment and over-diagnosis are quite small when considering your patient (Fig. 2-21A).

You decide that you will treat the patient with penicillin without any further testing, but the patient's mother pleads with you to do that new rapid strep test. You realize that the rapid strep test, if positive, will do nothing to change your plan to treat. A negative rapid test will not lower your pre-test probability enough to keep you from treating the patient based on your clinical exam.* You explain this to the mother and she accepts your reasoning.

Your second patient keeps wiping his runny nose with his sleeve. As you examine his throat, you notice only a mild redness. He has no palpable lymph nodes and is without fever. You set his pre-test probability for strep at 10% with the same decision thresholds (Fig. 2-21B). You tell the mother that you are comfortable sending the patient home without antibiotics and follow-up with his pediatrician in two days to ensure the resolution of what is likely a viral illness. The mother pleads with you to do a strep test. As you think about the test in this situation,

---

*Rapid strep test: sensitivity = 80%, specificity = 99%, LR+ = 80, LR– = 0.2. The likelihood ratio negative would not drive your post-test probability to below your accept threshold. In a later section, the mathematics necessary to do these calculations will be discussed.

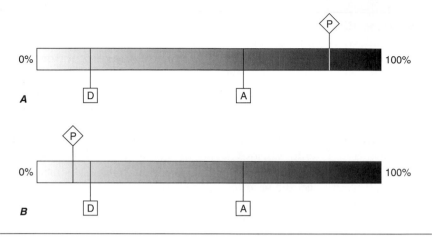

— FIGURE 2-21 — *A The pre-test probability crosses the accept threshold: no testing is necessary.* **B** *The pre-test probability is below the discard threshold: no testing should be necessary.*

you realize that a negative result will do very little to change your thinking, but a positive result would actually make you strongly consider "Strep." Pharyngitis as the false positive rate of this test is low. You perform the rapid test; the patient's mother feels quite relieved to hear it is negative.

If we do order a test, even when the pre-test probability would allow action without testing, we should only use tests that can change our decision to treat or discard a diagnosis.

Entrapment Bias

If halfway through a movie we realize that we are not enjoying ourselves, we have two choices. We can stay to the end or we can get up and leave. The rationale often raised for the first choice is that, since we have already spent the money for the ticket, we might as well stay through until the end, as we cannot get our investment back. Of course, this choice guarantees that we waste additional time, which could have been used for other entertainment. This misconception is an example of entrapment bias. This bias is pervasive in medicine as well; if we start a work-up and then realize it is not needed, we do not need to continue the work-up.

EXAMPLE

One of your residents is presenting a 25-year-old male with chest pain. He details his thorough history and physical and tells you that ordinarily he would send the patient home now, with primary care follow-up. However, a set of cardiac enzymes was sent before he got to the patient. He tells you that now we will have to admit the patient, because one set of enzymes is not enough to rule-out a myocardial infarction, and since the work-up has already begun, it must be completed. You inform him that since he did not feel the evaluation was necessary before sending the enzymes, the work-up does not need to be completed. You document your thought process in the chart and send the patient home.

Errors in the Interpretation of Test Results

How we determine what a test result means to the diagnosis of our patient is also error-prone.

Forced Dichotomy

This bias refers to a desire to see results as positive or negative even when the true result may be indeterminate. Many clinicians find it easier to think of tests in this manner, but as we have discussed above, even tests that are normally reported as positive or negative actually are scalar with predetermined cutoffs. The bias is especially operative with tests that do not easily fit into a dichotomous means of reporting, such as radiological studies.

EXAMPLE

You send a 28-year-old female for a CT scan of the abdomen and pelvis for severe right lower-quadrant abdominal pain. After she returns, you pull the radiology report up on the computer. You quickly scroll down to the bottom of the report, which reads: "No evidence of appendicitis noted." You interpret this as a negative and send the patient home. She comes back eight hours later with generalized abdominal pain and a rigid abdomen. The operative report after the completion of her surgery describes a perforated appendix with peritonitis.

You return to the original CT report, which has the line: "Appendix not visualized; no contrast in cecum." In retrospect, this CT result is not positive, nor is it negative; the patient needed further diagnostic testing in order to determine her diagnosis.

One possible means of avoiding this bias is the assignment of individual likelihood ratios to clinically indeterminate results. This strategy was successfully used for the low and intermediate results of a V/Q scan as we mentioned in the prior section.

At times, even the proper assignment of likelihood ratios does not prevent this bias from causing poor decisions. At times, a test branded positive or negative will cause acceptance of a diagnosis regardless of the actual test result characteristics.

EXAMPLE

One of your residents is evaluating a patient with shortness of breath. Due to the patient's history and physical exam, your resident assigns a low pre-test probability to this patient for the diagnosis of pulmonary embolism. He appropriately orders a d-dimer (Elisa LR $+ = 1.73$, LR $- = 0.11$). When the result comes back positive, he decides to admit the patient and start heparin. Even though the results of the test were positive, the likelihood ratio of this result does almost nothing to change the previously low assessment of pre-test probability.

Avoiding Cognitive Error

Biases such as the above are integrated into our thinking processes. Though sometimes useful, they can lead to missed diagnoses. Research in cognitive psychology indicates that biases can be unlearned by awareness and deliberate analysis of our behavior. One form of this process of cognitive debiasing is provided by metacognition.[51]

Metacognition

This branch of cognitive psychology deals with the awareness and understanding of our own thoughts.[61] Metacognition allows us to analyze our behavior and search for mental processes that predispose us to error.[17,51,62] Experience brings the ability to know what we do not know and makes us aware of when we are not processing information well. Metacognition is difficult for the novice, both because of a deficiency in clinical knowledge as well as a lack of past mistakes to draw upon.[17]

Cognitive Forcing Strategies

Often, an awareness of factors that predispose us to error can aid in their avoidance. Some biases are so entrenched in our thought processes that, even with the awareness of metacognition, we are still prone to error. There are strategies that we can use to lower the potential risks even further, such as cognitive forcing strategies.

This process evaluates consistent cognitive errors and creates solutions, which force the avoidance of these errors.[51] An example is a small sign placed in the physician charting area during the autumn and winter months reading: "Is this carbon monoxide poisoning?" Similarly, cognitive forcing is operative when we enter the complaint of chest pain radiating to the back into an electronic charting system causing a small box to pop up on the screen. The box has a message urging the physician to consider thoracic aortic dissection. In both examples, the physician is forced to consider adding a diagnosis to the differential. Even if in the vast majority of cases the physician would have already considered the diagnosis prior to the cognitive forcing, the combination of exhaustion, a busy department, and the juggling of numerous simultaneous tasks can lead to occasional misses. These forcing strategies attempt to prevent missed diagnoses even when our decision-making process is clouded.

EXAMPLE

When a patient presents in extremis with crushing substernal chest pain, we must rapidly make the diagnosis and treat with numerous medications. Realizing that this is a situation where contemplative critical thinking is difficult for the nurses and physicians, the director of the emergency department decided to develop a cognitive forcing strategy with the help of the pharmacy. All bottles of nitroglycerin have a sticker placed on top of the cap reading "Pt on VIAGRA?" This action was motivated by the knowledge that, in the chaos of treating a sick patient, it is easy to forget the severe hypotension that can be caused when nitroglycerin is administered to patients taking sildenafil and similar agents.

Algorithms

Diagnostic algorithms, such as Advanced Cardiac Life Support (ACLS) and Advanced Trauma Life Support (ATLS), provide another form of debiasing. If a patient presents with pulseless electrical activity (PEA), the ACLS course teaches the eight most common diagnoses along with mnemonics to aid in memory. The difficulty with this form of debiasing is that these algorithms are only as effective as a clinician's ability to remember them.

It is interesting that reluctance to adopt an algorithm can itself serve as a cognitive forcing strategy. ATLS advocates a film of the pelvis on all trauma patients; this is against the practice of many emergency physicians, when the patient has undergone only mild trauma. When we consciously discard the algorithm's recommendations, it still forces us to consider the possibility of pelvic trauma. If we decide not to obtain the radiograph, we know we are flouting the surgeons' standard of care and may apply increased diligence to assure that there is no pelvic injury.

Summary

Diagnostic error is a looming threat during every shift in the emergency department. By carefully screening our thinking for bias and false assumptions, we have an opportunity to reduce these errors. In particularly error-prone circumstances, cognitive forcing strategies can further limit the potential for error and harm. Algorithms and literature support, in the form of clinical guidelines and prediction rules, give us a springboard to developing our own ideal diagnostic plans.

PUTTING IT ALL TOGETHER

We have presented a structured approach to evidence-based diagnostic decision-making in emergency medicine. This approach brings evidence and quantitative information to bear on areas that traditionally involve purely "clinical" reasoning. While the process may seem daunting and unwieldy on first inspection, this approach of critical thinking quickly becomes intuitive and fully integrated into practice. We are convinced that you will ultimately find that the pain of acquiring these skills is compensated many fold by virtue of having become a smarter, more insightful, and also quicker emergency physician.

The alternative is to make non-critical diagnostic decisions. It may seem clinically intuitive that a patient with a negative CT scan of the head does not have a subarachnoid hemorrhage, until we miss one. It may make sense clinically that a patient with a normal WBC does not have a surgical abdomen, until she returns with a perforation. These two misjudgments were probably pointed out to us as problematic during the nascent stages of our training, but what of the scores of slightly flawed assumptions we do not even know exist within our biased thinking?

These methods do not require the abandonment of clinical judgment. In fact, as we have discussed, clinical judgment is essential to all parts of the process of evidence-based decision-making. Further, we build our clinical judgment on experience, and the foundation of experience is often the mistakes we have made. Evidence-based diagnostic decision-making offers another path to developing our clinical judgment by allowing the examination of seemingly logical diagnostic plans before we make a mistake.

More than anything else, this strategy forces us to think through our plans. This process of critical evaluation allows us to avert errors and avoid causing harm to our patients.

CASE: THE CLOT THICKENS

It is a busy Monday at 3 p.m., and Dr Wayne is signing out his patients to you. You both walk over to bed #10 where a young woman looks up from the gurney. He tells you that he picked up the chart of this 25-year-old woman just 15 minutes ago, but the case is an easy one. She has just returned home after an eight-hour plane ride and is now complaining of a "little" shortness of breath and some reproducible chest pain. He goes on to tell you that he ordered a V/Q scan, which has not yet been done. He advises: "If it comes back normal or low probability, send her home. If it comes back intermediate or high, just put her on heparin and admit her as a confirmed PE." He finishes sign-out and leaves the department to you. You decide to start over with bed #10.

After a brief history and physical exam, you gather the following information.

Clinical Exam

Chief Complaint   I took a plane flight yesterday and now my chest hurts.

History of Present Illness   The patient is a 25-year-old female, who flew from California back to New York yesterday. This morning, around 10 a.m., she experienced the sudden onset of right-sided chest pain described as constant, respirophasic, without radiation or alteration with changed position. She is also complaining of mild dyspnea.

Past Medical History   None.

Past Surgical History   None.

Family History   Paternal grandfather died of myocardial infarction at age 78.

Social History   No tobacco or drug use, including cocaine.

Medications   Oral contraceptives.

Allergies   None.

Physical Exam   Well-kempt 25 y/o female appearing her age. Temperature 99.2°F; pulse 96/min; BP 110/72 mmHg; respiration 24/min; SaO$_2$ 98% on room air.

- HEENT normal
- Neck: No jugular venous distention, trachea is midline.

- Lungs: Clear to auscultation bilaterally. Mild tenderness right chest wall which reproduces the patient's pain.
- Heart: S1 S2, regular rate and rhythm and no murmurs, rubs, or gallops.
- Abdomen: Benign.
- Extremities: Normal exam. No calf tenderness, masses, or cords.

You send Cindy, the medical student rotating in the department, in to interview the patient as well. After Cindy's interview, the two of you discuss the diagnostic plan.

Differential Diagnosis

When you ask Cindy her differential diagnosis, she proceeds to do an extremely thorough job of listing every known cause of chest pain that has ever plagued a human being. Her list has little connection to the patient's age, risk factors, or circumstances.

You then relay to her your own list: Pattern matching brought up the diagnosis of pulmonary embolism as soon as you read the chief complaint on the nurse's triage note. Upon interviewing the patient, you mentally reviewed many of the diagnoses on Cindy's list but discounted almost all of them except spontaneous pneumothorax, costochondritis, or musculo-skeletal pain.

Pre-test Probability

Pulmonary embolism (PE) remains at the top of your list of differential diagnoses. You know of quite a few different clinical prediction rules in the literature, which can aid in the calculation of pre-test probability for pulmonary embolism. You are most familiar with the Wells' criteria and decide to use them in this case.[63] You know this clinical prediction rule has been validated and has proven to be accurate in the emergency department population.

Your patient scores 3 points for pulmonary embolism being more likely than any alternative diagnosis; she has none of the other Wells' criteria (Fig. 2-22). A score of 3 points translates into a moderate pre-test probability, or quantitatively, a 21% pre-test probability.

Though they are not part of the Wells' criteria, you decide to adjust the pre-test probability due to the use of oral contraceptives and the plane flight. This alteration of pre-test probability in light of the patient's unique circumstances is based on your clinical experience. You decide to raise the pre-test probability of pulmonary embolism to 30%; you write this number in the chart.

Wells' Criteria for PE

Criteria	Points
Suspected DVT	3.0
An alternative diagnosis is less likely than PE	3.0
Heart rate >100 beats/min	1.5
Immobilization or surgery in previous 4 weeks	1.5
Previous DVT/PE	1.5
Hemoptysis	1.0
Malignancy (on treatment or treated within past 6 months)	1.0

Score	Mean probability of PE	Risk
<2	3.6%	Low
2-6	20.5%	Medium
>6	66.7%	High

— FIGURE 2-22 — *Wells' criteria for estimating quantifying the pre-test probability of pulmonary embolism.*[63]

You do not know of any decision aids for the assignment of probabilities for the other diagnoses on the list, so you use your clinical judgment. You assign a pre-test probability of 5% to spontaneous pneumothorax and 65% to costochondritis or musculoskeletal pain. The ROWS heuristic leads you to pursue the diagnosis of pulmonary embolism first, even though it is not the most likely diagnosis based on pre-test probability.

Decision Thresholds

Next, you pick your discard and accept thresholds for pulmonary embolism. Missing a clot can be life-threatening, not because of the current situation, but because of the risk of a subsequent larger embolism. Falsely diagnosing a pulmonary embolism is also problematic. If the patient is erroneously given this diagnosis, it will expose her to the risks of anti-coagulation, affect insurance premiums, and forever brand future medical interactions.

You decide to set the discard threshold at 2% and the accept threshold at 80%. To illustrate for Cindy what these numbers mean, you decide to draw the threshold diagrams for your work-up of pulmonary embolism.

You ask Cindy how she would go about working up this patient for pulmonary embolism. She tells you she wants a chest x-ray, an arterial blood gas, and an EKG.

Chest Radiograph You tell Cindy that the chest x-ray very rarely will help with the diagnosis of pulmonary embolism, but it may be useful to evaluate other conditions. You decide that you will get a chest x-ray as it will allow you to drive the probability of spontaneous pneumothorax below the discard threshold. You could have easily argued that, in the course of further studies for pulmonary embolism, the chest would be imaged and therefore hold off on the chest x-ray.

Electrocardiogram The EKG is also rarely useful in modifying the pre-test probability of PE. If acute coronary syndrome was in the differential, it would certainly be worth getting an EKG to evaluate for this possibility as well as other cardiac disorders, but in this patient, this is not a consideration given the absence of any risk factors. Supposedly, pathognomonic signs such as S1 Q3 T3 are neither sensitive, nor specific for pulmonary embolism.[64]

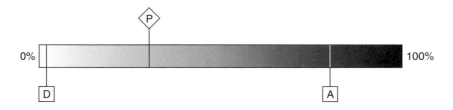

Arterial Blood Gas (ABG) As a field, we are moving towards a consensus that, aside from assessing a patient after intubation, this test is not useful in the emergency department. When we look at the data from PIOPED, the test has little utility in the workup of pulmonary embolism.[65]

The ABG is at its most sensitive when the criteria for an abnormal test are a $PaCO_2 < 35$, a $PaO_2 < 80$, or an Aa gradient >20. The LR negative using this criterion is 0.9.[65] This likelihood ratio has no ability to change our pre-test probability.

While you continue to discuss further diagnostic workup, you ask the nurse to take the patient over to get her x-ray, if her urine pregnancy test is negative.

You continue to barrage Cindy with questions about other diagnostic tests for pulmonary embolism. Digging deep into her first two years of medical school, she suggests a d-dimer and Dopplers of the legs to look for DVT.

D-Dimer This test has revolutionized the work-up of low-risk patients presenting to the emergency department with suspected DVT or PE. Unfortunately, the institution you are working in has a first-generation latex d-dimer as its only assay. The characteristics of this test are a likelihood ratio positive of 2.9 and negative of 0.39.[66] We see that it would do little to alter our pre-test probability. If we had an ELISA d-dimer, a negative result would have a more significant effect. The likelihood ratio negative of an ELISA assay is 0.06. You elect not to order the d-dimer assay.

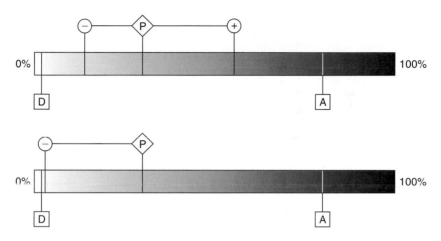

Dopplers of the Legs A positive DVT in a patient with chest symptoms virtually rules-in the diagnosis of pulmonary embolism. However, in a patient without leg symptoms or signs, the diagnostic yield of this exam is quite low. A negative ultrasound exam for DVT would do little to alter our pre-test probability for pulmonary embolism.

You tell Cindy that since a conventional pulmonary angiogram is not available at your hospital, there are two remaining choices: V/Q scan or CT angiogram.

Ventilation/Perfusion (V/Q) Scan We have discussed the likelihood ratios of the interval results of the V/Q scan in the prior sections.

RESULTS OF V/Q SCAN	LIKELIHOOD RATIO
Normal	0.1
Low	0.4
Intermediate	1.2
High	18.3

From these values, we can see that only a high-probability scan will have the ability to allow us to stop the diagnostic process without further testing.

Results of V/Q scan	Post-test probability
Normal	4%
Low	15%
Intermediate	34%
High	89%

The most common results of a V/Q scan are low or moderate probability.[67] Even a normal result will not drive our post-test probability below the discard threshold.

CT Angiogram of the Chest   A year ago, you only ordered CT angiograms for pulmonary embolism when your patients had severe underlying lung disease. You worried about the poor sensitivities for subsegmental clots and questioned the ability of your radiology department to interpret these scans. Two things have changed in your institution in the past few months. All scans are now performed on a new multidetector machine capable of 1-mm cuts and imaging of the entire pulmonary vasculature during a single breath. In addition, an outside group with fellowship training in CT imaging of the body now reads all CT angiograms of the chest.

These two factors have made multidetector spiral CT angiogram your first test of choice for pulmonary embolism. The most recent studies of this level of technology give a LR negative of approximately 0.05 and LR positive of 45.[68,69] These levels of accuracy are only achievable if poor quality scans, which do not achieve good visualization of subsegmental branches, are read as inconclusive and not as negative.

Not only are the testing characteristics of CT superior, but there is actual patient-oriented outcome data for this test. The risk of recurrent venous thromboembolic disease (PE or DVTs) in patients sent home after a negative CT angiogram and without anticoagulation is 0.5–1% at 3 months.[69–71] These data are as compelling as the excellent likelihood ratios. Your viewpoint is supported by the clinical policy of the British Thoracic Society, which accepts a negative new-generation CT angiogram as sufficient to rule out the diagnosis of PE (Fig. 2-23).[72]

If your institution had older machines or a radiology department inexperienced with this exam, then the likelihood ratios would have to be

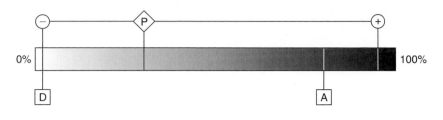

— FIGURE 2-23 — *The CT angiogram has the ability to both rule-in and rule-out the diagnosis of pulmonary embolism in your patient.*

adjusted. In this case, the *test characteristics* in the above-mentioned studies would not be *applicable* to your patient.

Testing

You put the order for CT scan in the computer. The patient has returned from x-ray; you pull the radiograph up on the point-of-care radiology system. The chest film appears completely normal. This does not affect the probability of pulmonary embolism, but you discard the diagnosis of spontaneous pneumothorax.

Cindy asks if we need renal function laboratory tests before the CT scan. You tell her that, in the absence of any risk factors such as preexisting problems or a history of diabetes, the pre-test probability for renal disease is almost nil.[73]

Post-test Probability

Your patient returns from radiology; a few minutes later, you get a call from the attending radiologist. He first discusses the technical quality of the scan. This is of vital importance as, if no clot was visualized on a poor quality scan, then the result is not negative, it is indeterminate. This scan was of excellent quality, with good timing of the dye bolus and visualization of the entire pulmonary vascular tree. No clot was visualized, nor was any additional lung or chest pathology noted.

Action

You explain the results to your patient with Cindy listening in. You tell them both that a negative CT scan is sufficient to drive the post-test probability of PE below the discard threshold. You believe she is suffering from a musculoskeletal condition and tell her to buy and take ibuprofen for the pain and inflammation.

You also explain that complete diagnoses are often difficult in the emergency department. You want her to follow-up with her private medical doctor in the next few days for a check-up.

CHAPTER 3

TREATMENT DECISIONS

CASE: THE CLOCK IS TICKING

Eight hours into your 12-hour shift you have finally found a couple of minutes to sit down and eat your now cold pad thai. That is until the triage nurse pops her head into the break room to tell you that she has just placed a Code Stroke into the resuscitation room. **To be continued** . . .

TREATMENT CHOICES

When a patient is truly sick, the immediate steps of treatment are second nature to us. The resuscitation of the critically ill is the sine qua non of an emergency physician. However, most of our treatment decisions require more thought than those made during the first few minutes of a code. We often place greater emphasis on evidence-based diagnostic decisions than treatment decisions. This emphasis makes sense: when the problem is less serious, if we make the proper diagnosis, any of a range of treatments will lead to an acceptable outcome, if not the ideal one.

But there are a number of treatments, which, if not used appropriately, can lead to grave outcomes. Thrombolytics, cardiac medications, intubation, and invasive procedures all require careful consideration of risks, benefits, and patient values. Beyond just these interventions, our patients deserve the best care we are capable of providing; we should strive for the ideal management rather than the acceptable.

TREATMENT DECISION-MAKING

In emergency medicine, all the factors that conspire to make our diagnostic decisions difficult also work towards complicating our treatment decisions. Our field's *ill-structured domain* makes cognitive treatment errors a constant threat to our performance.

We use recognition-primed decision-making for treatment choices, just as we discussed in the diagnostic section.[17] Figure 3-1 demonstrates this process.

When presented with a treatment decision, we determine if the situation is familiar or an anomaly. If the situation is familiar, we will use *rules-based* processes to formulate a treatment plan.

- *Rules-based decision-making:* We create this plan using precompiled responses from treatments we have used in the past. These pre-compiled responses take the form of *treatment scripts*; they provide a subconscious mental map, just as our illness scripts offered for diagnosis.

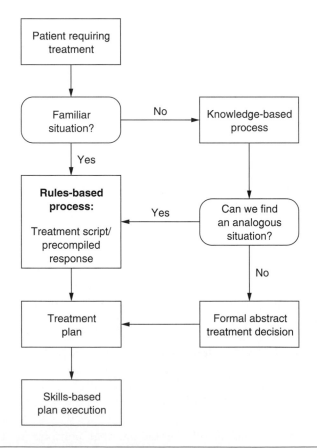

— FIGURE 3-1 —   *Recognition-primed treatment decisions.*

- *Knowledge-based decision-making:* If the situation is *atypical,* we first search for an *analogous situation* we have treated in the past. If we can discover a situation that is sufficiently similar, we may revert to rules-based decision-making, with slight alterations of the treatment plan given the unique circumstances of the atypical situation. This combines knowledge-based and rules-based decision-making.
- *Formal decision-making:* If we cannot find an analogous situation, then we resort to this least cognitively desirable situation. We say "least desirable" because the more we have to think, the more predisposed we are to error.[54,74]

Once we have created a treatment plan, we utilize *skills-based behavior* to carry it out.

Cognitive error can occur anywhere along the process of treatment decisions and execution. At the end of this section, we discuss the types of cognitive treatment error and the means to prevent them.

Formal Treatment Decision-making

In the next few sections, we describe the formal process of evidence-based treatment decisions. In order to use this process, we need to answer certain key questions:

- Do I have a treatment to offer for this condition?
- Do I have evidence for this treatment?
- Is this evidence sound?
- Is there a measurable treatment effect?
- Is this treatment effect measured in terms that matter to my patient and that I can interpret?
- What are the costs of the treatment (both monetary and societal)?
- What are the risks of the treatment (both short- and long-term)?
- Is the evidence supporting the treatment applicable to my patient?
- How does this treatment compare with or add to alternatives?
- How does this treatment compare with doing nothing?
- What are my patient's feelings about the proposed treatment?

We can distill these questions into the equation shown in Fig. 3-2. This equation embodies the process of critical thinking as applied to treatment decisions. We consider the benefit to our patients: a summation of the quantitative treatment effect and the analysis of the real-world value of that treatment effect. We examine the risk the treatment might have for the patient. We modify both of these values based on the individual characteristics of our patient; i.e., the applicability of the risk/benefit evidence. We now have the potential impact of the proposed treatment and we must

**(Benefit – Risk) Applicability =
Impact ± Patient Values =
Treatment Decision**

— FIGURE 3-2 —   *An equation for treatment decisions.*

bring this to the patient and elicit his or her views. We can then arrive at a treatment decision and act on this decision.

TREATMENT PARAMETERS

If the treatment we are considering has been studied, then its benefit can be represented quantitatively. The parameters that represent this benefit can be confusing and at times even misleading. Sorting through the various treatment parameters is the first step of determining benefit (Fig. 3-3).

While there are many permutations of study designs to evaluate treatment, almost all of them will compare a control group to a treatment or experimental group. The control group might receive standard therapy or a placebo. We discuss the different forms of treatment studies in Part II.

Note to readers: The mathematical formulations for each of the parameters are included as an aid for our left-brain dominant readers. If you are conceptual in your learning style, feel free to ignore the mathematics and concentrate on the underlying theories.

All of the treatment parameters we are about to discuss are the *point estimates* derived from studies. We discuss all of the intricacies of point estimates in Part II. For now, what is necessary to understand is that these parameters are the most likely estimates of the benefit of a treatment derived from a study. However, there is always an important degree of uncertainty associated with these estimates; investigators are expected to provide information regarding the extent of this uncertainty.* We discuss this concept in great detail in Part II; the rest of this discussion assumes that we have assessed the degree of uncertainty and believe it to be acceptable.

Link to Page 187

---

*This uncertainty is quantified by *confidence intervals*. They too will be explained in Part II.

> # (Benefit – Risk) Applicability =
> # Impact ± Patient Values =
> # Treatment Decision

— FIGURE 3-3 —

Event Rates

An event rate (ER) is the probability that an event will occur in a defined population. We can break the event rates of a study into the rate in the control group and the rate in the experimental group. Many treatment studies have dichotomous events (e.g., survival or death). Treatment studies may also use a range of values. For instance, in a study on asthma the researchers can look at the difference in FEV_1 between a treatment group and a placebo group. We use event rates to report dichotomous data.

- **Control event rate (CER):** In the control group, this is the number of patients who had the event divided by all of the patients in the control group.

$$CER = \frac{\text{Control group patients with the event}}{\text{All control group patients}}.$$

- **Experimental event rate (EER):** This is conceptually the same idea as CER, but in the experimental or treatment group.

$$EER = \frac{\text{Treatment group patients with the event}}{\text{All treatment group patients}}.$$

Just as with sensitivities and specificities, we express these rates as decimals or as percentages depending on the situation. To convert the decimal value to a percentage, we just multiply it by a hundred.

EXAMPLE

A trial of Inspire™, an imaginary new drug for the treatment of status asthmaticus, was performed. The study placed 400 patients in the treatment group and 450 in the placebo group. The endpoint for the study was the need for intubation during the first 24 hours of treatment. In the Inspire^{TM} group, 200 patients were intubated, while 300 patients were intubated in the control group.

$$CER = \frac{300 \text{ intubated patients}}{450 \text{ placebo-group patients}} = 0.67 = 67\%;$$

$$EER = \frac{200 \text{ intubated patients}}{400 \text{ Inspire-group patients}} = 0.50 = 50\%.$$

Absolute Parameters

Using the control event rate (CER) and the experimental event rate (EER), we can calculate the differences between the groups.

Absolute Risk Reduction (ARR)
This is the difference between the control group's and experimental group's rates. It represents the true difference found for the treatment in the study population:

$$ARR = CER - EER.$$

EXAMPLE

The absolute risk reduction in the Inspire^{TM} study is 17%. This means that 17% fewer patients with severe asthma attacks were intubated if Inspire^{TM} was administered:

$$ARR = CER - EER = 67\% - 50\% = 17\%.$$

Number Needed to Treat (NNT)
We can also express the absolute risk reduction as the number of patients that would have to be given the treatment in order for one of the patients to achieve the outcome measure in a given amount of time. NNTs are best understood in relationship to dichotomous outcomes, such as death, admission to the hospital, or myocardial infarction. The form NNT expressions take is:

NNT = (Insert number of patients) would have to be treated with
(Insert treatment in study) to prevent one (Insert outcome from study)
over the course of (Insert time period from study).

Or with the blanks filled in:

NNT = 30 patients would have to be treated with the new imaginary drug
Nephronic™ to prevent one additional death from renal failure
over the course of three months.

We can calculate the NNT from the ARR; we round the results to the
nearest patient:

$$NNT = \frac{100}{ARR}.$$

Example

The number needed to treat in the Inspire™ study would be six patients.
This means for every six patients treated with the drug, one patient
would avoid an intubation, during the 2 hours following treatment,
which they would have needed if they had received the placebo:

$$NNT = \frac{100}{17} = 5.9(6)\, patients$$

The number needed to treat provides practitioners with a direct measure
of patient-important impact of a therapy and has the added benefit of
allowing easy comparisons with other treatments.

Relative Parameters

Relative parameters express treatment effect as proportions of rates.

Relative Risk Reduction (RRR)

Relative risk reduction is one of the most common ways to report the
results of studies of treatment. It reflects the proportional reduction of
risk in the treatment group when compared to the baseline risk. It does
not reveal the actual reduction in risk; we can therefore be misled regarding the importance of a therapy to patients if only this value is
reported. Commonly used synonyms for relative risk reduction include
"effectiveness" and "efficacy" (even though these terms properly have
different meanings).

$$RRR = \frac{(CER - EER)}{CER}.$$

EXAMPLE

In the Inspire™ study, the relative risk reduction is 25%.

$$RRR = \frac{(67 - 50)}{67} = 0.25 = 25\%.$$

This means 25% fewer patients were intubated when Inspire™ was given than when placebo was given. Notice how easy this is to confuse with the absolute risk reduction. In this example, the difference between the two values is 8%. When the likelihood of the target outcome over the time period in question is low, the difference between the RRR and ARR becomes larger.

Relative Risk (RR)

This is the proportion of the control event rate (CER) represented by the experimental event rate (EER). This value expresses the degree of treatment effect compared to no treatment:

$$RR = \frac{EER}{CER}.$$

EXAMPLE

In the Inspire™ study, the relative risk is 75%.

$$RR = \frac{50}{67} = 0.75 = 75\%.$$

In other words, the intubation rate of the experimental group is 75% of the rate in the placebo group.

The relative risk (RR) and the relative risk reduction (RRR) when added together will always equal 100%. This means that we can easily convert one value to the other.

Odds Ratios

In addition to the parameters already mentioned, we will occasionally come across treatment effects expressed as *odds ratios*. This is somewhat unfortunate, because parameters based on risk, such as absolute risk reduction, relative risk reduction, and number needed to treat are often intuitively grasped by readers. We rarely have an innate comprehension of odds; we must resort to pondering in order to grasp this parameter.

$$\text{Odds ratio} = \frac{\text{Odds of event in experiment group}}{\text{Odds of event in control group}};$$

$$\text{Odds of event} = \frac{\text{Number of patients with event in group}}{\text{Number of patients without event in group}}.$$

When can one think of an odds ratio in the same way as you think of a risk ratio? The answer is when the event rates are relatively low; i.e., less than 10–15%. When this is the case, the odds ratios will be very close to the risk ratios.

Otherwise, an odds ratio of 2 does not mean that you are twice as likely to have the outcome, and an odds ratio of 0.5 does not mean that you are half as likely to have the outcome. The odds ratio, when less than one, will underestimate the relative risk; and when greater than one will overestimate it. The degree of this misestimation increases as the degree of baseline risk increases. We advise the interpretation of odds ratios only qualitatively and not quantitatively. If the true relative or absolute risk is needed, then they may be calculated either from the original data of the study or by using complex formulas.[75]

EXAMPLE

In the Inspire[TM] study, the odds of the experimental group for intubation are 1 (remember from the diagnostic decision section, odds of 1 are the same as a probability of 50%):

$$\text{Odds of intubation in experimental group}$$
$$= \frac{200 \text{ intubated patients}}{200 \text{ patients not intubated}} = 1.$$

The odds of intubation in the control group are 2:

$$\text{Odds of intubation in control group}$$
$$= \frac{300 \text{ intubated patients}}{150 \text{ patients not intubated}} = 2.$$

The odds ratio for the intubation between the experimental and control group is 0.5:

$$\text{Odds ratio} = \frac{1 \text{ in experimental group}}{2 \text{ in control group}} = 0.5.$$

If we look back to the example in the relative risk description above, we can see the relative risk using the same values is 75%. If odds ratios were considered equivalent to relative risk in this study, we would have thought that the risk of needing intubation is reduced by 50% in the experimental group when actually the risk is reduced by only 25%.

Odds ratios, although not intuitively clear, are a fact of life.* Their statistical properties make them appropriate when event rates are very high and authors of meta-analyses frequently prefer them.

Link to Page 207

Benefit Parameters

In the above discussion of treatment effects, we concentrated on treatments that reduced the risk of an undesirable outcome. Studies also use treatment effects that increase the chances of a beneficial outcome. For example, survival to hospital discharge is a treatment effect, which researchers hope is more prevalent in the treated group. In these studies, instead of risk reduction, we speak of *benefit increase*:

$$\text{Absolute benefit increase (ABI)} = \text{EER} - \text{CER};$$

$$\text{Relative benefit increase (RBI)} = \frac{\text{EER} - \text{CER}}{\text{CER}}.$$

Treatment Parameters for Continuous Outcomes

If instead of dichotomous treatment outcomes, researchers report study results in the form of continuous data, such as the increase in oxygen saturation on a pulse oximeter, then we do not use CER and EER. In these situations, usually the mean increase or decrease of the continuous values is used.

Absolute Parameter
The absolute parameter for a continuous outcome treatment would be the absolute difference between the change in the experimental group and the

---

*We do have the option of converting odds ratios to number needed to treat (NNT). This allows an easier comparison with other treatments. This formula can be used to make the conversion:

$$\text{NNT} = \frac{\{1 - [\text{CER} \times (1 - \text{OR})]\}}{[(1 - \text{CER}) \times (\text{CER}) \times (1 - \text{OR})]}.$$

CER represents the *control event rate* from the control group in the study. Even easier is to go to www.nntonline.net where you will find an online calculator.

change in the control group.

Absolute change = Experimental group change − Control group change.

We do not routinely calculate NNT for continuous outcomes.

Relative Parameter

Relative changes would be expressed as the *absolute change* (which we just calculated above) over the control group's change:

$$\text{Relative change} = \frac{\text{Absolute change}}{\text{Control group change}}.$$

EXAMPLE

If the Inspire™ study measured changes in FEV_1 instead of need for intubation, we would find the mean FEV_1 in the control group was 1.3 L and the mean FEV_1 in the experimental group was 1.9 L. There was an absolute change of 0.6 L between the two groups.

When expressed in relative terms, there was a 46% increase in FEV_1 in the experimental group:

$$\text{Relative change} = \frac{1.9 - 1.3}{1.3} = 46\%.$$

Relativity and Absolutism

You may now be wondering why we need both relative and absolute parameters to represent the effects of a treatment from a study. Each of these types of treatment parameters is vitally important to evaluate and use the new treatment.

- *Absolute parameters:* The absolute parameters listed in a study, such as ARR and NNT, reflect the *impact* of a therapy on the average patient in the study population. We can use this as a gauge of the importance of a new therapy.
- *Relative parameters:* The relative parameters, RRR and RR, reflect the potential effectiveness of the therapy across a broad range of patients, characterized by varying levels of risk for the outcome in question.

Relative parameters, in tandem with estimates of individual patient's risk, allow us to *apply* the treatment effects to our individual patient. Using our patient's baseline risk and a relative parameter, we can calculate an *individualized absolute parameter*, allowing us to assess the impact of a therapy on our patient. We discuss this more extensively in the applicability section below. In summary, the absolute parameters from a study allow us to gauge the importance of a therapy, while the relative parameters allow us to apply the therapy to our individual patient.

A Review of Treatment Parameters

You may find it useful to see a summary of the treatment parameters we have derived for the imaginary Inspire^{TM} study.
The numbers in the study were:

	NOT INTUBATED	INTUBATED	TOTAL PTS
Experimental	200	200	400
Control	150	300	450

Event Rates

$$CER = Event/Total = 300/450 = 67\%$$
$$EER = Event/Total = 200/400 = 50\%$$

Absolute Parameters

$$ARR = CER - EER = 17\%$$
$$NNT = 100/APR = 6 \, Patients$$

Relative Parameters

$$RR = EER/CER = 75\%$$
$$RRR = (CER - EER)/CER \, or \, 1 - RR = 25\%$$
$$OR = (Exp. \, group \, event/No \, event)/(Cont. \, group \, event)/No \, event)$$
$$= (200/200)/(300/150) = 0.5$$

PATIENT-ORIENTED EVIDENCE

"Not everything that can be counted counts, and not everything that counts can be counted." – Albert Einstein

If, after examining the treatment parameters, we decide that there is a solid quantitative treatment effect, we then must go further and ask whether this treatment benefit actually matters. In order to answer this question, we must examine the qualitative nature of the benefit (see Fig. 3-3).

In the past, clinicians administered interventions based on assumptions regarding their mechanism of action and the biology of disease, without necessarily knowing the *patient-important* outcomes of their treatments.

EXAMPLE

Patients with severe traumatic brain injury often have elevated intracranial pressure (ICP). It was standard practice to hyperventilate these patients down to a low $PaCO_2$, because the induced cerebral vasoconstriction would lower ICP. This intervention was performed even in the absence of signs of herniation. While ICPs were indeed lowered, the patients who received routine hyperventilation had worse neurological outcomes.[76,77]

Further studies showed that hyperventilation actually reduced cerebral blood flow at the same time it decreased intracranial pressure.[77] This is the problem with treating based on presumed pathophysiology; there may always be one more crucial piece of information we do not yet grasp. Practitioners of evidence-based decision-making should avoid treating based upon our understanding of presumed pathophysiology.

Instead, we should make our treatment decisions using the best available evidence. Evidence-based medicine traditionally breaks the evidence into two types: disease-oriented evidence and patient-oriented evidence. A large number of treatment studies published in the literature use disease-oriented evidence (DOE); this is just *pathophysiologic observation* brought beyond the scale of one patient to many patients. While DOE is a step up from individual observation, what we truly yearn for is patient-oriented evidence (POE).

Disease-oriented Evidence

Disease-oriented evidence examines parameters such as blood pressure or PaO_2 and draws treatment effect conclusions based on these physiological markers. It is a boon to researchers, as studies based on DOE often require fewer patients and shorter follow-up. It can serve as interesting background knowledge for clinicians; the danger is when we use this DOE as a stand-in for meaningful treatment outcomes.

EXAMPLE

Nesiritide (aBNP), a new treatment for decompensated heart failure, was compared to nitroglycerin in a prospective trial. The main outcome measures were a decrease in pulmonary capillary wedge pressure (PCWP) and changes in the patients' perceived dyspnea. At three hours, the nesiritide group had a mean decrease PCWP of 5.8 mmHg compared with a decrease of 3.8 mmHg in the nitroglycerin group. There was no decrease in subjective dyspnea in the nesiritide group. When we calculate the absolute reduction, there was an absolute mean decrease of 2 mmHg more with the nesiritide treatment. Many viewed this as a positive study and as an indication to replace nitroglycerin with aBNP.[78]

PCWP is a known marker for heart failure with cardiogenic pulmonary edema. Will a difference of 2 mmHg in the PCWP at three hours make a difference in true patient outcomes? We do not know; this is the problem with disease-oriented evidence. While decreasing the PCWP is seemingly a good strategy for the treatment of decompensated heart failure, how much of a change makes a difference in the real outcomes: the need for intubation, the need for ICU level care, and patient mortality. Beyond these questions, we must consider the fact that nesiritide is far more expensive than nitroglycerin and takes much longer to wear off if there is an adverse event.

We can analyze studies such as the above and conclude that the statistical analysis and methods are sound, but we do not intuitively know the clinical significance. When we have to pontificate on the clinical importance of a treatment, rather than immediately grasping it, we are dealing with DOE. Reduction of the PCWP is DOE; we do not know if nesiritide really changes our patients' outcomes.

Surrogate Endpoints

A recent systematic review looked at the use of nesiritide from the perspective of a useful endpoint: *patient mortality*.[79] The data from this study indicate that this medication may actually increase the risk of death. This demonstrates the danger of DOE; when real endpoints are examined the benefits of the treatment may look much different.

A slightly more useful form of DOE is its use as a surrogate endpoint. This refers to a disease-oriented piece of evidence, which has been clearly linked in past studies to a true patient-oriented outcome. If the surrogate endpoint has not been so linked, which is the case more often than not, then it remains an example of plain DOE.

EXAMPLE

Suppose we wanted to develop a new treatment to slow the heart rate in patients with acute coronary syndromes (ACS) with the goal of lowering mortality. If it has been proven in previous studies that a decrease in heart rate is clearly linked to a reduction in mortality, then if a new drug is proven to lower heart rate, it is possible to assume that it will lower mortality in ACS patients.

The danger is that in the original studies that linked heart rate and mortality, there may have been other factors in addition to the heart rate which led to the mortality benefit. If the heart rate studies were originally performed with beta-blockers, even if a new calcium-channel blocker can lower the heart rate as effectively, it may not have the same mortality benefit. There may be some unique feature of the beta-blockers besides their ability to slow the heart that lead to the decreased mortality.

Patient-oriented evidence is stronger than surrogate endpoints because it limits the possibility of false conclusions. Generally, surrogate endpoints are safer to apply to members of the same class of drugs, rather than applying them to disparate drug types with a similar treatment effect.

Patient-oriented Evidence

Patient-oriented evidence (POE) consists of outcomes that matter to us as clinicians: mortality, admission to the hospital, disease recurrence, etc. When clinicians look at a study with a POE outcome, they immediately grasp how it will affect their patients. POE is harder to produce; it takes many more patients and longer follow-up to see if a treatment for septic shock actually causes a reduction in mortality (POE) as opposed to an increase in blood pressure (DOE).

EXAMPLE

When a patient presents with a severe exacerbation of chronic obstructive pulmonary disease (COPD), the emergency physician must contemplate the dismal prospect of intubation. When we consider the difficulty of weaning these patients and the high rate of ventilator-associated pneumonia, an alternative to intubation becomes very desirable. Bi-level positive airway pressure, a method of non-invasive ventilation (NIV), offers an attractive alternative. The question, of course, is whether this NIV actually benefits our patients. A meta-analysis from the Cochrane Group shows that NIV clearly reduces $PaCO_2$ and respiratory rate and increases pH.[80] While this sounds attractive, this information is DOE; it is intriguing, but it does not definitively tell us that NIV is clinically useful. However, the meta-analysis also reveals that the treatment reduces mortality and the need for intubation; these outcomes are POE. If we believe the results of the meta-analysis, then NIV will truly help our patients with COPD exacerbations.

We should base our treatment decisions on POE, whenever it is available. Treatments that look attractive when the DOE is published often do not prove themselves when POE outcome trials are later performed. Guyatt et al. also refer to this form of evidence as "patient-important."[81] This stresses the point that our patients understand and care about outcomes such as death and rates of myocardial infarction, but not a two-point change in their systolic blood pressure.

Patient-oriented Evidence that Matters

We can take our need for patient-oriented evidence one-step further. A beautifully done study, using treatment criteria that matter, but examining a condition we may see once in our careers, is certainly patient-oriented evidence, but does not matter much to our daily treatment decisions. We need POE that directly ramifies on our practice, causing Shaughnessy and Slawson et al. to create the term POEM*: Patient Oriented Evidence that Matters.[82,83] These authors describe POEMs as evidence that:

- Addresses a question that doctors encounter
- Measures outcomes that doctors and their patients care about: symptoms, morbidity, quality of life, and mortality
- Has the ability to change the way doctors practice.

We would add one more criterion to declare evidence a POEM: the study must demonstrate a reasonably useful change in these patient-important outcomes. In other words, the outcome must exceed a *treatment effect threshold*.

Treatment Effect Thresholds

We can go beyond simply demanding a demonstrable treatment effect and set a level for a new treatment that would make it worth the effort to change practice. A new drug that reduces admission rates by 0.5% (ARR) is fairly worthless to our clinical practice. With a NNT to prevent one

---

*The authors have also adopted the term to describe a collection of articles on the web they deem to be POEM evidence. These articles are also published in the *British Medical Journal* and the *Journal of Family Practice*. Here, we use the term only in the *generic* sense.

admission of 200, the drug's effect on any individual patient is miniscule. Clinically, we would observe very little difference in our patients with the use of this drug. We might demand that a new drug reduce admission rates by 5–10% before we would deem it useful.[84] At the same time, if a drug is created that has a small effect, but has rare side-effects and is inexpensive, it is worth lowering the treatment effect threshold.

Unfortunately, POEMs are scarce. One study deemed that fewer than 3% of the articles published in major journals of internal medicine were POEMs; i.e., articles that could change practice.[85]

System-Oriented Evidence (SOE)

This category of evidence is implicit when discussing treatments, but it is often far from the forefront of our considerations. While our focus is the individual patient, our actions always have ramifications on the healthcare system. Small actions repeated by thousands of clinicians have a huge cumulative effect. We must at least consider the cost and consequences of every treatment we provide.

Diminishment of Our Treatments

An example of an SOE question we deal with on a daily basis is whether to prescribe antibiotics to patients with viral illnesses. It is often easier to write the prescription than to offer an explanation as to why these medications are not needed. Even if we put aside the issue of wasted monetary resources, we are still destroying the future utility of this treatment, without any demonstrable benefit.[86]

When we consider this choice from the perspective of SOE, we realize that the problem of antibiotic resistance is rampant. While this unnecessary treatment may lead to a low risk in the individual patient, it hurts our ability to care for the system.

Diminishment of Our Resources

Our healthcare resources are not expanding but actually static and often shrinking. Any expenditure is a lost opportunity to provide another form of treatment, which might yield a greater good. Economists refer to this concept as the *opportunity cost* of an action. This runs counter to most physicians' value system: we care about our patient's welfare, costs be damned. Evidence-literate clinicians take a longer-term view and realize that treatment choices for individual patients have effects on our healthcare system as a whole.

EXAMPLE

Glycoprotein IIb/IIIa agents have a beneficial treatment effect when given to patients with acute coronary syndromes (ACS) going to cardiac catheterization.[87] A few current studies have shown a treatment effect, albeit an extremely small one, on subsets of patients with ACS not going to catheterization. Patients stratified to high-risk groups derive the most benefit from the medication. There may be some benefit in lower risk patients, but currently the data do not show anything but a minor effect.[87] If we discount the risks, and the medication were inexpensive, then perhaps we should administer it if there is even a chance of some benefit. However, this medication is both expensive and not without risk. When we add the SOE to the analysis, there would be an enormous cost to a strategy of giving IIb/IIIa agents in all ACS patients not going to catheterization. We can make similar comparisons for the medication clopidogrel for ischemic stroke.

Patient Values in a Healthcare System

Another system-oriented evidence issue to consider is patient values. We will discuss how to apply the individual patient values to our treatment decisions shortly; what we are alluding to here are treatments that affect large groups of patients without offering them choices.

Resuscitative drugs for cardiac arrest or unresponsive patients embody this category. These are treatments that may prevent death, but not create life; i.e., they may bring back a pulse, but leave patients in a vegetative state. In addition to the cost and resource utilization, as well as the trauma to the patient's family, we must consider if this form of treatment violates the values and desires of the patients in our healthcare system.

EXAMPLE

High-dose epinephrine was once routinely used for patients in cardiac arrest. While this treatment increases the percentage of patients with return of spontaneous circulation (ROSC), it does not increase the chances that a patient will leave the hospital alive.[88]

When evaluating this treatment in terms of the individual patient, it may seem an obvious decision to give high-dose epinephrine. Increased return of spontaneous circulation is definitely a patient-oriented outcome. However, if patients are surviving cardiac arrest only to remain in the hospital in a vegetative state, this is not an acceptable treatment from the perspective of SOE. We can raise similar questions for the use of Amiodarone™ in patients with ventricular fibrillation and pulseless ventricular tachycardia.

We need system-oriented evidence to examine the ethics, risks, benefits, and opportunity costs of the treatments for our healthcare system as a whole.

APPLICABILITY OF TREATMENT EFFECTS

Up to this point, we have discussed the meaning of the measures of treatment effect and the evaluation of the import of these effects. Now we must decide if these values are directly relevant to our patient. We must ask if he or she will derive the same level of benefit as the studied population (Fig. 3-4). The NEEDLE for the treatment we are evaluating provides the information we need to make this determination (Fig. 3-5).

Is my patient sicker than the study population?

The first question to answer is whether our patient has the same baseline risk as those patients in the study. If our patient is much sicker or much healthier, we may need to adjust the benefit they will receive from a treatment.

All of the following are patient characteristics that we should compare to the study population:[4]

- Age
- Gender
- Severity of disease
- Stage of disease
- Comorbidities.

Knowledge of these characteristics may allow us to estimate our patient's baseline risk. Literature support can also be found in articles on _prognosis_, which assess patient risk in a given disease state. We can also use the control event rate from other _treatment studies_ with populations

(Benefit – Risk) Applicability =
Impact ± Patient Values =
Treatment Decision

— FIGURE 3-4

Treatment NEEDLE:
tPA for acute ischemic stroke
Benefits/Downsides

- 0.9 mg/kg (10% as bolus, 90% as infusion over 60 minutes)
- ABI 13%, RBI 50% compared to placebo for minimal/no dysfunction at 3 months
- ARI 5.8%, RRI 900% compared to placebo for symptomatic intracerebral hemorrhage at 36 hours
- 90% probability of cost savings due to decreased hospitalization and rehabilitation costs

Applicability

- NIH Stroke Scale 5-21
- CT without signs of bleed or early infarct; read by neuroradiologists
- BP <185/105; may give labetolol × 2 doses if BP <220/140.
  If BP still >185/105 patient is not a lysis candidate
- Standard tPA contraindications

Original Study: *N Engl J Med.* 1995; 333:1581.
Cost Data: *Neurology.* 1988 Apr; 50(4):883-90.
–Valid RCT (ABI 95% CI 8.9-23.7)

— FIGURE 3-5 —   *An example of a treatment NEEDLE; we can use the information it contains to make applicability determinations.*

similar to our patient. However, the reality is that, most of the time, we will qualitatively adjust the baseline risk depending on the individual characteristics of our patient.

Once we have an idea of our patient's baseline risk, we can use the relative risk reduction we discussed above to obtain the absolute risk reduction for our patient.

Finding the Absolute Risk Reduction in Individual Patients

Absolute parameters reflect the benefit to the average patient in the study. With most treatments, the relative risk will stay approximately the same even in populations with higher control event rates; i.e., sicker patients.*

---

*One interesting exception is the emergency treatment of asthma. Medications such as magnesium sulfate have been shown to benefit patients with severe asthma, but have demonstrated no benefit in mild asthma.

This allows us to use the relative risk reduction to directly adjust a patient's baseline risk and derive the new risk after treatment.[89]

EXAMPLE

We examine a study of a new treatment, which reduces mortality from a baseline of 5% (CER) to 2.5% (EER). The relative risk reduction in this case is 50% and the absolute risk reduction is 2.5% (Fig. 3-6A).

If we wanted to use this treatment on our patient, who is sicker than the average patient in the study, we would start with a higher baseline risk, say 20%. If we apply the relative risk reduction (50%) to our patient's baseline risk, we can see that our patient will achieve an absolute risk reduction of 10%, quadruple that of the study population (Fig. 3-6B).

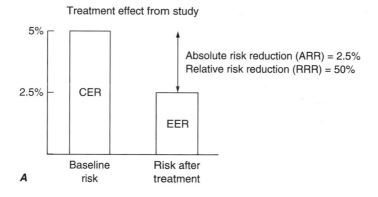

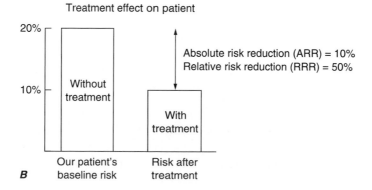

— FIGURE 3-6 —

The relative risk reduction stays constant, but the absolute risk reduction changes depending on whether the patient is sicker or healthier than the study population.

We can now see why we need both absolute and relative parameters to use the results of a study. Absolute parameters help us determine if the treatment is meaningful, whereas relative parameters allow us to use the study's results to calculate our individual patient's treatment effects.

This is identical to the reasoning we discussed in diagnosis, when we adjusted our pre-test probabilities by the effects of the likelihood ratio of a test. While the pre-test probability varied from patient to patient, the LR stayed constant. We could get our patient's post-test probability by combining the two. In treatment decisions, our patients will have different baseline risks and the relative risk reduction of a treatment will stay constant. We can combine the two to yield our patient's absolute risk reduction.

In addition to adjusting for our patients' baseline risk, there are circumstances in which we must directly alter the degree of treatment effect.

Patient Disease Etiology

Sometimes the cause of a patient's disease will lead us to reject a treatment that ordinarily would be effective.

EXAMPLE

A 24-year-old male comes to the emergency department with crushing substernal chest pain. His electrocardiogram reveals 4 mm ST elevations in the anterior leads. After going through the diagnostic process, we are sure the patient is having a myocardial infarction. Ordinarily, we would use thrombolytics or send the patient for angioplasty; however, the patient reveals that he stayed up all last night snorting cocaine. We decide not to administer thrombolytics or send the patient to the cath lab. In this particular patient, very little treatment effect would be experienced by these treatments despite the fact that they are extremely effective in most patients with myocardial infarctions.

Adapting our Assessment of Treatment Effect

The two factors which may cause us to alter the degree of expected treatment effect for an individual patient are:

- We are different from the clinicians in the study.
- Our practice setting is different than the one in the study.

Are We the Same as the Study Clinicians?

If the study physicians received training in order to perform a treatment, we may not be able to perform the treatment as well as them.

EXAMPLE

We read about a new nerve block that reduces the pain of a humeral fracture by 75% using just a few milliliters of lidocaine; we are eager to utilize this procedure on our next patient. However, when we read beyond the abstract, we find that the four physicians who participated in the study spent a month with anesthesiologists learning the technique. If we attempt this nerve block for the first time, we may not achieve such an impressive reduction in pain. Our adverse event rate may also be higher, because of our relative lack of experience.

Longitudinal Learning

Even if the study clinicians did not have training before the study, in the act of performing the treatment on patients during the course of the study, they may gain prowess. We call this development of additional skill in the process of clinical study *longitudinal learning*, and it can contribute to a smaller than expected treatment effect during our initial use of a treatment.

Can We Duplicate the Treatment in Our Setting?

The setting of the emergency department is quite different from an outpatient clinic or a general medical ward. We must always assess whether the clinical setting ramifies on the application of the study data to our patients in the ED. Even if the study was performed in an emergency department, there are centers that can provide a level of care or equipment unobtainable in our own department.

EXAMPLE

Rivers et al. published a study on early goal-directed therapy for severe sepsis and septic shock patients in the emergency department.[90] They showed a significant benefit in mortality when aggressive monitoring and treatment are used early in a patient's clinical course. However, to obtain these benefits, they used central venous pressure monitoring, invasive blood pressure monitors, and continuous central venous oximetry. If in our emergency department we would have to substitute intermittent blood gases from a central line for the continuous monitoring and standard blood pressure cuff readings for the arterial line, would the study results still be applicable to our patient?

When either our practice settings or we as clinicians differ from those in the study, we may need to adjust the degree of treatment effect. This is necessarily a qualitative adjustment; it is part of the art within the science of evidence-based medicine.

The final issue we must discuss under applicability is the patient that does not fit into our standard treatment plan.

Individualizing Care

We may alter the treatments we generally use for a disorder due to the unique circumstances of an individual patient. Treatments that have only a small benefit or that are too expensive in aggregate may occasionally still have a role given certain unique circumstances.[91]

EXAMPLE

A 24-year-old female patient comes to the emergency department complaining of a sore throat and a runny nose. You recommend fluids, rest, and ibuprofen for this obvious viral illness. Your patient then tells you that she is getting married in eight hours; she asks if there is anything else you can do? Because of these unique circumstances, you devise a treatment plan far in excess of your norm. You give her 40 mg of prednisone to relieve some of the discomfort of her sore throat. You prescribe a couple of tablets of acetaminophen/hydromorphone to provide a maximum of analgesia. You tell the patient to take pseudoephedrine and use neo-synephrine nasal spray, both available over the counter. You also prescribe ipratropium nasal spray, a very expensive medication, because it may have minimal additive effects to the neo-synephrine spray. This treatment regimen is far more than you would offer to most patients with a viral illness and most of it is unsupported by good evidence. However, in this instance it may make a huge difference in this patient's life, with a minimum of risk.

RISKS OF TREATMENT

Much of the harm in medicine is perpetrated in the space between Can and Should.

(Benefit – Risk) Applicability = Impact ± Patient Values = Treatment Decision

— FIGURE 3-7 —

Harm is one of the four primary categories of evidence discussed in evidence-based medicine.* Evidence on harm can range from the dangers of a medication to the effects of living next to high-power lines. The type of harm we deal with most in emergency medicine is the harm caused by our treatments and procedures. We often specifically refer to this type of harm as "risk" (Fig. 3-7). The risks of every treatment must be given at least as much consideration as the benefits.

While one of the tenets of our profession is *first do no harm*, exposing our patients to some degree of risk is usually unavoidable. It is therefore imperative that we carefully weigh the benefits and risk to maximize the former and reduce, as much as possible, the latter.

Just as with the benefit parameters we have discussed, when we look at treatment studies there will be a rate of complications or adverse events in both the control and experimental groups.

■ Risk Parameters

Absolute Risk Increase
This is the difference between the rates in the control group and the experimental group:

$$ARI = EER - CER.$$

Number Needed to Harm (NNH)
Just as number needed to treat (NNT) gave us an easily understandable measure of treatment effect, NNH expresses risk in a way that makes it intuitive:

$$NNH = \frac{100}{ARI}.$$

*The other three categories are diagnosis, treatment, and prognosis.

The NNH is the number of patients we would need to treat before we see a side-effect in one patient during the described time period. If the number is high, then the treatment is safer than one with a lower NNH.

Nature of the Risk

The above parameters give us an idea of the frequency of adverse events with any given treatment. We must also take into consideration the significance of the actual side-effect or adverse event. An NNH of five patients to get a mild rash is very different from an NNH of five patients for a cardiac dysrhythmia.

In emergency medicine, we are very cognizant of the potential side-effects of our treatments that occur in the department. We are also made aware of the adverse events that occur once a patient has gone home, as these patients often return for a revisit. The risks we do not sufficiently consider are from treatments initiated in the emergency department on patients we admit to the hospital.

Of course, the reason for this lack of awareness is that we do not get feedback on these side-effects. The patient we sent home on oral pro-chlorperazine who develops akathisia will often return to the department and let us know. The patient with central-line–induced sepsis often does not come downstairs to lambaste us for the lack of sterility during our insertion technique.

EXAMPLE

A patient with poor peripheral access requires intravenous medications and fluids. You place a central line via the femoral vein, because you wish to minimize the risks of pneumothorax. You consent the patient, warning him of the risks of bleeding or arterial puncture. Four days later the patient develops a deep venous thrombosis at the site of the catheter; the clot embolizes to his lung. You must consider non-immediate adverse events, such as this DVT or line sepsis, just as carefully as immediate events. You must also present these risks to the patient. When we factor all of the risks, both short-term and long-term, a subclavian or internal jugular vein placement may be a safer procedure.[92,93]

It is unfortunate, but the medico-legal risks of a treatment play a role in our decision as well. Some treatments, despite solid evidentiary backing of their efficacy and safety, can still expose us to liability.

EXAMPLE

Droperidol is a medication with numerous uses in the emergency department. It has great utility for sedation, the amelioration of nausea, and the treatment of headache. The FDA placed a black box warning on droperidol; i.e., a warning printed on each medication box. This warning was placed despite very little evidence to support the assertion that droperidol is any more dangerous than are a host of other drugs we use routinely.[94] Even though droperidol presents little risk when analyzed from an EBM perspective, many emergency physicians will no longer use the medication. The decision-making equation is altered by the external medico-legal risk, despite the lack of supporting evidence of actual risk.

Evaluating Evidence on Risk

Often, the benefits of a treatment are publicized more extensively than the risks. Sometimes a treatment's risks will not become apparent for months or years after it is adopted into common use.

EXAMPLE

Some practitioners felt that rofecoxib (Vioxx[TM]) and other COX2 inhibitors were superior to the earlier generation of NSAIDs because of decreased gastrointestinal side-effects. However, years after its FDA approval, a study revealed that there was an increased incidence of cardiovascular risk.[95] Merck subsequently withdrew rofecoxib from the market amidst widespread allegations that they had suppressed early evidence of harm. Even more frightening is the fact that there were suggestions, but not clear proof, of this cardiovascular risk in earlier trials of rofecoxib.

The question we must ask ourselves is what to do when there is no clear proof a drug is dangerous, but there is also insufficient proof that it is safe.

The Kehoe Principle
Kehoe was a toxicologist who vigorously defended the safety of leaded gasoline, despite many early indicators that this form of fuel posed dire risks to public health. Dr Kehoe's rationale for supporting leaded gasoline was that there was no good published evidence of harm to humans.[96] Evidence-based medicine warns of the dangers of the Kehoe principle, which can be summarized as:[97]

The absence of evidence of risk = Evidence of the absence of risk.

The number of treatments that initially appeared safe, but that have subsequently been proven to be dangerous (and the absence of leaded gas at the pump) can be taken as reflections of the risks of premature assumptions regarding safety.

The Precautionary Principle

The safer path is the use of the *precautionary principle*.[98] This can be summarized as:

$$\text{The absence of evidence of no risk} = \text{The possibility of risk}$$
$$\text{until proven otherwise.}$$

Applicability of Risk

Just as we need to alter the treatment effects depending on the characteristics of our individual patient, we need to do the same for the risks of treatment. Some of the factors to consider when adapting the risk to our individual patient are:

- Age
- Gender
- Severity of disease
- Comorbidities
- Stage of disease.

Any comorbidity not present in the study population will require an adjustment of the risk if it is present in our patient. A patient with hepatic, renal, or cardiovascular failure will have a higher risk for most treatments than a study population without these disorders. Patients at the extremes of age also require risk adjustment. There are populations that will have increased risks with specific drugs; e.g., sickle cell patients with acetazolamide.

PATIENT VALUES

Once we have established the impact of a treatment, we need to present our plan to the patient (Fig. 3-8). A patient's viewpoint can completely alter our decision-making. When we present a treatment plan, the responses can run the gamut from:

"Whatever you think is best, doctor."
to
"I don't like the idea of you popping my lung, but if you think I need this central line procedure, then I guess we'll have to do it."

(Benefit − Risk) Applicability =
Impact ± Patient Values =
Treatment Decision

— FIGURE 3-8 — *A patient's values will alter our estimate of a treatment's impact.*

to

"Doctor, you say I will get much sicker without this blood transfusion, but I still do not want it."

to

"I understand I will die if you do not intubate me and place me on the ventilator, but I do not want these procedures and I'll sign the papers attesting to that."

As long as they are capable of making decisions, patients' views trump even the most beneficial, low-risk treatment plans. This is why it is so essential that, whenever possible, we discuss the plan with our patients prior to initiating a treatment.

Consent

For invasive and experimental procedures, we obtain written consent. The patient signs a document stating that we have discussed and that they understand the risks, benefits, and alternatives of a treatment. Even with treatments that do not require written consent, we must exert the same effort to explain and get a patient's verbal permission to go through with a treatment.

The only time this does not apply is when the patient is unable to give consent and we cannot locate a proxy for decisions. It is sometimes difficult to discern whether a patient is able to give informed consent. Obviously, mind-altering drugs may cause patients to fall into this category, but medical illnesses can make a patient unable to give consent as well. The extreme stress of illness can distract a patient and prevent him or her from concentrating on the choices. Conditions such as hypoxia or shock may also leave us with a verbal patient who is not truly in the correct mental state to decide on the desirability of a treatment. One study estimates that as high as 20% of patients with acute myocardial infarction are not able to give informed consent.[99]

It's Not What We Say, It's How We Say It   When presenting the risks and benefits of a treatment to a patient, we must be scrupulous about offering an unbiased discussion. If we discuss consent for a central line in a way that emphasizes the risks and we mention the benefits only in passing, then any sane patient would refuse this treatment. The same discussion with the risks minimized would obtain a very different patient reaction. The goal is to always present as accurately as possible the potential risks and benefits.

Conversely, we cannot merely present the likelihood of each risk and benefit and then put the onus of decision-making entirely on the patient. We must express our opinion as well; patients come to us for treatment because of our medical expertise and knowledge. It is sometimes quite a difficult balance between paternalism and patient autonomy.

As a group, we are quite adept at our presentation of the technical medical issues. Where we often fail is in our discussions of a patient's values, fears, and alternatives.[100]

While mathematical systems exist to quantitatively factor in a patient's utility versus risks and benefits, they are unwieldy; a qualitative approach in the emergency department is more workable. If a patient understands our treatment plan but refuses it, then we must work together to find another treatment plan that is acceptable and still has a positive impact.

Literature Support

There is no substitute for a face-to-face conversation with the patient about his or her values and opinions regarding the treatment choices. Sometimes, due to severity of illness, our patients cannot talk to us. In these circumstances, the literature can aid us by providing the opinions of the emergency department population. This evidence often takes the form of a qualitative study; this form of literature takes a multidirectional path to gleaning the thoughts and feelings of a study population. We discuss qualitative literature more extensively in Part II.

Link to Page 236

SOURCES OF ERROR

Just as with diagnostic decisions, when we treat patients emergently, there is a potential for error. Numerous sources have discussed the system-based causes for error, such as overcrowding and understaffing. Personal issues such as exhaustion, burnout, and circadian disruption also contribute

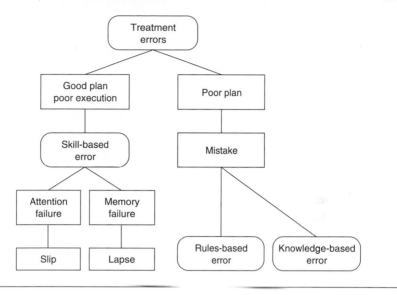

— FIGURE 3-9 — *Cognitive treatment errors.*

to treatment errors in emergency medicine.[101] What we will concentrate on in this section are the cognitive factors that can cause error.

Cognitive treatment errors can be broken into three types. *Skills-based* (SB) errors are the result of a good plan which nevertheless goes awry, resulting in an inappropriate action. We can further divide SB errors into *slips* and *lapses*, as can be seen in Fig. 3-9. Skills-based errors are *errors of execution.*

Rules-based and *knowledge-based* errors are the result of a poorly conceived plan, which then results in inappropriate action. These two forms are *errors of intention.*

Skills-based Errors

Skills-based errors are the result of a good plan that is executed poorly. When we make a medical error because of skills-based behavior, cognitive psychologists refer to it as either a slip or a lapse.[54] Both slips and lapses cause us to make a mistake while performing treatments we normally do automatically. When we are driving, we can make it from the hospital to our home with a minimum of conscious thought; this is skill-based behavior.

Lapses

A lapse is an error of memory. In the midst of stressful situations or during the juggling of numerous tasks, we forget information, which ordinarily is easily recalled and readily available.

EXAMPLE

You have just cardioverted a patient with ventricular tachycardia and a thready pulse. You shocked him at 200 joules with the machine synchronized. There was no change in the rhythm after the first shock, so you shock again at 300 joules, but you forget to press the synch switch this time. This lapse has the potential to cause ventricular fibrillation if the unsynchronized shock is delivered at a vulnerable point in the cardiac cycle.

We can devise *cognitive forcing strategies* to avoid lapses, similar to the ones we discussed in the diagnostic errors section.

EXAMPLE

Often in the emergency department, apneic patients are ventilated with a bag–valve–mask (BVM) without the use of an oral airway. This is despite the fact that most emergency physicians know that BVM ventilation is far more effective with the oral airway. They are underutilized because of a lapse in the midst of the complex situation of emergent airway management. If we tape an oral airway to the mask portion of the BVM when setting up the resuscitation bay, this lapse is avoided.

The lapse of forgetting to reset the synchronization switch when cardioverting seems ripe for a forcing strategy. While this lapse could be avoided by having the machine stay in synchronized mode over the course of many shocks, this would leave the potential for a more dangerous lapse. If while cardioverting a patient the rhythm degenerates to ventricular fibrillation, a machine in synchronized mode will not be able to shock this lethal rhythm. The designers of the machine appropriately concentrated their forcing strategies to eliminate the possibility of this latter lapse, instead of the less dangerous one in the example above.

Slips

Errors of this domain often take place during procedures or in the course of medication administration. Slips are the result of inattention or interruption; any stimuli that disrupt what would ordinarily be an automatic progression of steps can cause a slip. Unlike lapses, slips are not the result of forgetting information, but instead they are a diversion of a subconscious process by a disruption of concentration.

EXAMPLE

In the midst of placing a central venous catheter, we are interrupted by a medical student who is worried about another patient. The portion of the task we are in the middle of is the threading of the catheter over the wire. Ordinarily, we would always make sure we grasped the wire protruding from the proximal end of the catheter before advancing it. We have performed the procedure so many times, that we do not even have to consciously think of the rule: *always have a hand on the wire*. Instead, this has been incorporated into our subconscious performance of the skill. But this time, due to the interruption, we start to advance the catheter prior to grasping the wire. Luckily, we quickly realize this slip and recover by withdrawing the catheter and rescuing the wire.

Debiasing Techniques

The most fertile area of research for the elimination of errors secondary to slips is in the field of medication errors. A large number of techniques have been created to decrease slips. Techniques such as placing similar sounding drugs in separate areas of a medication room or forcing drug manufacturers not to pick new medication names that sound similar to old ones are effective techniques.[102]

EXAMPLE

Acetazolamide is often confused with acetahexamide, because of medication slips. These drugs must now have their names printed on vials using Tall Man Letters (Fig. 3-10).

Single-use vials can decrease slips related to dose calculations. If only 10 units of insulin are placed in each vial, it would be difficult for the

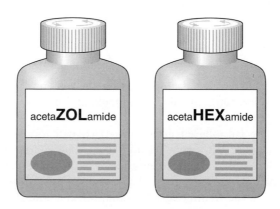

— FIGURE 3-10 — *Two pill bottles using tall-man lettering. This method reduces the potential to confuse the two medications.*

nurse drawing up the medication not to realize that 1000 units is an inappropriately large dose. It is a very different scenario when a nurse inadvertently draws up 1000 units drawn from a multi-use vial, when all this requires is that 10 mL of the medication is drawn into a syringe.*

It is more difficult to avoid slips during procedures, but obviously keeping interruptions of concentration to a minimum should be beneficial, if not often realistic.

Mistakes

Both rules-based and knowledge-based errors are the result of a poor plan. In the field of cognitive psychology, these types of error are referred to as *mistakes*.

Rules-based Errors

This form of error occurs when we create a treatment plan without the requirement for large amounts of consideration or pondering. When we find that, after diagnosis, we have a treatment plan within moments, we are utilizing rules-based behavior. The benefits of this method are obvious: we can make treatment decisions rapidly and immediately move our cognitive resources to the next patient.

The reason for rules-based behavior is that we do not like to think about decisions.[54] This is the case not just with emergency physicians, but all across the spectrum of human thought processes. This desire to avoid the cognitive strain of abstract decision-making leads to the use of *precompiled responses* in treatment scenarios. This reluctance towards rationality is usually beneficial. When we pick treatments by rules-based behavior, we are *less* likely to make errors than when we actively consider a plan.

These precompiled responses are very similar to the illness scripts we mentioned in the diagnostics section. They are a host of treatment responses, which we have used numerous times in the past. We are familiar with the risks and benefits of these treatments and have seen the responses they normally generate.

We can divide rules-based errors into two categories: application of flawed rules and misapplication of good rules. The common root of both of these types of error is the presentation of an anomaly not accounted for by the precompiled response. These misclassifications of situation may make our routine treatment scripts inapplicable and dangerous.[74]

---

*In most multi-use insulin vials, 1 mL = 100 units.

Example

A patient comes in with chest pain with a history suggestive of cardiac etiology. The EKG shows small inferior ST segment depression; the patient is hemodynamically stable. You go through the diagnostic process outlined earlier and decide that this patient has an acute coronary syndrome (ACS). You barely have to think about how you will treat this patient as you have seen hundreds of similar patients and have created a *treatment script* outlining the therapeutic plan:

- Administer aspirin
- Administer SL nitroglycerin
- Administer a beta-blocker
- Send labs, including cardiac enzymes
- Admit to a monitored bed.

However, in this particular patient, after administration of SL nitroglycerin, his blood pressure drops precipitously. You now must rapidly move to knowledge-based treatment to correct this problem.

In the future, your mental rule for treating ACS includes:

- Consider right ventricular infarction, prior to administering nitroglycerin.

Disregarding New Treatments

When we use familiar treatments, we can operate automatically using rules-based decision-making. In order to integrate a new treatment into our practice, we must shift to knowledge-based decision-making. The reluctance to make this transition can lead to the rejection of any new therapies, simply to avoid the consideration involved. The first time a new treatment is used requires a formal consideration of benefits, risks, and procedure; some clinicians feel it is easier to stick with what they know. This reluctance is an error if it causes the rejection of proven and efficacious new treatments.

Avoiding Errors

As we will discuss shortly, experience leads to superior precompiled responses and therefore less treatment error. Case reports in the literature and institutional exposure from conferences such as morbidity and mortality also allow the internal testing of rules-based responses.

The field of *knowledge translation* attempts to bridge the evidence gap between new, proven treatments and their adoption by clinicians.[103] If we inform our treatment scripts by being evidence-literate, we decrease the chances of making cognitive errors.

Knowledge-based Errors

When we face a treatment decision for which we do not have a precompiled response, we move to abstract or *knowledge-based* decision-making.

Search for Analogous Situations

Of course, our minds do not give up on the reluctance to think that easily, so the first set of thought processes we utilize are attempts to generate an analogous situation for which we already have a treatment script. In this way, we can convert a situation requiring knowledge-based consideration into a situation in which rules-based treatment is applicable. The process is often an attempt to convert a unique treatment situation (an anomaly) into a more generic one with which we have experience.

Errors in this stage of treatment decisions emerge from *forced analogies*. When faced with an anomalous condition, forced rules-based behavior can cause serious harm.

EXAMPLE

Our generic response to patients with breathing abnormalities is to protect the airway and take over the job of respiration mechanically.

EMS brings a patient into the emergency department complaining of rapid breathing and extreme thirst. His respiratory rate is 48/min, but he has clear lungs and no difficulty moving air. Your resident is not sure what is going on, but decides that any patient breathing this quickly needs to be intubated immediately. He performs RSI, successfully intubates the patient, and places him on mechanical ventilation. Moments later, the patient loses his pulse with the monitor showing ventricular fibrillation. The loss of respiratory compensation for the extreme acidosis in this patient with diabetic ketoacidosis was caused by intubation without full consideration of the situation.

If we cannot find an analogous situation, then we resign ourselves to a formal decision-making process.

Errors of Formal Treatment Decisions

In the preceding sections, we have outlined the steps of formal treatment decision making. At each stage, biases can cause flawed evaluation of the situation. Just as in diagnostic decisions, our thought processes may be tainted by flawed heuristics.

Commission bias can lead us to treat a condition, which may respond better to inaction. The consideration of doing nothing should be an option we consider in every treatment plan.

EXAMPLE

When a physician prescribes an antibiotic for a viral upper-respiratory infection, he is exposing a patient to all of the risks of a treatment without any of the benefits. The fact that this is an unacceptable treatment is in no way ameliorated by the fact that the patient is asking for the antibiotics.

Conversely, **omission bias** can cause us to allow indecision or fear of consequences to lead to inaction when the situation dictates a viable treatment.

There is a built-in incentive to choose treatments that provide immediate results. This **instant gratification bias** makes us less likely to give treatments that have no immediately demonstrable results, even though they have large benefits in the long term.

EXAMPLE

When a patient with an acute coronary syndrome complains of chest pain, we almost uniformly administer nitroglycerin, but we might forget to give aspirin. Though aspirin results in a much greater mortality benefit than nitroglycerin, it is easier to ignore because, unlike with nitroglycerin, there is no immediate effect.

When our treatment plans are based on faulty evidence, we are in danger of making dangerous decisions. This error is infinitely worse when we take our treatment guidance from sources that do not have the patients' best interests as their first priority.

EXAMPLE

If we change our practice based on the advice of the pharmaceutical company representative who just bought us lunch, we are prone to make false decisions. Only slightly better is taking our assessment of treatment risks and benefits solely from the company-selected literature reprints provided by this drug representative.

The evaluation of the risks of a procedure is also prone to error. Emergency physicians, like all people, are cognitively predisposed to underestimate large risks and overestimate small ones. Further, we tend to minimize the risks of treatments that we are performing ourselves.[104,105]

When we consider the risks of a treatment, but not the risks of the auxiliary therapies that go along with it, we are also falling prey to error. The risks of the secondary treatments **hitch a ride** on the first; we must consider them as well.

EXAMPLE

Cardioversion is a safe and effective treatment for tachycardia.[106,107] When considering the risks of electrical shock, they are probably lower than many of the medications we use to control tachycardias emergently. However, in all but the direst of cases, we want to offer sedation and analgesia for the cardioversion procedure. These medications increase the risk of cardioversion; we must add the risks of sedation to that of cardioversion when comparing shock versus medical management for the treatment of tachycardias.

Errors Due to Lack of Feedback

The lack of effective feedback on the quality of our decisions is another factor that predisposes us to treatment error in emergency medicine. While an obvious poor outcome will often result in a change in practice and an evaluation of the cognitive processes resulting in error, when there is no obvious bad outcome there is little impetus for change.

EXAMPLE

A 65-year-old male is brought in with severe shortness of breath. He has rales up to the nipple line and a blood pressure of 190/110. Your resident already is setting up the intubation equipment. If you intubate this patient, it will definitely stabilize his condition. If the rapid sequence intubation is performed flawlessly, you will probably congratulate your-self on excellent treatment of the patient. You admit the patient to the cardiac care unit, administer some lasix, and move on to the next patient.

However, by administering high-dose nitroglycerin and a sublingual ACE inhibitor, this patient may have been managed with CPAP or no ventilatory assistance at all. We would not expose the patient to the risks of intubation and mechanical ventilation.

Intubating this patient may have been a poor treatment choice, but there is no possibility for feedback. The cardiac care unit physician will receive an intubated patient with pulmonary edema and presume the intubation was necessary. It is rare to have a second emergency physician present during these cases to offer real-time feedback. This lack of feedback offers no impetus to change this behavior in the future.

Avoiding Error

The key to avoiding knowledge-based errors is to critically examine each step of the process. We must choose and utilize the best-available evidence for each stage of decision-making.

The Benefits of Experience

The avoidance of knowledge-based errors comes from a diligent pursuit of evidence, but also from the gathering of clinical experience. Experience offers many cognitive advantages when dealing with difficult treatment decisions.

- *More and better treatment scripts:* As we advance through our careers, we gather more precompiled treatment responses. We can therefore treat a greater number of conditions without having to perform formal decision-making; this leads to fewer errors. Our treatment scripts are also more substantial and durable; they incorporate anomalous situations and thereby minimize rules-based errors.
- *Greater breadth of knowledge:* If we do encounter situations for which our experience has not offered a precompiled response, we have more knowledge to perform abstract decision-making. We are also more capable of creating an analogy to an existing treatment script.
- *Recognition of error:* Experience also allows an earlier perception that a treatment is erroneous and allows a more rapid correction. We are more apt to avoid **fixation error**: the steadfast maintenance of a treatment plan despite indicators that it is not working.

In short, novices are forced to make most of their decisions by knowledge-based practice. Further, their knowledge bases are limited, leading to an even greater predisposition to error. Lastly, they are less likely to recognize an error in its early stages and therefore avert it.

PUTTING IT ALL TOGETHER

The equation we have been using in the previous sections considers one treatment at a time. Of course, for most situations we are actually considering a number of treatments. We should also compare these treatments to the risks and benefits of doing nothing. Instead of the equation in Fig. 3-11, we can make alterations as shown in Fig. 3-12.

We now have a comprehensive process for treatment decisions in the emergency department. By evaluating the benefits, risks, and patient values as they apply to our patient, while checking our thought processes for error, we can make the best possible therapy choices.

$$\begin{array}{c} \textbf{(Benefit} - \textbf{Risk) Applicability} = \\ \textbf{Impact} \pm \textbf{Patient Values} = \\ \boxed{\textbf{Treatment Decision}} \end{array}$$

— FIGURE 3-11 —

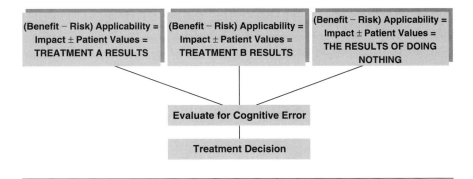

— FIGURE 3-12 —

CASE CONTINUED: THE CLOCK IS TICKING

Eight hours into your 12-hour shift you have finally found a couple of minutes to sit down and eat your now cold pad thai. That is until the triage nurse pops her head into the break room to tell you that she has just placed a Code Stroke into the resuscitation room.

You rapidly gather a history and perform a physical exam.*

Clinical Exam

Chief Complaint   "Suddenly, I could not move my right side."

---

*For didactic purposes, we have broken down the treatment decisions in this scenario into discrete steps. In an actual patient encounter, all of these steps would be performed simultaneously, with most of the cognitive load sifted through before the patient ever arrived.

History of Present Illness Mr Smith is a 68-year-old man who, until today, was in his normal state of health. At 11 a.m. (30 minutes ago) he felt weak all along his right side; his arm was affected more than his leg. He was sitting in a chair at his kitchen table at the time; he did not fall. His wife, who witnessed the event, noticed that the right side of his face seemed slack as well. She noted no seizure activity, nor loss of consciousness. Mr Smith denies chest pain, shortness of breath, headache, neck pain, or fever. In answer to your querying, Mr Smith reports that he is left-hand dominant.

Mr Smith's wife is an emergency charge nurse at a neighboring emergency department. She immediately recognized her husband's symptoms and drove him to your department herself. As to why she chose to come to your ED as opposed to her own, you choose not to dwell on now.

Past Medical History Hypertension, hypercholesterolemia.

Past Surgical History Cholecystectomy 15 years ago.

Family History Mother and maternal uncle had type II diabetes.

Social History No tobacco or drug use. He drinks five beers per week. He is able to perform all activities of daily living for himself.

Medications Atenolol, aspirin, and lipitor. While his wife steps out of the room to call their daughter, Mr Smith confides that he does not like pills so he only takes them when his wife is around.

Allergies None.

Physical Exam Well-kempt 68 y/o male appearing his age. Temperature 98.8°F; pulse 88/min; BP 140/92 mmHg; respiration 16/min; SaO_2 99% on room air.

- HEENT normal.
- Neck: No jugular venous distention. Trachea is midline.
- Lungs: Clear to auscultation bilaterally.
- Heart: S1 S2, regular rate and rhythm and no murmurs, rubs, or gallops.
- Abdomen: Benign.
- Extremities: Normal exam. No calf tenderness, masses, or cords.
- Mental status: A & O × 3; GCS 15; serial 7s intact.

- CN: PERL; Gaze deviation to the left; V_{1-3} normal; right-sided facial droop with sparing of forehead; no aphasia. Articulation normal. Remainder intact.
- Motor: R UE 1/5; R LE 2/5; L U & LE 5/5; R pronator drift. F to N intact on left. RAM normal on left. Gait not assessed.
- Sens: Decreased pain and touch on the right side.
- DTR: 2+ throughout. Babinski downgoing B.

32 Minutes from Symptom Onset

You immediately have an intravenous line started by the ED technician. The nurse is already performing a fingerstick glucose determination with results of 110 mg/dL. Having established IV access, the technician now works on a 12-lead EKG; blood work has already been sent to the lab.

As per hospital protocol, after obtaining a normal blood glucose, the nurse calls the operator to announce a code stroke. The operator pages the neurology team, the radiologist, and the CT technician.

38 Minutes from Onset

You quickly consider the differential diagnosis for the patient, using the steps outlined in the previous section. It would be easy to jump to the diagnosis of acute ischemic stroke, but this can cause missed diagnoses. Your differential is:

- Ischemic stroke
- Hypoglycemia
- Hemorrhagic stroke
- Transient ischemic attack (TIA)
- Migraine
- Todd's paralysis
- Carotid dissection.

Due to the patient's bedside testing, history, and physical, you are able to narrow the list to ischemic stroke, hemorrhagic stroke, and TIA. Due to the timing and the lack of any change in the patient's symptoms, you are almost certain this is an ischemic stroke. You would put a pre-test probability of 75% on this diagnosis. However, before you consider treatment, you want to raise this probability to at least 95%. You therefore rush the patient to the CT scanner for a non-contrast scan of his head.

44 Minutes from Onset

The on-duty general radiologist reads the CT of the head as negative for signs of hemorrhage or ischemic stroke.

46 Minutes from Onset

At this point you would put the probability of ischemic stroke at above 95% and are ready to consider treatment decisions. The neurology resident arrives; the two of you begin to discuss whether the patient is an appropriate candidate for the administration of tPA. At that moment, a nurse tells you that one of the residents wants to intubate a patient and needs you at the bedside. You ask the neurology resident to start talking to the patient about tPA.

You return to the resuscitation room four minutes later to overhear the neurology resident discussing consent with the patient:

"So, if we give you this drug, there is a good chance you will have a full recovery. There is a very small chance of side-effects, but I think you should give it a shot. So just sign right here so we can get started."

53 Minutes from Onset

You wince at this "informed" consent. You take out your PDA and pull up a program called HandiStroke.[108,109] It allows the rapid assessment of the NIH stroke score, one of the essential screening values in order to use tPA for stroke. You hand your PDA to the neurology resident and ask him to assess the stroke score. This distraction tactic will keep him occupied while you take a moment to solidify your recollections of the risks and benefits of tPA for ischemic stroke.

You start by considering the benefits from the one study, which showed clear treatment effect from the use of tPA. The NINDS study investigated the use of tPA for ischemic strokes treated within three hours of the onset of symptoms.[110,111]

You access your personal emergency medicine database on the web and refresh your memory on the actual numbers from this trial. You also print out the NEEDLE you created from the NINDS study (see Figure 3-5).

Benefits   In patients treated with tPA, the risk of having minimal or no dysfunction at 3 months was 39%.* In this study, the patients who received standard care without tPA (placebo), 26% had minimal or no dysfunction. This translates to an absolute benefit increase (ABI) of 13%:

$$ABI = EER - CER = 39 - 26 = 13\%$$

---

*These numbers were from the evaluation of a Rankin score (a measure of functional status) of 0 to 1. Similar, but slightly different, ABI were obtained on each of three other scales used in the study. The ABIs ranged from 11% to 13%.

You calculate a number needed to treat: $NNT = 100/ABI = 100/13 = 8$ patients. This translates to the requirement that eight patients be treated with tPA to achieve one additional patient with minimal or no dysfunction at 3 months over placebo care alone.

You can also calculate the relative benefit increase: $RBI = (EER - CER)/ CER = 13/26 = 50\%$.

tPA offered no statistically significant mortality benefit.

The next step in deriving the benefit is deciding whether the benefit is patient-oriented or disease-oriented (DOE or POE). In this case, the return to a fully functional life is definitely patient-oriented evidence.

Risk   Unfortunately, the use of tPA for stroke is not without risk. The primary risk from the use of this medication was a dramatic increase in the number of symptomatic intracerebral hemorrhages. 6.4% of patients treated with tPA had a symptomatic intracerebral hemorrhage within 36 hours; only 0.6% of the patients treated with placebo had symptomatic hemorrhages.

We can use these numbers to calculate the absolute risk increase:

$$ARI = EER - CER = 6.4 - 0.6 = 5.8\%$$

If we calculate the relative risk increase, we can see that this number is even more dramatic:

$$RRI = EER - CER/CER = 6.4 - 0.6/0.6 \times 100 = 900\%$$

The number needed to harm can also be calculated: $NNH = 100/5.8 = 17$ patients. For every seventeen patients treated with tPA, one additional patient will have a symptomatic hemorrhage compared with placebo.

Is the risk qualitatively meaningful? Obviously, this is a risk that matters; it is not a mild rash, but worrisome amounts of blood in the brain sufficient to produce symptoms.

Applicability   *Entrance criteria:* When assessing applicability, the first issue to consider is whether our patient would fit into the entrance criteria of the NINDS study. The NIH stroke scale was used to determine strokes that were too mild or too severe to be entered into the study. The values of 5–21 were considered as entrance criteria for the study. By this point, the neurology resident has derived a stroke scale score of 8 for our patient.

This means that our patient would have been eligible for the NINDS study protocol. This score also indicates that Mr Smith may be at a lower risk for symptomatic hemorrhage than patients with higher scores.

Reading of the CT scan: Signs of intracerebral hemorrhage or a large ischemic stroke on the initial CT scan would contraindicate the use of tPA. In the NINDS study, neuroradiologists, using an explicit set of study criteria, read the CT scans. At your institution, you are lucky enough to have 24-hour attending radiology coverage, but these physicians are general radiologists. This fact may make the risks of tPA greater in your patient. You decide that, despite not having fellowship training in neurological radiology, the attending reading CTs today is quite familiar with the NINDS criteria. She has been reading at your institution for years; you make the clinical decision not to alter the risks of tPA based on this fact.

Time from stroke onset: While NINDS allowed up to three hours from symptom onset to enter the study, our patient is in a unique group. He will be eligible to receive thrombolytics less than 90 minutes from stroke onset. Our patient has a much greater potential benefit from TPA as compared to patients presenting later. This increased benefit comes without additional risk. While it is difficult to determine an exact quantitative shift of our NNT of eight, we can say that the benefit is at least this good in our patient, and probably better.

Blood pressure control: One of the unique aspects of the NINDS trial was the option for clinicians to pharmaceutically lower hypertensive patients' blood pressures and still administer thrombolytic agents. You reason that while this was an allowable intervention, the fact that your patient is not hypertensive may lower his risk of hemorrhage. Again, this decreased risk is difficult to quantitate, but it makes you feel more confident that your patient's risk is equal to or less than the standard risk reported in the study.

Impact   At this point, you can consider the entirety of the impact of tPA for the patient. The quality of the benefit is enormous; a patient can go from needing care for a persistent neurological deficit to being fully self-sufficient. The quantity of benefit is significant, but not overwhelming. The risks are also significant: patients can go from the baseline deficit associated with their stroke to having an intracerebral bleed leading to no function at all. This has led to a simplification of the use of tPA to a choice between walking and bleeding.

Patient Values and Consent   You then bring the result of your treatment impact analysis to your patient. You try to keep your discussion on the level of a layperson. You tell Mr Smith if we use standard care for his stroke, he has about a 1 in 4 chance of recovering fully. If we use tPA, it will raise his chances for a full recovery to 2 in 5. To put it another way, without tPA, 5 in 20 patients will recover fully; with tPA, 8 in 20 will recover.

This benefit is balanced by an increased risk of a bleed in his head. The risk is at least 10 times greater than if tPA were not given. However, the number of patients who die is the same in patients who received tPA and those who did not.

You also tell the patient that because his wife brought him to the hospital so quickly, his chance of deriving benefit from the tPA is probably greater than the numbers above.

You are lucky to have your patient's wife present during the conversation; she helps to relay this information to your patient. They ask if they can have a minute or two to discuss the decision. While you know time is of the essence, this decision is too crucial to rush, so you step away for a moment.

61 Minutes from Onset

In the meanwhile, you quickly review your actions to see if there is any possible cognitive error.

Search for Error   *Skills-based:* On a skills-based level, tPA can be dosed improperly or given through a non-functional IV line. You have the nurse assure the patency of the IV line. The HandiStroke PDA program allows an exact calculation of tPA dosing for ischemic stroke if the patient's weight is inputted.

Rules-based: Because of the extreme risks and controversial benefits of tPA for stroke, it is never a treatment that is considered merely at the rules-based level. We inevitably will treat using knowledge-based considerations.

Knowledge-based: The entire process of administering tPA is a rushed affair. This makes knowledge-based errors even more prevalent. You review the relative and absolute contraindications to administration of a thrombolytic agent to make sure your patient is free of contraindications, which you might have forgotten. You also reexamine your thought processes to assure yourself that nothing has been missed.

You return to the bedside to find out your patient's decision. He tells you that he wants to take the tPA, because his desire to increase his chances of walking and using his right arm is greater than the fear of the risks. You are lucky to have a patient who can understand and process the information you have offered. Having his wife, a medical professional, present certainly helped as well.

If your patient could not as readily comprehend the risks and benefits, you would be forced to decide whether this is a choice that you can make for the patient. You would probably err on the side of caution and not administer tPA. This decision is not clear-cut enough to make a paternalistic choice.

65 Minutes from Onset

You administer tPA by bolus and infusion and admit the patient to the hospital's stroke unit. You make a note in your PDA to follow-up on Mr Smith to find out the results of the treatment.

CHAPTER 4

DECISIONS ABOUT PROGNOSIS

THE ART OF PROGNOSTICATION

Prognosis deals with predicting the future progression of disease. Prognostic decisions in emergency medicine occur in a very different context from those faced in other specialties. The stakes of our prognostic decisions are often very high. In the emergency department, when a *major therapeutic decision* hinges on a prognostic assessment (i.e., one dealing with mortality or long-term function), we often have the back-up of a consultant. At this stage, the diagnosis has generally already been agreed on and we are no longer "on our own."

EXAMPLE

A patient presents after a motor vehicle collision with severe traumatic brain injury. Before telling the family that the injury is non-survivable, most of us would obtain the consultation of one of our neurosurgical colleagues.

The decisions we must make on our own often revolve around *disposition*. Can we discharge a patient or does he or she need to be admitted? If we do discharge a patient, do we need to start medication or can this wait for follow-up? These determinations are the subject of the prognostic literature most relevant to emergency medicine.

ED prognostic questions we ask on a daily basis are:

- Can we send a patient home after two negative troponins?
- Do we need to start patients with first-time seizures on a medication prior to their neurologic follow-up?
- What is the likelihood of HIV or hepatitis C seroconversion after a needlestick injury from a positive patient?
- What is the likelihood of getting rabies after a rodent bite?
- Is it safe to discharge a patient with a transient ischemic attack (TIA)?

We can discuss prognostic decisions in the context of this last question.

EXAMPLE

If a 65-year-old female reported to the emergency department with right-sided weakness and slurred speech, but has now returned to her baseline, can we send her home? After a negative CT of the head and some basic lab work to rule-out other conditions, we have a prognostic decision to make.

PROGNOSTIC EVIDENCE

Evidence useful in addressing issues of prognosis is characteristically drawn from *cohort studies*. A cohort is just a group of patients; in this case the group would be a number of patients with the condition in question. We can follow these patients over time and observe what percentage experience the outcomes of interest. We can also try to determine the factors that influence the likelihood of those outcomes in individual patients. We discuss the *evaluation* of these studies in Part II.

Link to Page 228

Evidence necessary to make decisions

Prognostic NEEDLEs provide the information we need to make decisions about prognosis. A NEEDLE for prognosis should include the following information:

- Risk of an Outcome
- Condition
- Population
- Setting
- Citation

If we return to the decision of what to do with our patient with a TIA, our attending hands us the NEEDLE in Fig. 4-1.

Results

Since prognostic evidence concerns the natural history of a condition, what we want to know is what happens to the patients. The main results of a prognosis study can simply be reported in percentages of patients with the studied outcomes.

EXAMPLE

In the study above, patients were followed to see if they had a stroke. Approximately 10% of patients did have a stroke. Even more

Prognosis Evidence:
Prognosis of patients sent home from ED after TIA

Results

- Patients with TIA discharged from ED: 10.5% had a stroke in following 90 days, half of these within two days of discharge

Prognosis worse if:

- Age >60 years
- Diabetes mellitus
- Longer duration of TIA
- Signs or symptoms of weakness, speech impairment, or gait disturbance
- Patients with symptoms still present upon arrival to the Emergency Department

Applicability

- Adult patients (~80% >60 y/o), many with comorbidities
- HMO patients: hospital use discouraged; may represent a sicker population
- Academic Emergency Department
- Ninety day follow-up important, 2 day data especially relevant

Brown MD et al. Annals Emerg Med 2002;40(2):133-144
-Valid Prospective Cohort Study, (Risk of stroke at 90 days 95% CI 9-12%)

— FIGURE 4-1 — *A NEEDLE for prognosis.*

relevant to our practice, half of these strokes occurred within two days of ED discharge. It is this latter piece of information which makes this prognostic study so important to our practice.

Follow-up

Emergency medicine prognosis is different from other specialties largely because of the limited time span during which we retain *active responsibility* for a patient. We are therefore particularly concerned with *short-term outcomes*. If a patient coming to the emergency department with chest pain has a high likelihood of cardiac ischemia and of having a myocardial infarction (MI) within a year, but a very low likelihood of bad events and outcomes within the time frame of a few days to a week, it may be

To create a CPR, researchers first derive a set of prognostic factors from an initial study, just as in the TIA study we have been discussing. They then perform a second study to see if these prognostic factors are truly independent predictors of outcome; this is the validation study. If the factors are validated, we can then use them to guide our prognostic decisions.

The following are some of the prognostic clinical predication rules we use routinely in emergency medicine:

- PORT pneumonia score
- Goldman's triage rule for ACI
- TIMI score for acute MI.

We can illustrate the use of these rules to help us make prognostic decisions by discussing the PORT score.[114] This CPR was developed in 1997 to identify patients at low risk of death from pneumonia. The first part of the study was a derivation of factors that increased the risk of death from pneumonia. Using these factors, the researchers developed a CPR, which they believed would predict the patient's likelihood of mortality within 30 days of diagnosis. This rule was then tested against two different populations of patients with pneumonia in order to validate the rule. Figure 4.2 demonstrates the completed rule.

If the patients are aged less than 50 years they are first assessed for the absence of any high-risk factors by means of the flow chart. If they have none of these high-risk factors, they are placed into risk class I. Patients older than 50 or with high-risk factors are assigned a point score. This point score allows assignment to risk classes II–V. Each of the risk classes is associated with a mortality percentage. We can see that patients in risk classes I–III are at very low risk for death, while classes IV and V have a much higher mortality. We would want to admit patients in these latter two risk classes.

This rule does not tell us *not* to admit patients in the first three risk classes, if there are clinical factors, which make us worried.* Instead, it just tells us that, on average, these patients have a very good prognosis in terms of mortality. It also is probably *not applicable* to certain patient groups. For example, patients with AIDS probably deserve admission even if they are PORT class I or II.

Clinical prediction rules such as the PORT score give us the best available evidence for integrating prognostic information into decision-making. When they are available, we should use them to augment our assessment of a patient's potential outcome.

---

* Many emergency physicians have used a low pulse oximetry reading as one of these factors.

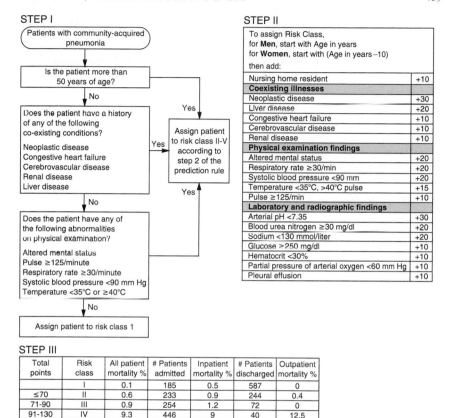

STEP I

Patients with community-acquired pneumonia

Is the patient more than 50 years of age?

↓ No

Does the patient have a history of any of the following co-existing conditions?

Neoplastic disease
Congestive heart failure
Cerebrovascular disease
Renal disease
Liver disease

↓ No

Does the patient have any of the following abnormalities on physical examination?

Altered mental status
Pulse ≥125/minute
Respiratory rate ≥30/minute
Systolic blood pressure <90 mm Hg
Temperature <35°C or ≥40°C

↓ No

Assign patient to risk class 1

Yes →
Yes →

Assign patient to risk class II-V according to step 2 of the prediction rule

↑ Yes

STEP II

To assign Risk Class, for **Men**, start with Age in years for **Women**, start with (Age in years –10) then add:	
Nursing home resident	+10
Coexisting illnesses	
Neoplastic disease	+30
Liver disease	+20
Congestive heart failure	+10
Cerebrovascular disease	+10
Renal disease	+10
Physical examination findings	
Altered mental status	+20
Respiratory rate ≥30/min	+20
Systolic blood pressure <90 mm	+20
Temperature <35°C, >40°C pulse	+15
Pulse ≥125/min	+10
Laboratory and radiographic findings	
Arterial pH <7.35	+30
Blood urea nitrogen ≥30 mg/dl	+20
Sodium <130 mmol/liter	+20
Glucose >250 mg/dl	+10
Hematocrit <30%	+10
Partial pressure of arterial oxygen <60 mm Hg	+10
Pleural effusion	+10

STEP III

Total points	Risk class	All patient mortality %	# Patients admitted	Inpatient mortality %	# Patients discharged	Outpatient mortality %
	I	0.1	185	0.5	587	0
≤70	II	0.6	233	0.9	244	0.4
71-90	III	0.9	254	1.2	72	0
91-130	IV	9.3	446	9	40	12.5
>130	V	27	225	27.1	1	0

— FIGURE 4-2 — *The PORT prognostic store for patients with community-acquired pneumonia.*

MAKING THE DECISION

If there is good prognostic evidence, it makes our decision-making easier. Given the evidence provided by the Kaiser TIA study, we would have to consider carefully the potential downsides of a plan to discharge our 65-year-old woman presenting with a TIA. Based on the study results, she has a large risk of having a stroke in the next couple of days. If she is admitted, she will get an expedited work-up for stroke risk factors; and if she does experience an ischemic stroke, she can receive immediate thrombolysis in the hospital.

A patient with a PORT score placing him in class II is probably safe to discharge, even if he is 75 years old, assuming nothing else in his exam worries us. Without the use of the clinical prediction rule, we might have admitted the patient simply because of his age.

SOURCES OF ERROR

The effects of cognitive bias and heuristics on prognostic decision-making have been explored far less extensively than on diagnostic and treatment decisions. As a profession, physicians' prognostications are often inaccurate.[112] We are not aware of any studies on the accuracy of our prognostic decisions in emergency medicine.

If our diagnoses are correct, we can make the proper admission decision on a large percentage of our patients. Prognostic errors arise in the small number of patients in whom we overestimate or underestimate the risks of bad outcomes.

In studies of patients with cancer, experienced physicians were more capable of accurately predicting patients' outcomes.[113] It is logical (though unproven) that experience would also lead to greater prognostic ability in emergency physicians.

The use of prognostic evidence also aids in the avoidance of misestimations of the potential for bad outcome. Prognostic cohort studies and especially clinical prediction rules can augment our clinical judgment to help us make good decisions.

PUTTING IT ALL TOGETHER

In emergency medicine, the more difficult prognostic decisions are those in which the stakes are very high and the evidence is scarce. In these situations, it is reasonable to return to the *precautionary principle*. If we are in doubt whether a patient is safe for discharge, we should probably admit.

Housestaff often dichotomize emergency attendings into *walls* or *sieves*. Walls stereotypically admit any patient who walks through the door, while sieves send home any patient who is not actively dying. While these terms make for enjoyable mealtime chatter in the medicine call rooms, they do point out that we must walk a fine line between over-admitting patients who will be safe in their homes and sending home the potentially sick. We must therefore endeavor to find a balance in our practice in the best interests of our patients.

ONWARD

We have described the process of making decisions in the emergency department in a way resistant to error. The process was predicated on our possession of the best available evidence. It is now time to explain how we decide if a study is the best available evidence and how to seek out such studies. The rest of the book is split into two parts:

- Part II: *Evaluating the Evidence*. We describe how to evaluate a study and decide if it approximates the truth.
- Part III: *Finding the Evidence*. We outline the process of searching for the best evidence through the wide variety of modalities.

PART II

EVALUATING THE EVIDENCE

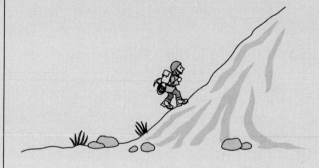

CHAPTER 5

GOOD EVIDENCE

All of our discussion to this point has dealt with decision-making. We analyzed the application of trusted evidence to our individual patients in unique clinical situations. Early in our careers, this trusted evidence may have been given to us by our attendings. As our training progressed, we may have sought out distilled evidence-based resources such as clinical guidelines. We then begin to assimilate evidence from myriad sources. While a good number of decisions can be made with evidence from preappraised literature sources and provided by colleagues who have devoted their careers to evidence-based medicine, at some point we will have to evaluate a piece of literature and decide for ourselves whether we can trust its results.

In this part of the book we delve into the process of analyzing a study. We explain how to decide if the results represent and adequately approximate the truth. There are two primary factors that may cause the literature to fall short of this goal:

Bias and random error

We intend in the next sections to offer the tools necessary to search out and identify each of these potential errors.

BIAS

Bias is the injection of systematic error into a study. A *valid* study is one that is relatively unlikely to be subject to such error. Increasing study size will not compensate for this systematic error.

Bias is the enemy of validity

Each type of study has unique characteristics that make bias more or less likely. Evidence-based medicine has established a hierarchy of study types based on their potential for bias. In Fig. 5-1 we can see the hierarchy of study types for therapy studies. At the top of the pyramid is the study type least likely to be associated with bias.

Detractors sometimes accuse evidence-based medicine (EBM) of worshiping randomized trials to the exclusion of all other study types.

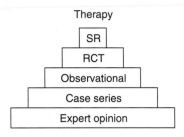

— FIGURE 5-1 — *Treatment study hierarchy.*

This criticism is untrue; each type of literature has merits and disadvantages. If we place the randomized trial on a pedestal, it is only because, when rigorously performed, it is the individual study type least susceptible to bias.

RANDOM ERROR

Just as we must examine the internal design of a study to weed out bias, we must examine the study results to determine statistical significance and precision.

- *Significance* in a study does not relate to *import* as the word is commonly used. Instead, it refers to the likelihood that the result observed in a study can be accounted for by true effect and not by chance.
- A study's *precision* represents the range of possible results within which the true estimate of whatever we are trying to measure is likely to reside. If this range is narrow, we can be confident that the true effect is close to the study's results.

Error in the realm of statistics takes the form of chance masquerading as true differences. A significant study gathers enough patients that the risk of random error creating false effects is minimal. If there are large numbers of patients in the study, the results will be associated with a minimum degree of uncertainty regarding where the true effect is likely to lie; this is a precise study. Unlike systematic error, the potential for random error and imprecision can be ameliorated by increasing study size.

Small study size is the enemy of precision

Before we believe a study's results to represent the truth, there is one final assessment that we must make.

DELIBERATE MISREPRESENTATION

The last and perhaps most difficult threat to assess for is deliberate misrepresentation. In a world free from deception and greed, we would not need this category. At times, the authors of a study or the groups they represent will attempt to manipulate the facts or presentation of a study to create false results and conclusions. While some of these methods are *discoverable* by careful analysis of study methodology, other techniques of misrepresentation are *undiscoverable*.

Even the potential for misrepresentation may then diminish our trust in a study.

Misrepresentation is the enemy of trust

We can therefore believe a study provides a reasonable estimate of the truth if we determine that it is valid and precise. We can examine the results to make sure they are trustworthy. In the following pages, we hope to offer a means to make this determination for any of the study types we may encounter in the literature.

CHAPTER 6

INITIAL EVALUATION OF A STUDY

Before we even begin to analyze a study, we must decide whether it is worth reading. If we decide the study has the potential to be useful, how we go about reading it can influence our perceptions.

FOREGROUND AND BACKGROUND KNOWLEDGE

Our first assessment is whether an article provides foreground or background knowledge. Background knowledge is the foundation of our understanding of a disorder or issue. It is the knowledge of historical context, the physiology, and the traditional means of diagnosis and treatment. Background knowledge fills the pages of most textbooks and is the fodder of narrative reviews. Case reports and case series, because they have no inherent comparisons to other patient groups, contribute to our knowledge of disease and only rarely to our knowledge about the risks and

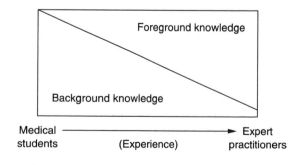

— FIGURE 6-1 — *Progression of the type of knowledge we need throughout our careers.*[118]

benefits of therapy. Sources that provide background knowledge are very useful for students and tyros; even experienced practitioners will sometimes turn to background sources for conditions that are seen less frequently.[1]

Answers to foreground questions are provided by clinical studies. These sources are the essential fuel for evidence-based decision-making. As we progress in our careers, we yearn for greater proportions of foreground to background knowledge (Table 6-1).

TABLE 6-1   BACKGROUND AND FOREGROUND KNOWLEDGE

BACKGROUND KNOWLEDGE	FOREGROUND KNOWLEDGE
Narrative review	Clinical trial
Case report	Systematic review
Case series	Meta-analysis
Monographs	Qualitative research
Textbook chapters	Clinical prediction rules
	Clinical practice guidelines

We categorize the literature into these two groupings because our approach to each is different. We read background literature with an eye towards learning. Our perusal is more relaxed, as we are trying to establish some familiarity with the subject; but we know that for most clinical questions we will have to seek foreground knowledge. Studies that provide foreground information, because we will use them directly for the care of our patients, must be approached analytically and systematically. We must make crucial decisions about the worth and utility of the information from a foreground study.

The distinction between background and foreground knowledge and the sources of such knowledge are discussed further in Part III.

Link to Page 263

THE FIRST PAGE

A wealth of information is included on the first page of any study. From this page alone we can often decide if the article is worth reading.

The Abstract   Many journals are competing for our extremely limited time, so if a study is flawed or not written on a subject of particular interest to us, we can find this out by a perusal of the abstract. The abstracts of most articles are sufficient to assess study design and potential relevance and applicability to our practices. We must then read the *entire study* to decide whether we believe the results.

Who Funded the Study?   In the next few sections we will extensively discuss bias, both conscious and unconscious. If a company that stands to gain from the results funds a study, it creates bias. We are at a point in the history of medical research in which a dizzying proportion of studies are funded by the pharmaceutical industry.[2] Whether an author chooses to acknowledge this bias or not, if an outside interest is funding a study, it may have ramifications on study design and execution. This *pecuniary bias* should be in the forefront of our thoughts when analyzing a funded study.

Many of the methodological flaws, biases, and spin of industry-funded studies speak for themselves to the evidence-literate reader. Unfortunately, some of the present tactics of industry-funded research are undiscoverable from merely reading the study. It is because of these *undiscoverable biases* that we advise the reader to be cognizant of the funding source of a study. We will shortly discuss these issues in detail.

Link to Page 239

AVOIDING PRECONCEPTIONS

Preconceived notions garnered from the opinions of others can affect our perceptions of a study's worth. The best way to analyze a study is to come to our own conclusions after reading the methods and results section. Only then should we delve into the opinions of the authors and editors, but only for the purposes of assuring our own reasoning has not omitted consideration of important issues of knowledge of disease, alternative therapeutic options, and patient issues that affect appliczability.

Do Not Judge a Study by its Authors   Emergency medicine is a small world; often, we may know one of the authors of a study. We should strive not to let our feelings, positive or negative, alter our analysis of a study.

While we should avoid evaluating the article based on our recognition of the authors, we *should* check to see if there is mention of outside interests that can result in bias. Any reputable author should disclose financial interests that have even the slightest potential to influence their work. If the author is a paid consultant for the manufacturer of the study drug, it does not mean we automatically discount the findings of a study, but it certainly may sharpen our skepticism.

Beware of Spin in the Discussion Section The discussion section of a study allows the authors to give their interpretation of the study. Ideally, the discussion section would be a *systematic review* of all of the literature that preceded the current study.[3]

Link to Page 207

The discussion section may also serve to highlight relevant issues of applicability. However, oftentimes this section includes the authors' spin and may falsely influence our assessment of a study's value. It is a good policy to first assess a study's worth by reading only the methods and results section.

Watch Out for Spin in the Editorials and Letters Major articles are often published with editorials or commentary from experts in the field. Their interpretations of the study may be extremely helpful or they may falsely alter our evaluation of a study. It is always safer to come to our own conclusions prior to reading these additions.

VALIDITY OF INDIVIDUAL STUDIES

UNDERSTANDING VALIDITY

Studies take a *sample* of patients, observe them, and then derive results that can apply to a broader population. We can therefore split our discussion of the validity of a study into two parts.

- *Internal validity:* This reflects whether there was systematic bias in the choosing and analyzing of the sample of patients included in the study. If a study lacks internal validity, we cannot believe the results and we cannot use the evidence to help us make decisions.
- *External validity:* We perform studies to find answers we can use for a target population. Since we cannot study the entire *target population,* we analyze sample of patients in the *study population.* External validity relates to whether the study population accurately represented the target population intended by the investigators.

EXAMPLE

A researcher wants to prove the value of a new drug to treat vertigo in the emergency department. He tests the medication on 120 emergency department patients. If the study of these 120 patients is free from systematic bias, then we can say the study is internally valid. We then can assess if these 120 patients adequately represent vertiginous ED patients in general. If they do, then we can say the study is externally valid.

External validity asks whether the conclusions drawn from the study population can be applied to a larger population of interest. If the study is not usable in ED patients, then it will not help us make decisions.

Applicability

Applicability was one the main points of Part I; it goes beyond external validity, as defined by the investigators, by asking: "Does the *population* of the *study* and the population for which we determined the study to be *externally valid* accurately represent *my patient*?" (Fig. 7-1).

DIAGNOSTIC STUDIES

The standard format for a diagnostic study is a *cross-sectional analytic study*. These studies examine a single group (cohort) of patients to see the performance of a test. This study type can be *retrospective* or *prospective* (Fig. 7-2).

- **Retrospective** studies look backwards using data already gathered in a chart or medical record.
- **Prospective** studies look forward; they often use information gathered specifically for the study at hand (Fig. 7-3).

Unlike studies of treatment, retrospective diagnostic studies, if they are performed meticulously, are not inherently inferior to prospective studies.[4]

We will discuss specific points to evaluate in retrospective diagnostic studies in a subsequent section. In this section we discuss key issues common to both study types.

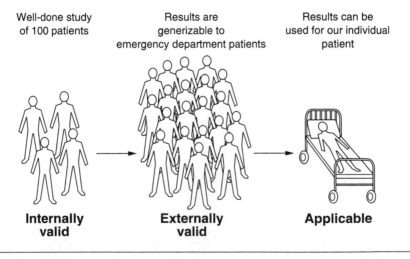

Well-done study of 100 patients	Results are generizable to emergency department patients	Results can be used for our individual patient
Internally valid	**Externally valid**	**Applicable**

— FIGURE 7-1 —

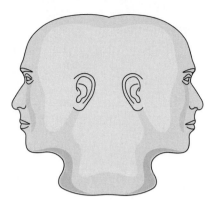

— FIGURE 7-2 — *The different perspectives of retrospective and prospective studies.*

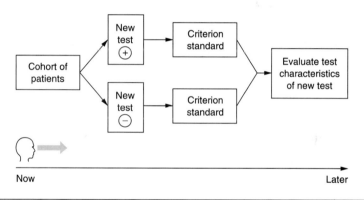

— FIGURE 7-3 — *Prospective diagnostic study.*

Internal Validity

Our first step to analyzing a diagnostic study is to assess its internal validity. We search for systematic bias in the analysis of the study population by examining the following points:

- Criterion standards
- Blinding
- Spectrum of disease.

Criterion Standards

The study authors want to compare their new test to the diagnostic *truth*. Unfortunately, we have no access to the truth; instead, we use the inferior substitute of a criterion standard: the closest to the truth we can get.

Acceptability of the Criterion Standard

We must examine the suitability of the criterion standard: is it an accurate means of diagnosing the disorder? The criterion standard should have been validated in the past and, ideally, it is the best available means of diagnosing the disorder. If a diagnostic test is compared to an inferior criterion standard, then all we can take from the study is that the new diagnostic test is as good as this sub par standard.

EXAMPLE

A study is performed to evaluate the ability of emergency physicians to use ultrasound to evaluate for pancreatitis. The gold standard in the study is elevations of lipase. Lipase is not an overly accurate evaluator of pancreatitis; therefore, we cannot make definitive statements of the diagnostic quality of the pancreatic ultrasound.[5]

Was the Criterion Standard Applied to All Patients?

An ideal diagnostic study would apply the valid criterion standard to every patient in the study, regardless of the results of their experimental diagnostic test. If the criterion standard is applied only to some of the test subjects, then bias is created.

Referral Bias   This bias is also referred to as *work-up bias or verification bias*. If we send only subjects with a positive result on the experimental diagnostic test to further criterion standard testing, we are introducing potential error into our study. By referring only the positives, we potentially miss the patients with the disease, but with a negative experimental diagnostic test. This overestimates the sensitivity and underestimates the specificity of the test.

EXAMPLE

An imaginary researcher (not an emergency physician) hypothesizes that an erythrocyte sedimentation rate (ESR) can predict high-grade coronary stenosis. He sets up a study in which any patient with an elevated ESR is sent to cardiac catheterization, but the patients with a normal ESR are not catheterized.

   If the patients with normal ESR were sent too, some of them would have had positive caths (false negatives) and some would have had negative caths (true negatives). But the study did not include any of the patients with a negative ESR, they were not enrolled (Fig. 7-4). This eliminates both the true negatives and the false negatives; the sensitivity

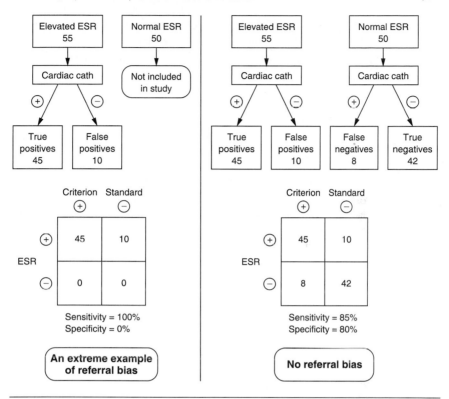

— FIGURE 7-4 — *Referral bias.*

will therefore be falsely increased and the specificity will be falsely decreased.

If instead of sending only patients with positive or negative diagnostic test results for the criterion standard, we allow the clinicians to determine who needs it, this bias will still be operative, but less predictably. Inevitably, the patients to whom the clinicians assign higher pretest probabilities will be more likely to get further work-ups. The only way to avoid this bias is to perform a criterion standard on *every* patient in the study.

EXAMPLE

The NEXUS study established criteria which allowed the reduction of the need for radiographs in the clearance of patients with potential cervical spine fractures.[6] Patients were only enrolled in the trial if they had a cervical spine x-ray ordered. During the study period, clinicians were already using the NEXUS criteria to determine who needed x-rays. Patients deemed to be low risk never had x-rays ordered and were therefore never enrolled in the study. Only patients believed to be at higher risk for a cervical spine injury were referred for the criterion standard of x-ray. This *referral bias* would be expected to falsely lower the specificity and falsely raise the sensitivity of the criteria. This expectation was borne out when the criteria was revalidated in a study in which *all* patients with potential cervical spine injury received a criterion standard.[7]

In some studies this form of bias is unavoidable, because of the ethical problems of exposing patients, unnecessarily, to invasive testing. In that case, another criterion standard, that we also deem acceptable, must be applied to this second group of patients with negative diagnostic tests. A study with multiple criterion standards is more subject to bias than a study with only one criterion standard.[4]

EXAMPLE

We wish to study the new generation of helical CT scanners for the diagnosis of appendicitis. All patients with a positive CT scan are sent to the operating room for appendectomy. To apply this same criterion standard, surgical pathology, to patients with a negative CT scan is deemed unacceptable. Instead, these patients are observed for 24 hours and then followed up at one-week intervals for a month. Though the latter criterion standard seems acceptable, the study would be stronger if *all* patients had their appendix examined by a pathologist.

Of course, the patients with normal CT scans and normal appendices would rightfully object to the researcher's zeal to eliminate bias through these unnecessary surgeries. In this example, two criterion standards are an unavoidable evil.

Patients Lost to Follow-up If follow-up is part of a criterion standard used in the study, then patients lost to follow-up can affect the validity of the study. Ideally, every patient in the study should be accounted for. If patients are lost, the percentage should be very low if we are to trust the study results.

Independence of the Criterion Standard

Even more grievous than the use of the diagnostic test for referral to the criterion standard is when the diagnostic test is actually made part of the criterion standard. The two must be independent for the study to be an adequate assessment of the new diagnostic test's validity.

EXAMPLE

A study examined the role of brain natriuretic peptide (BNP) for the diagnosis of decompensated heart failure.[8,9] The criterion standard was the opinion of cardiologists that the patient had congestive heart failure. One of the factors on the checklist used by the cardiologists to render their opinion on whether or not the patient had the disease was a positive BNP level. Any test measured against itself will appear to perform perfectly.

A valid study of a diagnostic test will always have a clear separation between the criterion standard and the experimental test.

Blinding

The manner in which the experimental test and the criterion standard were assessed can inject significant bias into a diagnostic study. The examiner of the experimental diagnostic test should not know the results of the criterion standard, nor should the assessors of the criterion standard have access to the experimental diagnostic test results. The interpretation of either test can be influenced by knowledge of the other, leading to bias. All test interpreters should be blinded to the other test results in the study.

Review Bias

This bias comes in two flavors, depending on which test a reviewer is interpreting:

- *Index-test review bias:* This refers to the bias created when an investigator has prior knowledge of the results of the diagnostic test being studied when interpreting the criterion standard.
- *Gold-standard review bias:* This bias occurs when the investigator has knowledge of the results of the criterion standard when interpreting the experimental diagnostic test.

EXAMPLE

If the radiologist has already seen a pneumothorax on the CT scan of the chest (which is being used as the criterion standard), it is much easier to subsequently pick out the pneumothorax on the supine plain film.

Whenever possible, the assessors of both the diagnostic test and the criterion standard should be also be blinded to the nature of the study itself. If a radiologist knows that the CT scan he is reading is being used as a criterion standard for a study on pneumothoraces, he will more avidly search for a pneumothorax. Assessors should be blinded to the intent of the study and given only the amount of clinical patient information as they would receive in the course of their normal duties.

Spectrum of Disease

For almost every diagnostic test, sensitivity will be greater when it is performed on patients with severe disease than when it is performed on patients with mild disease. Specificity will be higher when the test is performed on healthy patients with no symptoms or comorbidities. Since the patients we see in the emergency department may be anywhere on the disease spectrum, in order to assure validity, the study sample must also represent a range of disease severity.

Diagnostic Uncertainty   The first way to assess for an adequate spectrum of disease is to assure that the study population represented a source of *diagnostic uncertainty*.

We perform diagnostic tests to determine whether a patient has a disease. Patients who *obviously* have a disease do not need a diagnostic test; obviously well patients do not need a test either. It is in the middle ground of diagnostic uncertainty where diagnostic tests become useful. If a diagnostic test is studied only on the very ill and the entirely healthy, its accuracy may appear falsely high. When we evaluate diagnostic studies, we want to see a group of patients who run the gamut of clinical disease presentation.

EXAMPLE

Many clinicians are now measuring brain natriuretic peptide (BNP) as a means of diagnosing exacerbations of congestive heart failure. A large international trial of BNP yielded a sensitivity of 90% and specificity of 76% using a cutoff of 100 pg/mL.[10] While these numbers may be initially impressive, most of the patients enrolled in the study were at opposite ends of the disease spectrum; they either obviously had CHF or they obviously did not.[11] Hohl et al. reanalyzed the testing parameter of BNP in the patients in which the diagnosis was *clinically uncertain*.[12] Their derived sensitivity of 79% and specificity of 71% demonstrate that BNP would be much less useful than it originally appeared in the patients for whom we need the test most (Fig. 7-5).

Subgroup Variation   In some studies, the patients' clinical presentation will not be an accurate gauge of their disease severity. In these cases, the

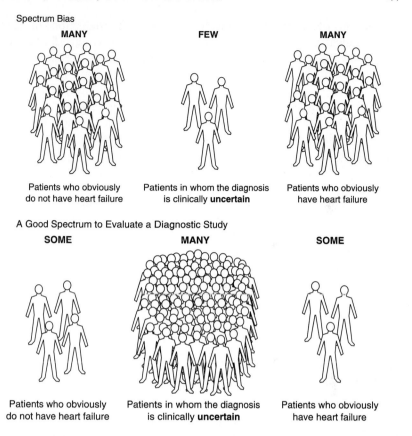

Spectrum Bias

MANY	FEW	MANY
Patients who obviously do not have heart failure	Patients in whom the diagnosis is clinically **uncertain**	Patients who obviously have heart failure

A Good Spectrum to Evaluate a Diagnostic Study

SOME	MANY	SOME
Patients who obviously do not have heart failure	Patients in whom the diagnosis is clinically **uncertain**	Patients who obviously have heart failure

— FIGURE 7-5 —   *The sensitivity and specificity of the BNP assay change depending on the spectrum of disease.*

criterion standard may give us an idea of whether the study population represented the entire spectrum of disease or just certain subgroups. In a similar manner to the spectrum effect we have just discussed under diagnostic uncertainty, different subgroups of disease severity may have different diagnostic test characteristics. This *subgroup variation* can bias study results if applied to patients with disease severity different from the subgroup in the study.[13]

EXAMPLE

Pulmonary embolism can present with wide variety of clot sizes and locations. The CT angiogram is extremely sensitive for the detection of large clots and less so for the detection of smaller subsegmental clots. In a hypothetical study evaluating CT scan with a criterion standard of pulmonary angiogram (PA), we are surprised to see that the PA criterion standard reveals that all the patients with positive results had only large clots. The study sensitivity of the CT angiogram is 100%. We would be hard pressed to apply this derived sensitivity to our patients because we do not know what size clot they may have. We would therefore question the validity of this study.

To allow us to assess for adequate disease spectrum composition, the study should report age distribution, sex, presenting signs, disease stage, and any other available markers of disease severity.[14] When we try to apply the results of studies with inadequate disease spectrums to patients with disease severity not included in those spectrums, our decision-making will be falsely influenced by *spectrum bias*.

External Validity

If we believe the study is internally valid, we next must decide if the study is generalizable to the patients that we routinely see in the emergency department.

Target Population
We can identify from the abstract or introduction the target population the study authors hoped to represent. We then need to analyze whether the study results are truly generalizable to this population.

Inclusion and Exclusion Criteria
A diagnostic study must explicitly detail inclusion and exclusion criteria so that we may evaluate not only whether it was performed on patients conforming to a valid clinical spectrum of disease but also whether the results of the study are otherwise applicable to our own patients.

EXAMPLE

Malignancy was one of the exclusion criteria in a diagnostic study establishing the accuracy of a d-dimer for pulmonary embolism. Many of the emergency patients we suspect of having a pulmonary embolism have a history of malignancy; we may not be able to use the study results to represent all of our patients.

Results
_____

The results of a diagnostic study are usually expressed in terms of sensitivity and specificity. Far more useful, as we discussed in Part I, are results expressed as *likelihood ratios*.

Link to Page 35

Indeterminate Results

If the study had patients who tested neither positive nor negative on their diagnostic test, it is important that we review how these equivocal results were handled. We should take note of the frequency of these non-diagnostic results; if they are frequent, it is a strike against the new diagnostic test. If indeterminate results were excluded from the analysis of accuracy, then we must note this and disregard indeterminate results when they occur in our patients. If, instead, the study authors included these indeterminate results as either positive or negative, then the sensitivities and specificities will be falsely skewed.[14]

The ideal solution is for the study authors to report the indeterminate results with attached *likelihood ratios*, as we discussed in Part I.

Link to Page 35

Does It Cause a Change in Patient-oriented Outcomes?

This question takes diagnosis to the next level, beyond accuracy, to the examination of whether testing actually makes a difference. To examine this issue, not only the performance of the new diagnostic test must be studied, but also its effect on patient-oriented outcomes such as mortality, morbidity, and hospital length of stay. In other words, the *utility* of the diagnostic test is studied in the same way we would analyze new therapies.

EXAMPLE

Recent studies on CT angiogram for pulmonary embolism have used a criterion standard of 3-month follow-up for mortality or recurrent thromboembolic events. If patients with a negative test result did not receive anticoagulation, did not die, and did not have additional PE or DVT, then CTA has proven itself against important outcomes instead of against a less than perfect gold standard such as pulmonary angiogram.

TREATMENT STUDIES

In the emergency department, a percentage of what we do is immediately recognizable as efficacious. When we find a comatose patient has a blood sugar of 26 mg/dL, we give dextrose. We do not require a trial to know that this will help our patient; we see it before our eyes as the patient becomes alert and oriented. If the hypoglycemia was caused by sulfonylurea overdose, should we now administer octreotide?[15] This question is more difficult to answer intuitively. We need studies to demonstrate the effects of many of the treatments we use during a shift.

Study Designs

Clinical Trials

In order to perform a clinical trial, patients must be assigned to a treatment group and a comparison group. It is this deliberate assignment and the presence of a comparison group which defines a clinical trial. For the reasons we will discuss shortly, the ideal study of a treatment is the *randomized controlled trial* (RCT). A representation of a well-done RCT is shown in Fig. 7-6.

At times, the patient assignments to the treatment or placebo group are not randomized. These non-randomized controlled trials are prone to a greater degree of bias than the RCT (Fig. 7-7).

Prospective Observational Studies

Instead of a clinical trial, we may choose to prospectively observe the patients who in the course of normal care receive a treatment as well as those patients who do not (Fig. 7-8). In these studies, also known as

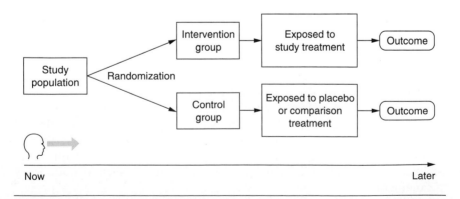

— FIGURE 7-6 — *Randomized controlled trial.*

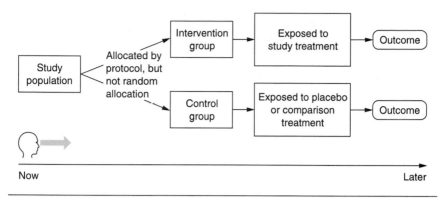

— FIGURE 7-7 — *Non-randomized prospective trial.*

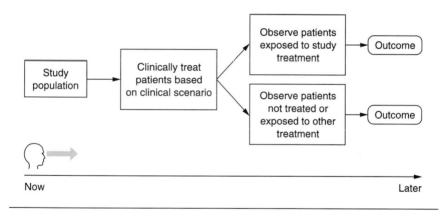

— FIGURE 7-8 — *Prospective observational study.*

prospective cohort trials, there is a large potential for a biased selection of patients. Since researchers can merely observe the patient group assignments made by clinicians, as opposed to assigning them, the validity is inherently lower. These studies can still be important; when both RCTs and prospective observational trials have examined the same treatment, the results are often *qualitatively* similar.[16,17]

Prospective observational studies *without* control groups are very difficult to evaluate. They can often be put on the same level as *case series*, which we will discuss below.

Retrospective Treatment Studies

This form of trial examines two groups of patients; one group receives the treatment and the other does not. By examining the outcomes, some indication of treatment effect can be gleaned. This form of treatment study is inherently biased and inferior to a prospective clinical trial. We discuss the means to analyze these studies in the next section.

Case Series and Case Reports

These studies are uncontrolled; they just report on patients who received a treatment without providing a comparison group. Uncontrolled trials are subject to a number of inherent errors which make interpretation of treatment effect difficult or impossible. All of the observed treatment benefit may be due to a *placebo effect* (discussed below), but we cannot make this determination without a control group.

Treatments such as antihypertensives may also be biased by the phenomena of *regression to the mean*. This describes the tendency of any grossly abnormal value to move towards normal over time. Regression to the mean can cause a false treatment effect if there is not another group who did not receive the treatment for comparison.

The lack of a control group as well as the fact that this form of literature is often retrospective makes any conclusions doubtful. There are a few circumstances in which these studies can provide information beyond background knowledge. If the treatment is being used for a disease whose outcome has in the past been *consistent*, then a case report or series that shows a *different outcome* is suggestive of a treatment effect.

EXAMPLE

Until November 2004, disseminated rabies infection in an unvaccinated host was uniformly fatal. Doctors in Wisconsin tried an experimental treatment regimen on a young woman with rabies infection from a bat bite.[18] She survived the infection and was discharged from the hospital. A case report of the treatment used in this patient can be regarded as much higher evidence than a routine case report. In fact, since a randomized controlled trial of this treatment versus a placebo will now be unethical, this case report established a new standard of care.

The other circumstance in which case series can be vital is when they demonstrate previously unrecognized treatment risks. Harm from treatments will often be reported in the form of case series prior to the publication of controlled trials. If the risks are severe, then we must regard and evaluate them even before further studies are performed.

EXAMPLE

A decade ago, when patients presented with very high blood pressures and the absence of symptoms, it was felt that this hypertension should be treated in the emergency department. A seemingly attractive treatment was the use of an oral nifedipine pill as a sublingual medication. By puncturing the pill and placing it under the tongue, it worked much more quickly. A case series revealed that the precipitous lowering of blood pressure using this method resulted in strokes and myocardial infarctions.[19]

Crossover Trials

In this study type, each patient in the study serves as his or her own control. Each patient is given the experimental treatment and a placebo or comparison treatment. Ideally, this is performed in a blinded fashion, so that neither the patient nor the clinician knows which treatment was administered. One of the advantages of this study type is that the treatment and control groups are automatically matched for baseline prognostic factors. Another plus is that a much smaller sample of patients can be used to achieve significant results (Fig. 7-9).

The disadvantage is that whichever treatment is administered first may still be affecting the patient when the second treatment is administered. To avoid this potential *carryover*, an adequate *washout period* must be allowed between the two treatments.[20] *Carryover bias* occurs if the period between the two treatments of a crossover trial is too short; the effects

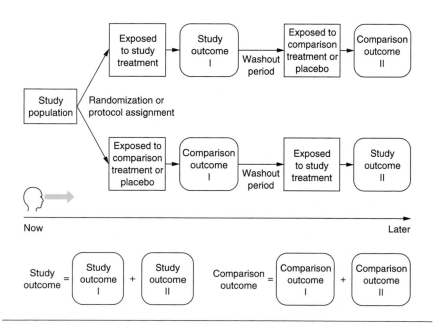

— FIGURE 7-9 — *Crossover trial.*

of the second treatment may be obscured by a continuing effect of the first treatment.

All of these types of treatment studies require thorough and systematic evaluation; we need to examine each of these studies for both internal and external validity.

Internal Validity

When evaluating the internal validity of a treatment study, we must assess the following points to determine its susceptibility to systematic error or bias:

- Randomization
- Baseline group similarity
- Intention to treat
- Blinding
- Appropriate control treatments
- Outcome assessed in all patients.

Randomization

Why Is Randomization so Important?

The ideal for a study on treatment is to have two groups identical in every way except for the presence or absence of the treatment being evaluated. In practice this is impossible, but a well-done study will strive to come as close to this ideal as possible. We call the myriad variables we wish to match between the two groups *baseline prognostic factors*.

Randomization of the study participants gives researchers the best chance of matching these baseline prognostic factors. Non-randomized trials may attempt to match the groups for all of the characteristics that the researchers hypothesize may matter. What this study type cannot do is match the two groups for factors that the researchers, prior to the start of the study, did not realize would be important. By their nature, randomized trials will match for these unforeseen factors as well.

Selection Bias If the study is *observational* (group assignments occur by clinician's choice), then there is a reason a patient is placed into one group or the other. This reason may be clinician preference, disease severity, or patient request. The problem is that the reasons patients are assigned to each group may cause one group to be systematically different from the other in terms of baseline prognosis; this leads to bias.

Was the Randomization Method Acceptable?

Some studies claim to be randomized, but they are actually *pseudo-randomized*. Pseudo-randomization is any method of group assignment that does not allow pure chance to pick the assignments. Examples include group assignment by days of the week, medical record number, hour of day, etc. The problem with these methods, known as *deterministic* assignment, is there may be subtle, unforeseeable reasons why the groups will be different.

EXAMPLE

A new therapy is being studied in a "randomized" controlled trial. Group assignments between placebo and treatment group are done by days of the week. At the end of the study the placebo group had an extra Monday and Friday as compared to the treatment group. At this particular institution, a large volume of sick nursing home patients are treated in the department on Mondays and Fridays. This put a disproportionate number of patients with a greater severity of illness in the placebo group, falsely elevating the treatment effect of the studied drug.

The process of randomization must be truly random. Acceptable means of randomization include any method of generating a random number such as computerized randomized number generators, dice, or even a coin toss.

Pseudo-randomization also usually precludes clinician concealment, a vital concept which we will discuss shortly. We can think of pseudo-randomized trials as another form of non-randomized controlled clinical trials, and analyze them accordingly.

Was the Randomization Concealed?

If clinicians can defeat the randomization procedure, then past instances show that they will often try to do so. We should never underestimate the zeal of physicians to regain control over their patients' care, if given even the slightest opportunity. When randomization is not concealed, patients with different severity of disease may be selectively allocated. As a result, the trial groups may start the trial with different baseline prognoses, creating systematic error.

EXAMPLE

Researchers used a random number generator to pick treatment from assignments for a clinical trial. Depending on whether the number was odd or even, they typed treatment A or treatment B on a piece of paper and sealed it in a blank envelope. Five hundred of these envelopes were placed in the emergency department. Clinicians were given instructions that when an eligible patient arrived, an envelope should be chosen and the paper inside would dictate group assignment. What the researchers did not realize is that the clinicians kept opening envelopes until they got the treatment they wanted to give their patient.

Sequential lists are another example of this phenomenon. This method uses a printout with one line, which reads "treatment A," the next line reads "treatment B," the next line reads "treatment A," etc. Clinicians are expected to use whichever treatment is next on the list and then cross it out. This method is easy to tamper with; a clinician who wishes to offer his patient one treatment even though the opposite one is next on the list can simply cross out two lines.

The safest means of randomization is offsite assignment (outside of the emergency department). Ideally, a clinician calls a geographically diverse location and is provided with the group assignment. Concealment can also be guaranteed by using a website that gives a clinician the group assignment after the entry of the patient's data.

Baseline Group Similarity

Were key prognostic factors similar between the groups? Even with a well-performed randomization method, chance will sometimes lead to unmatched groups. In non-randomized trials, the potential for group mismatching is even greater. In a properly done study of treatment, researchers will provide a table comparing the two groups for every important *baseline factor* they hypothesize will be relevant. Using this table, we can easily compare the treatment groups.

EXAMPLE

We are examining a randomized-controlled trial of a new medication for the treatment of upper gastrointestinal bleeds. The outcome measure in this study is mortality. We examine the chart of baseline factors:

	PLACEBO GROUP	TREATMENT GROUP
Average age	68 y/o	46 y/o
Hepatic disease	50%	26%
HIV positive	43%	10%
Initial Hemoglobin	6	11

We can see that, despite the randomization, there are many reasons why the treatment group may have a better mortality irrelevant of the new treatment. If there was a treatment effect for the new medication, it would be difficult to say whether it was intrinsic to the drug or due to baseline mismatching.

Baseline Mismatching

If the treatment groups are imbalanced with respect to prognostically important characteristics, then there are a variety of methods which attempt to remedy the situation.* Such methods are, at best, stopgap measures; they may corrupt the overall effectiveness of randomization. Ideally, if these methods are used, the authors will show us an analysis of the data with and without the statistical fixes.

Regardless of how the study authors dealt with the problem, we must decide if we believe the results. We must ask qualitatively which direction the results would go were the imbalance not present and decide if the results are still valid.

Differences in baseline frequency of prognostically important factors are one form of *confounders*.

Confounders A confounder is any variable that, if present with different frequency between the two groups, would lead to different overall outcomes. The combination of strict randomization and large study size is a powerful means of avoiding their influence. Other techniques can be used in particular trials to guarantee equal distribution of key prognostic factors between the groups. However, study design alone can never fully guarantee the absence of confounders.

Intention to Treat

Were the patients analyzed in the groups to which they were assigned? If for some reason patients did not take the experimental therapy, were they still analyzed in the treatment group? If patients died during the study, but other outcome data were available, were those data used in the analysis? If all of the assigned members of each of the study groups, whose outcomes were known, were included in the final analysis; this is known as *intention to treat analysis*. Usually, analyzing the patients in the groups to which they were originally assigned leads to the most valid study. When trials are not performed in this manner, bias may result.

EXAMPLE

A hypothetical study of ED thoracotomy for blunt trauma is performed at a major trauma center. Patients with systolic blood pressures <60 mmHg are randomized to either standard care or thoracotomy by random allocation. Some patients assigned to the ED thoracotomy

---

*These methods include direct adjustment of continuous values, multivariate analysis, and interim modification of group assignment. Discussion of these methods would only muddy the water; readers are referred to the sources mentioned in the additional reading section for more information.

group died before the procedure could be performed. Some members in the standard care group died as well. If the mortalities were included in the analysis of the standard group but excluded in the thoracotomy group, then thoracotomy will look falsely efficacious. Even worse, if the patients assigned to the thoracotomy group who died prior to the procedure were reassigned to the standard therapy group, then the overestimation of the treatment effect would be even greater.

If the placebo group inadvertently receives a treatment medication, this will also obviously bias the study and make group analysis extremely difficult. This *contamination bias* can be a mistake on the part of the researchers or due to the actions of the patient.[21] For instance, in a blinded study of aspirin for stroke, a patient in the placebo group may take his own aspirin tablet because he had a headache. Some researchers would argue that these patients should be excluded from the trial; doing so may upset the integrity and effectiveness of the original randomization.

Blinding
Blinding is one of the most effective means of reducing bias in treatment studies. We often hear the terms single-blinded or double-blinded, but these descriptions are ambiguous. It is better for designers of a study to simply report exactly who was blinded (or masked) and the methods used to accomplish the blinding.[22]

Were the Patients Blinded to the Treatment?
When possible, patients should be unaware of whether they are receiving a treatment or a placebo. The reason for this is to avoid a perceived treatment effect from the *placebo effect*.

The placebo effect is a well-known phenomenon in which patients improve, simply because they think they are receiving a treatment, regardless of any actual effect of the treatment. The terminology can be confusing, because if a placebo is not provided to the control group, then the patients in the treatment group will experience the placebo effect while the patients in the control group will not. However, if the patients are blinded to whether or not they received the treatment (i.e., the control group received a placebo), then both groups will undergo the placebo effect, hopefully canceling out this effect as a source of bias.

EXAMPLE

If a study is comparing two formulations of a medication, intravenous versus oral, the patients in the injection group may have a larger placebo effect than the oral. This is based on the supposition that patients perceive injections to be a stronger treatment than oral formulations. This bias can be avoided by giving one group a placebo pill/real injection and the other real pill/placebo injection.

In observational studies, the patients are not blinded to the treatment, leading to potential bias.

Were the Clinicians Blinded?

We want studies to succeed; it is inherent to our belief system as doctors that our treatments make a difference. If we know which patients are receiving the treatment and which are receiving placebo, we may treat them differently, whether consciously or unconsciously. Similarly, if we never believed in the treatment being studied, we might bias the study in the opposite direction.

Cointervention and Performance Bias While a well-done study will randomize patients to intervention groups, there are other treatments a patient may receive in the course of the study that can alter their outcomes. These cointerventions, if administered preferentially to one of the groups, are another form of confounding and therefore bias the study. Such imbalances may occur by chance alone in a small trial. However, they are much more likely when there is a lack of clinician blinding, especially in observational studies.

EXAMPLE

In a study of a new drug for congestive heart failure (CHF), patients are randomized to receive either a new injection medication or a placebo. If the placebo group get much higher doses of nitroglycerin than the treatment group, this might underestimate the treatment effect of the study drug. The nitroglycerin is a confounder, because it causes a difference between the two groups.

The most effective way to counter this bias is effective blinding of the clinicians. In blinded and unblinded trials, a method to counter the confounding bias is to devise a study protocol giving standardized treatments to both groups varying only on whether they receive the study treatment. A chart of the important cointerventions received by each of the groups should be included in the study.

Were the Assessors of Outcome Blinded?

In some studies, the assessment of outcome after the treatment/placebo is subjective. If the outcome is mortality, we do not have to worry about bias in the assessor; but in most other outcomes, it is possible for knowledge of group assignment to bias the determinations.

If the assessors of outcome are aware of group assignment, it may influence their determination of outcome. This bias can affect researchers and even patients, if the patients are assessing their own outcomes.[23]

Were the Statisticians Blinded?

Few trials go so far as to blind their data analyzers as to group assignment, but there is a potential for bias even at this level. Instead of unblinding the study, statisticians can analyze the data as treatment A and treatment B. The placebo and treatment group can be revealed only after the calculations are complete.

Were the Investigators/Authors Blinded?

Throughout the trial, the researchers should not have any access to interim data. During some trials, an interim analysis of the data is performed for patient safety.

Interim Analysis   During trials of some treatments, patient safety demands an analysis of the data before trial completion. This is to prevent either:

- Treatments with large risks to continue to be given to the treatment group
- Treatments with large effects to continue to be denied to the placebo group.

If interim analysis is undertaken, an *independent* assessor should perform it. The results should not be shared with the researchers, if the trial is allowed to continue.

Blinded Results Sections   In the interest of avoiding bias, ideally the study authors should continue to be blinded until after they have written the results section of the paper. They could simply leave blank spaces for the data. This would assure an unaffected portrayal of treatment effect. To our knowledge, this aspect of author blinding has not yet become commonplace.

Appropriate Control Treatments

Inherent in the structure of a clinical trial is the concept that the control group will provide a baseline with which to compare the new experimental treatment. However, if the control group is exposed to a detrimental or ineffective intervention, then the experimental treatment's effect may be falsely elevated.

Placebo-controlled Trials

The placebo treatment in a placebo-controlled trial should be identical in appearance to the experimental treatment, but it should have no effect either positive or negative. Occasionally, the placebo can actually cause harm, biasing the assessment of the experimental treatment.

EXAMPLE

In the 1980s, a randomized controlled trial was performed to establish the benefit of nebulized ribavarin treatment in infants with severe respiratory syncytial virus (RSV).[24] The placebo in this trial was nebulized distilled water. We now recognize that distilled water induces bronchospasm; this may have falsely inflated the trial's treatment effect for ribavarin.[25]

Comparison Controlled Trials

Many trials are performed by comparing two treatments rather than pitting an intervention pitted against a placebo. This might be for ethical reasons; i.e., the withholding of any treatment would be ethically unacceptable. These trials are also performed to compare the relative efficacy of two treatments. If the control treatment is ineffective, this will increase the perceived relative benefit of the experimental treatment.

Straw Man Comparisons If two treatments are compared, each treatment should be utilized at the standard dose or using the most common method. Comparing a new treatment to an inferior existing treatment is equivalent to setting up a *straw man*, destroying it, and then claiming victory against a real, flesh-and-blood opponent.[26]

Outcome Assessed in All Patients

If the outcome data cannot be obtained from all patients in the study, bias will be present if the true outcomes of the missing patients in one group differ from those in the others. If less than complete follow-up is present in a study, there are a few options:

- If the loss of follow-up is small, then it might not irreparably bias the study. In this case, we can analyze the study in the standard fashion.
- Assume that all patients not located are comatose on their floor and therefore cannot pick up the phone when the follow-up researcher calls. If the study still has a statistically significant treatment effect, then we can definitely believe the study.
- If the loss to follow-up is large, but the treatment effect would not persist if we assumed all patients lost to have a negative outcome, then we must make a qualitative judgment about the treatment effect. We can base this decision on the size of the treatment effect and the potential for bias in the patients who did not follow-up.

EXAMPLE

A study was performed to evaluate the use of hyperbaric oxygen to treat carbon monoxide poisoning.[27] One of the outcome measures was neurological function at 1-month follow-up. The study showed no benefit to hyperbaric therapy. However, greater than 50% of the patients never attended their follow-up appointment, despite the attempts of the researchers. It is difficult to draw conclusions from the data when over half of the patients could not be assessed for the outcome.

We must be especially wary of any study that does not attempt to account for every patient originally enrolled.

External Validity

Just as in diagnosis, once we have assured internal validity, we must ask if the study population is generalizable to a broader target population.

Inclusion and Exclusion Criteria
We must assess the inclusion and exclusion criteria to assure the study sample is representative of the general emergency department population.

Efficacy versus Effectiveness
There are two perspectives on the utility of treatments and therefore the way they are analyzed:

Efficacy measures whether a study generates an important treatment effect under idealized circumstances. Efficacy assumes that patients take their medication, clinicians do their job properly, resources are available when they are needed, and ancillary interventions are effectively administered. When performing a study, efficacy is what we care about. If a study does not work in idealized circumstances, then it will obviously never work.

Effectiveness measures whether a study will work in the real world. It is a representation of a study's external validity. If patients would be likely not to take their medication due to side-effects, then a treatment may be efficacious, but not effective. By the same token, if the resources needed to make a study treatment work are arduous, effectiveness may suffer.

EXAMPLE

The NINDs trial indicates that tPA for acute ischemic stroke is an efficacious treatment given a very narrow set of clinical circumstances.[28] However, when this treatment is taken from large, academic centers and tried in the community, effectiveness suffers.[29,30]

Results

In Part I, we argued that a clinician needs to understand the effect of a therapy on outcomes (relative risk reduction) and also a measure of impact on the individual patient (absolute risk reduction and number needed to treat), to be able to appropriately use the results in clinical decision-making. Both of these types of results should be reported.

Were Validated Outcome Measures Used?

When assessing results, study authors occasionally make up their own means of measuring outcomes such as pain or scar size. It is far more reassuring if previously validated instruments are used to assess outcomes. For instance, in the case of pain, a visual analog scale can be used. The advantage of this is we know what a 1-cm difference in visual analog pain scale means as opposed to an arbitrary author-generated scale of one to six (Fig. 7-10).[31]

The outcome scale should be a measure of clinically relevant effect. Validation of the outcome measure offers a gauge as to whether the treatment effect has any true importance.

EXAMPLE

The NASCIS II trial examined the effects of steroids for acute blunt spinal cord injury. In a post hoc subgroup analysis (we will discuss the

Validated scale

Mark below on the scale from 0 to 100 your level of pain/discomfort
with 0 being none and 100 being unbearable

Visual analog scale (VAS)

No pain   Unbearable

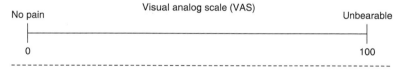

0   100

Arbitrary author-created scale

Rate your pain:

☐ 1	☐ 2	☐ 3	☐ 4	☐ 5	☐ 6
Don't feel a thing	I'm strong, I can take it	That's kind of annoying	Yeah, you can definitely stop doing that now	Can I have a stick to bite on	It's killing me

— FIGURE 7-10 — *Validated pain scale as compared to an arbitrary author-created scale.*

meaning of these terms in a few pages), neurological improvement was found in patients receiving steroids within eight hours of injury. However, this neurological improvement was measured using a scoring system that had not been shown to correlate with either functional or cognitive outcomes.[32] As a result, although steroids resulted in improvement in the neurological score, we cannot say whether this improvement is *patient-important*.[33]

Study Reporting

In an effort to standardize reports of randomized controlled trials and ensure validity, a group of researchers created the *CONSORT statement*. A consensus on the best methods of performing and reporting randomized trials is contained in the statement. It is available both in print and on the internet.[23,34] Almost all of the major American medical journals have adopted the CONSORT statement as the standardized form of reporting clinical trials.

Link to Page 129

PROGNOSTIC STUDIES

Evidence useful in addressing issues of prognosis is characteristically drawn from *cohort studies*. A cohort is just a group of patients; in this case the group would be a number of patients with the condition in question. We can follow these patients over time and observe what percentage experience the outcomes of interest. We can also try to determine the factors that influence the likelihood of those outcomes in individual patients (Fig. 7-11).

Prognostic studies can be retrospective or prospective; if well-performed, retrospective studies of prognosis are not inherently flawed.

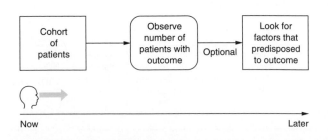

— FIGURE 7-11 —   *Prospective prognostic study.*

Internal Validity

We can discuss the steps of examining the internal validity of the prognostic studies using the example of the TIA study we discussed in Part I.

EXAMPLE

A prognostic study of discharged TIA patients was performed by the Kaiser-Permanente group in California.[35]

The Condition

The first step in assessing a prognostic study is to assure that the condition in question is clearly defined. If we wanted to know the prognosis of first-time seizure patients, then we have to make sure that patients entered into a study truly had a seizure. To this end, adequate diagnostic classification of patients must be discussed in the methods section.

EXAMPLE

In the TIA study above, patients were classified by emergency department diagnosis and a review by a neurologist blinded to patient outcome.

The stage of the disease for each patient in the study should also be documented. Comorbidities can alter a patient's prognosis, so researchers should obtain and report this information for the study population.

Outcome

We then need to determine what outcomes the study examined. Each of the study outcomes should have clear criteria for characterization.

EXAMPLE

In the TIA study, the outcomes of interest were repeat stroke, TIA, mortality, and hospitalization for cardiovascular events. Stroke was the primary outcome in this study. Outcomes were assessed by medical records and neurologist confirmation.

The means of outcome assessment are conceptually similar to the criterion standards of diagnostic tests, as we discussed in an earlier section.

Follow-up

The duration of follow-up can range from days to years in a prognostic study. As we mentioned in Part I, we are most concerned with short-term outcomes. A study that makes no mention of the period immediately following a patient's emergency department discharge is not readily used to help us make decisions.

A good prognostic study should also try to account for all of the originally enrolled patients. If patients are lost to follow-up, it may bias the validity of the results.

EXAMPLE

In the Kaiser TIA study, the follow-up period was 90 days. Of particular relevance to us, short-term outcomes were also tracked. Due to the setup of the hospital system in which the study took place, follow-up was extensive despite the large cohort (1707 patients).

External Validity

We next need to decide with which groups of emergency department patients we can use the study's findings.

Patient Population

The inclusion and exclusion criteria will give us some indication of whether the study's results relate to the prognosis of all ED patients, just adult ED patients, just elderly ED patients, etc.

EXAMPLE

In the TIA study, the mean age was 72 years and the mean symptom duration was 207 minutes. Most of the patients had a history of diabetes mellitus, hypertension, and known history of vascular disease.

From this information, we can determine that the results of this study are valid for *elderly* emergency department patients.

Setting

We would always prefer to use prognostic evidence obtained from emergency department settings. Prognostic studies performed in hospital clinics or outpatient physician offices may represent a very different spectrum of disease from those patients who choose to come to or are brought to an emergency department.

EXAMPLE

The population of the study consisted of only emergency department patients presenting with the signs and symptoms of TIA.

Results

The results of prognostic studies can be descriptive or analytic.

Descriptive results

Descriptive results can simply be reported as percentages of patients with the studied outcomes.

EXAMPLE

In the TIA study, 10.5% of patients had a stroke within 90 days of emergency department presentation. Even more distressing, half of these strokes occurred *within 2 days* of ED presentation.

Analytic results

Researchers will sometimes take prognostic findings one step further by analyzing factors that may predispose some patients to a different prognosis from the rest of the study group. These *prognostic factors* can suggest patients at particularly high risk.

EXAMPLE

In the TIA study, after the results were available, the researchers attempted to find independent prognostic factors that made patients more likely to experience the outcomes. Five factors were found to predispose patients to a worse prognosis:

- Age > 60 years
- Diabetes mellitus
- Longer duration of TIA
- Signs or symptoms of weakness, speech impairment, or gait disturbance
- Patients with symptoms still present upon arrival to the emergency department.

The important thing to understand is that factors are qualitative information. They do not have the power to be applied quantitatively to influence our decisions. They are also to be regarded as preliminary data, until they have been prospectively *validated*. If researchers decide to perform a second study to validate prognostic factors, then they are on the path to creating a clinical prediction rule; we will discuss this form of literature in a subsequent section.

RETROSPECTIVE STUDIES

Rather than expend the effort to perform a prospective clinical trial, it is tempting to use data that have already been collected. This means of data acquisition is quicker and less expensive than a clinical trial. Unfortunately, this ease comes with a price; a retrospective study is prone to a degree of bias far greater than prospective studies. If there is to be any value to retrospective studies, they must be performed meticulously. Even when well done, they usually can only be interpreted as suggesting an interesting possibility to pursue prospectively.

There are two sets of potential problems with retrospective data:

- Bias present inherently in even well-done retrospective studies
- Bias created from poor methodology.

First, we will discuss the inherent bias in retrospective studies of treatment and diagnosis, and then we will outline a methodology that minimizes further bias from flawed study design.

Treatment

Retrospective Cohort Studies

This form of study is also known as a non-concurrent cohort study. The key to understanding this study type is that it is identical to a prospective observational study, except we start the study in the past. The study still has two groups: one which received the treatment and one which did not (Fig. 7-12).

Finding the Patients

Retrospective study authors must first find patients who had the condition of interest. Examination of medical records can be used to split patients into two groups, based on the treatment they received.

EXAMPLE

You pick up a study assessing whether acyclovir has an effect on the duration of paralysis in patients with Bell's palsy. The study is a retrospective analysis, using the institution's medical records. The authors searched the electronic chart database of the emergency department for patients sent home with the ICD-9 code for Bell's palsy in the past five years.

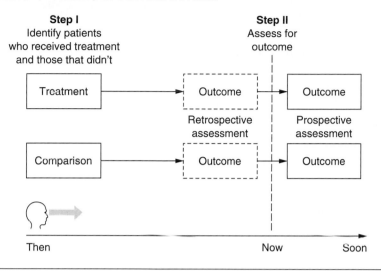

— FIGURE 7-12 — *Retrospective cohort study.*

Misclassification Bias Since chart review studies rely on medical records for the selection of patients, there is the potential to identify only patients with selective characteristics. Sicker patients may have multiple simultaneous diagnoses, but may be coded in a medical chart under only one of the diagnoses and not the others.[36] For instance, patients with decompensated heart failure may also have acute myocardial infarction (AMI). If they are coded under AMI and not under heart failure, then a retrospective study of heart failure will not include these sicker patients. If, instead, chief complaints are used as the entrance into a retrospective study, the patients giving multiple complaints or not knowing what is wrong with them may cause the misclassification.

Dividing the Patients into Groups

Patients are then separated into those who received the study treatment and those who received a comparison treatment (or no treatment at all). In this way, a treatment group and a control group are created.

We have no way of knowing why each patient was treated in either manner. We must assume that there was a reason that one treatment was chosen over another, but we have no way of obtaining this rationale. Instead, we can gather as many data as possible about the baseline characteristics of the patients. We can then compare the two groups to see how they match. Of course, we can only compare based on variables that we think of and that are available in the chart.

EXAMPLE

Patients who were sent home with Bell's palsy were split into two groups: those who received acyclovir and those who did not. Data on the patients' ages, comorbidities, severity of disease, and any cointerventions they received, such as treatment with or prescriptions for steroids. If the authors had not thought to examine whether or not a patient received steroids, a huge bias would have been introduced into the study.

Patient Outcomes

Next, the study authors must determine if patients had different outcomes in the two groups. The chart is reviewed to see follow-up, further diagnostic testing, mortality registers, etc. This introduces additional bias into the study.

Attrition Bias   Patients who achieved good effects with a treatment may be more likely to keep their follow-up appointments and diagnostic test dates. Patients who were not helped or had adverse effects might decide to pursue their care with another physician or at another hospital. This attrition of patients with negative effects can overestimate treatment effect. The converse is also possible; patients with no further symptoms may ignore their follow-up appointments, while patients with continuing complaints will come to clinic with greater alacrity. Either scenario can alter and bias a study's results.

EXAMPLE

Outcomes in the acyclovir study were the degree of facial paralysis at the 1-month neurology clinic follow-up appointment. These data are only recorded in the medical record for half of the patients in the study.

Prospective Follow-up

One means to attenuate bias at this stage is to contact all of the patients in the study. This allows for a more complete assessment of outcome. It also gives the researchers an opportunity to fill in any gaps in the patients' baseline characteristics that were not included in the original review of the medical record. This method blends some of the benefits of a prospective trial into the retrospective format.

EXAMPLE

All of the patients in the study population were called and asked how long their facial paralysis lasted. The researchers managed to contact 90% of the patients; this is much better than the 50% who came to their clinic appointments. They were also able to fill in gaps in baseline characteristics and co-interventions data.

Unfortunately, even this superior method of performing a retrospective study has associated bias.

Recall Bias   Since patients may be followed up at longer periods than in prospective studies, they must recall events that may be months to years in the past. Those with poor outcomes may have a better recollection of their events than those with good outcomes.

Data Analysis

Since patients in retrospective studies often have differing baseline characteristics and co-interventions, specialized data analysis is used to attempt to minimize these differences statistically.

When we discussed prospective treatment studies, we declared this process controversial and prone to bias; in a retrospective trial, there is no other way to control for *confounders*. It is a necessary evil and one of the reasons why retrospective studies of treatments can suggest, but not prove, effect.

EXAMPLE

The results of the study showed no difference in duration of facial paralysis with the administration of acyclovir. The authors did find that in the group who received the co-intervention of steroids there was a small benefit seen in the acyclovir group, not present in the steroids-alone group.

Wisely, instead of taking the results of this retrospective trial as definitive proof of the utility of these two medications in Bell's palsy, you await the results of a randomized trial of acyclovir in combination with steroids versus placebo.*

Diagnosis and Prognosis

Retrospective diagnostic studies are not innately inferior, unlike retrospective studies of treatment.[4] Retrospective prognosis studies can also supply important results that we can use for our medical decisions. The biases we have just discussed are also applicable to retrospective studies of diagnosis and prognosis.

*This trial has been performed; for more information see *Emerg Med J* 2002;19:326.

▨ Harm

Case–control Studies

This methodology is often used for studies on harm, risk, and etiology; it is especially useful for rare diseases or exposures. In emergency medicine, occasionally researchers will use this type of study to analyze treatment side-effects or procedural risks. When this type of study is used to analyze treatment *effects* or answer diagnostic questions, the conclusions are hopelessly biased.

While retrospective cohort studies start in the past and look forward, case–control trials start in the present and look backwards (Fig. 7-13).

The first step in a case–control trial is to find a group of patients with the outcome to be studied; this will be called the "case group." Next, a second group is gathered that is identical to the first in all baseline characteristics except the outcome. This latter population is known as the "control group." The researchers may then retrospectively determine how many members of each group were exposed to a risk factor. If significantly more members in the case group had the exposure than the control group, then this may indicate an *association*. Case–control studies cannot reliably demonstrate *causation*.

EXAMPLE

A pediatric emergency medicine researcher postulates that head CT scanning of infants may cause astrocytoma, a neoplasm of the brain. A case group of 500 patients with astrocytoma is assembled. Five hundred patients without cancer, but with matching baseline

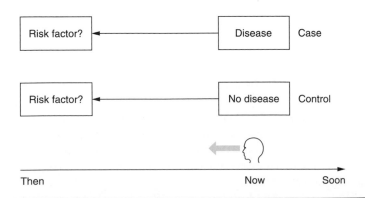

— FIGURE 7-13 —   *Retrospective case–control study.*

characteristics, are to be used as the control group. Both groups are then questioned to see if they were exposed to CT radiation as an infant.

Many of the same biases we discussed above are present in case–control trials. However, their effects are often magnified due to the longer time courses in case–control trials. There are also a few biases that are unique to this study type.

Equal Likelihood of Exposure

Many of the biases of a case–control trial relate to whether or not both groups had an equal chance of being exposed to the possible source of harm. The following two biases illustrate this concept.

Unmasking Bias If an exposure causes harmless symptoms that prompt a search for the disease outcome, then the exposure may falsely be believed to have caused the outcome.

EXAMPLE

We routinely send post-menopausal women with vaginal bleeding to follow-up with gynecology for further evaluation. We would make this clinic referral even if the vaginal bleeding is incidental to the emergency department complaint. A number of post-menopausal women will have symptomless endometrial cancer. Estrogen, often prescribed to post-menopausal women, can cause incidental vaginal bleeding. If a patient with symptomless endometrial cancer is taking estrogens, she may bleed because of the estrogen alone. These patients will be referred because of this vaginal bleeding and their cancer will be discovered. We will not refer the patient with symptomless cancer who is not bleeding. This results in a larger number of known endometrial cancer patients who are taking estrogen, even though the estrogen may have nothing to do with the etiology of the cancer. The unrelated side-effect of the estrogen caused the unmasking of the condition.

Diagnostic Suspicion Bias This bias is similar to unmasking, but relates to clinical suspicion rather than demonstrated symptoms. If an exposure raises our suspicion of an outcome, we may be more likely to perform a diagnostic work-up. If later a case–control trial is performed, we will therefore see more of the case group with the exposure.

EXAMPLE

A patient presents at the emergency department with very mild chest pain and a respiratory rate of 19/min. The rest of our history and physical reveal nothing out of the ordinary and no history of air travel. We decide to send the patient home on ibuprofen and have him follow-up with his primary physician. At one week, the patient has no further chest pain and feels fine. If a second patient, identical in every regard, arrived in the emergency department after a 14-hour plane flight, we may decide to evaluate for pulmonary embolism (PE). A PE is indeed found and the patient is sent home on anticoagulation. The first patient in this example had a clot as well, but it was never discovered. If a case–control trial was performed including these patients, it could falsely conclude that plane flights had a greater role as a risk factor for pulmonary embolism than exists in reality. The history of air travel only made us more likely to work-up the patients and therefore discover their clots.

Validity of Chart Review Methodology

Medical records such as patient charts, ambulance run-sheets, and triage notes were not designed to be used as a research tools. When retrospective studies are performed using review of medical records, additional errors can stem from the methods used to extract the data. Only with good methods of chart abstraction can we believe the results of a retrospective study.

Implicit Reviews

Implicit chart reviews make no mention of the methods use to glean data from the medical record. We have a difficult time determining whether we can believe the results of a study, if the methods are left to our imaginations.

Explicit Reviews

If there is an explicit description of chart review, then we look for the criteria, adapted from a review by Gilbert and Lowenstein:[37]

- *Case selection:* Were there explicit criteria for inclusion and exclusion of patients into the study? If not, then we can only imagine patients were selected for entrance in the midst of performing the study; this can lead to biased results.
- *Chart abstraction:* Ideally, trained chart abstractors, using pre-made worksheets, should perform the chart review. The researcher should not be one of these abstractors as this may introduce bias in the selection of the patients and interpretation of patient data.

Quality assurance should be performed during the abstraction period to assure adherence with the study design.

- *Definition of variables of interest:* A list of variables should be determined prior to the chart abstraction. This limits the subjective interpretation of patient data during the process of record review.
- *Blinding:* To prevent potential bias, the abstractors should not know the hypothesis of the study. This is one of the reasons why the researcher should not be a data abstractor.

CHAPTER 8

EVALUATING STUDY RESULTS

PRECISION AND SIGNIFICANCE

"There are three kinds of lies: lies, damned lies and statistics."
– Leonard H. Courtney

When we flip a coin, we expect there to be an equal chance we will get a head or a tail. If we flip the coin four times, obtaining three heads and one tail, we feel confident that we can attribute this discrepancy to chance. If we flip the coin 1000 times and obtain 750 heads, we may start wondering who has tampered with our nickel. When evaluating clinical studies, it is far more difficult to utilize our intuition to decide whether chance or true effect caused the results. Instead of intuition, we resort to statistics to make this decision.

Statistical Significance

The results of a study may seem to reveal an important benefit of a therapy, or more broadly, an important difference between a therapy of interest and a comparison treatment. When this is the case, before we recommend it to our patients, it is incumbent upon us to consider the likelihood that the observed difference was only the result of the play of chance. Researchers are obviously concerned with this as well.

The researchers who design and conduct a trial use statistical techniques to estimate the likelihood that the results they observed might have occurred by chance. This estimate is called a test of *statistical significance*. Researchers are often satisfied if it is simply *unlikely* that *all* of a study's results occurred by chance. For them, it is an all or none phenomena: either a study is significant or it is not.

Clinicians, on behalf of our patients, need more than this dichotomy. It is not enough for us to simply believe that some part of a study's results is real, i.e. not caused by random error. We need to know exactly how confident in a study's results we can be; further we need to be able to quantitate this level of confidence. The information we need is not whether a study is significant, but the *precision* of a study's results.

We will first discuss hypothesis testing and *p-values*, as the measure used by researchers to test for statistical significance. We do this owing to the ubiquity of the use of p-values in reporting clinical research. As we will shortly show, they are an inferior method of evaluating the results of a study when compared to the information we really need: *confidence intervals*. Hopefully, when we are creating the second edition of this text, we will not even have to discuss p-values, as all journals will be using confidence intervals exclusively.

Hypothesis Testing

The first step in the traditional method of assessing statistical validity is to establish hypotheses.

When trying to prove that a treatment works, we state two hypotheses. We must first state a *null hypothesis*, the proposition that there will be no difference between the new treatments and a comparison.

EXAMPLE

In Part I, we discussed the imaginary drug Inspire^{TM}, a medication that was shown to reduce the need for intubation in severe asthmatics. In the case of Inspire^{TM}, the null hypothesis would be that there is no difference in the need for intubation between this new drug and a placebo.

Along with the null hypothesis, we state the *alternative hypothesis*: that there is a difference between the two groups.

EXAMPLE

The alternative hypothesis in this example would be there will be a greater reduction in need for intubation if Inspire^{TM} is given when compared to the placebo.

If a study proves there is a true difference, we *reject* the null hypothesis and *accept* the alternative hypothesis.

Statistical Errors

Type I Error
If we accept that the treatment effect is real (i.e., accept the alternative hypothesis) when there is actually no difference, statisticians would declare we have made a *type I error* (Table 8-1).

TABLE 8-1

	STUDY SHOWS TREATMENT EFFECT	STUDY SHOWS NO TREATMENT EFFECT
Treatment effect actually exists	Truth	Type II error
Treatment effect does not actually exist	Type I error	Truth

Type II Error

A *type II error* is in stating there is no difference between the treatments (i.e., accepting the null hypothesis) when a difference actually exists.

Point Estimates

The point estimate is the result from our study data that is *most likely to be true*. However, this value is just an estimate; there is always a degree of uncertainty around any such result. It is possible that this perceived effect was just the result of chance. In our example, maybe the drug does not really reduce the need for intubation at all. The degree of uncertainty and the possibility that a point estimate was caused by chance alone is dependent on the size of the study.*

EXAMPLE

At the end of our Inspire™ study, we note that there was an *absolute risk reduction* (ARR) of 17% in the treatment group. This percentage value is the *point estimate* for the treatment.

P-values

In order to avoid making the assumption that effects caused by chance are real (type I error), we need a way to discern whether our treatment effect is

---

*The results we learned to interpret in Part I were a study's point estimates. These point estimates should always be interpreted in tandem with the degree of uncertainty surrounding them.

statistically significant; i.e., likely to be caused by true effect and not random error. The traditional (and inferior) way to make this determination is with the p-value.

The "p" of the p-value stands for "probability": the probability of chance alone causing the observed effects in a trial. Arbitrarily, in the setting of medical research, we are willing to accept a 5% risk that chance caused any observed effect in a study. Though this value does not have any firm foundation, it is the standard throughout clinical medicine. P-values are expressed from 0 to 1, so this 5% corresponds to a p-value of 0.05. The highest p-value we are willing to accept in order to believe the statistical significance of a study is known as the *alpha value* (α).

If we decide to use the standard alpha value of 5%, then when we examine a study, we need it to yield a p-value less than 0.05 in order for us to accept the alternative hypothesis. It is crucial to note that, with this level of assurance, there is still a 5% possibility of type I error. To state this another way, there is still 1 chance in 20 that the observed differences in a study were caused only by chance and not from any real effect. The p-value of a study is *directly proportional to the sample size*. If the study population is large, then the p-values will be small.

If a study's results have a p-value of 0.02, then we can conclude that there is only a 2% possibility, or 1 in 50, that chance caused the observed treatment effect. This lower p-value states nothing about the degree of treatment effect or the clinical utility of the treatment; it simply means that it is less likely that chance caused the perceived difference.

EXAMPLE

If the results of the Inspire^{TM} study were an ARR of 17% ($p = 0.02$), then with 98% assurance we can believe that the true results are greater than zero.

The *true ARR* may be 1% or it may be 29%; the p-value does not give us any indication of this. All it tells us is that there is only a 2% chance that the results are not greater than zero.

If our data yielded a p-value of 0.07, then we would state that the decreased intubation rate in the treatment group was not statistically significant. We reject the alternative hypothesis and accept the null hypothesis; i.e., there is no difference between our drug and the placebo. This p-value gives us no indication of whether we are making a type II error. Did we reject our alternative hypothesis because there really was no treatment effect, or was it because our study was just too small to show a statistically significant difference? P-values do not help us answer this question, they only assess type I error.

Despite the widespread reporting of *p*-values as our gauge of statistical validity, they are far from ideal. It often seems that when a *p*-value is greater than 0.05, clinicians immediately feed the study through a paper shredder without any further perusal. Conversely, if a *p*-value is less than 0.05 the study is accepted as gospel. This shows a true misunderstanding of the shortcomings of *p*-values. Gallagher terms this biased fixation on a $p < 0.05$ as "decerebrate genuflection."[38]

In case we were not hyperbolic enough about the reasons why *p*-values fail us as measures of statistical significance, let us repeat them one more time:

- They are often *misperceived* as an indication of the study's internal validity. A study rife with bias can produce a false treatment effect with a statistically valid *p*-value.
- They give no indication of the *precision of the point estimate*. *P*-values just tell us whether we can reject the null hypothesis. They do not represent how well the point estimate actually represents a true treatment effect.
- If the *p*-value is above the alpha value (above 0.05 in most studies), we have no indication of whether a *type II error* has been made. In other words, we do not know if there is really no treatment effect or if the study was just too small to demonstrate one.
- They do not gauge the *patient-importance* of the results of a study.

Confidence Intervals

Confidence intervals are a far more clinically salient means of reporting statistical values in medical literature. This method rejects the traditional precepts of hypothesis testing, while providing substantially more information than *p*-values. They can be used with any quantitative result in any study type. Confidence intervals should replace *p*-values in all journals, whenever the information is likely to be used in clinical decision-making.[23]

When using confidence intervals, we are presented with a point estimate as well as a range of values representing the confidence interval.

EXAMPLE

In our Inspire™ trial, we could represent our treatment effect as the ARR for intubations in the treatment group as 17% with a 95% confidence interval of 5–23%. This is often written as 17% (95% CI 5–23). We can also represent these values graphically, as in Fig. 8-1.

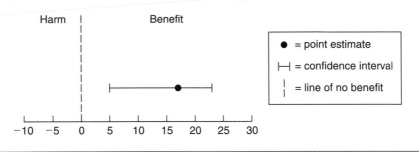

— FIGURE 8-1 —

What is the 95 percent?

The 95% is simply the degree of assurance that chance did not cause a study's effects. With *p*-values, we traditionally accepted a 5% chance of type I error. When using confidence intervals, the normal set point is to be 95% sure that chance did not cause the observed effect (represented as a 95% confidence interval). The 95% confidence interval is analogous to an alpha value of 5%. While other percentages can theoretically be useful, 95% is almost universally used in the medical literature.

A working definition of a 95% confidence interval is the range at which the true value will be found 95% of the time.* If every number in the range of the confidence interval still shows a treatment effect, then the results are *statistically significant*. This is synonymous with a *p*-value of less than 0.05. There is still a 5% risk that the true value will be outside the confidence interval and that chance alone caused the perceived treatment effect. In this way, the confidence interval has already provided the same information as the *p*-value offered.

Sample Size

The width of the confidence interval is *proportional to the sample size* of the study. A tight confidence interval indicates a sample size that is large enough to assure us that the point estimate is probably close to the true value.

EXAMPLE

If the Inspire^{TM} study enrolled 200 patients, the results would be ARR = 17% (95% CI 4-30) (Fig. 8-2A). However, if the study enrolled

---

*A working definition is presented because the true definition can be quite confusing and offers little additional utility. The actual definition of a 95% confidence interval is: if the trial were repeated thousands of times using thousands of similar patients, in 95% of these trials the 95% confidence intervals would contain the true value.

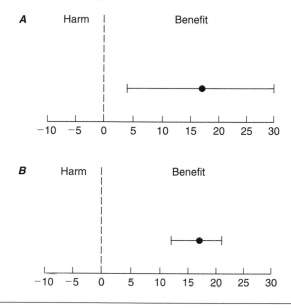

— FIGURE 8-2 —

2000 patients, the confidence intervals would be much narrower, even though the point estimate remains the same: ARR = 17% (95% CI 12–21) (Fig. 8-2B).

Statistical Significance

If the lower value of the confidence interval crosses the line of zero difference, then we can say the results are *not statistically significant.*

EXAMPLE

If the result of our Inspire™ study was an ARR of 17% (95% CI –2 to 28), then we cannot call the results statistically significant (Fig. 8-3). There is too great a chance that random error caused the perceived treatment effect.

When using confidence intervals, we must accept that, while the point estimate is the most likely value, any of the values within the interval may be the true treatment effect. This is why, if the confidence interval crosses zero, we must not deem the study to represent the truth.

We can take confidence intervals one step further using one of the precepts we discussed in Part I.

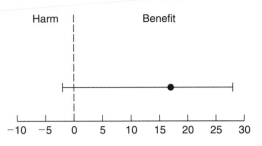

— FIGURE 8-3 —

Action Thresholds

Just achieving some minimal effect above the no-difference line is really not sufficient for patient-important decisions. If the lower border of the confidence interval were 0.000001, is this really much better than no effect at all? Earlier in the book, we mentioned the concept of *treatment thresholds*; they are the minimal difference of treatment effect a new treatment must achieve in order for it to be worth using.

Link to Page 96

A drug that caused an absolute risk reduction of admission to the hospital of 0.5% would not be useful unless it was dirt cheap and risk free. We can integrate this concept into our evaluation of confidence intervals to assure that a treatment is not just statistically significant in the world of numbers but patient-important.

EXAMPLE

Our new imaginary medication Inspire^{TM} is relatively side-effect free, but it costs $1000 a dose. We decide that it would have to absolutely reduce intubation rate by at least 4% (NNT = 25) in order to be a valuable new treatment option.

For the purposes of this discussion, we are concentrating on confidence intervals for treatments, but the concepts are applicable for any quantitative study result. For instance, we can think the same way for *likelihood ratios* in diagnostic tests. We may say a likelihood ratio must be greater than 5 or less than 0.5 in order to make a real difference in decision-making.

We can take these action thresholds and add them to our analysis of confidence intervals.

Patient-important and Statistically Significant Results

In the case of a study that observes an apparent benefit, if the confidence interval does not cross the no-difference line and is above our action threshold, then we can say that we are sufficiently sure that the true effect is patient-important.

EXAMPLE

For Inspire^{TM} to be statistically significant, its lower confidence interval must not cross zero; but for it to be patient-important, its confidence intervals must not cross 4%. If the results are ARR = 17% (95% CI 7–25) then the results are both (Fig. 8-4).

Possibly Not Patient-important but Statistically Significant Results

If the confidence interval does not cross the no-difference line, but does cross our action threshold, there is a chance that the true results are not patient-important.

EXAMPLE

If the results of the Inspire^{TM} study are ARR = 17% (95% CI 2–24), then we have a problem (Fig. 8-5). Since there is the possibility that the true result of the study is not patient-important, we cannot consider the study to be definitively positive. In this circumstance, the study suggests a patient-important effect, but it does not prove it. Further studies with larger sample sizes are needed before we can fully accept the results.

Rarely, we may alter our practice based on the results of a statistically significant, but possibly patient-unimportant, trial; but we must do so with a careful analysis of the risks and benefits.

Possibly Patient-important, Negative Result

If a treatment study observes a point estimate effect corresponding to harm, but the confidence intervals around the results crosses the line of

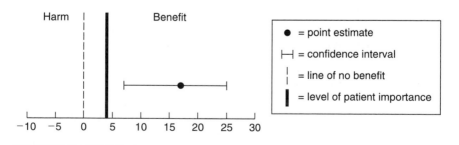

— FIGURE 8-4 —

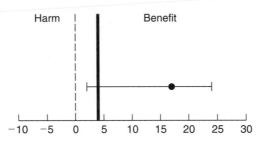

— FIGURE 8-5 —

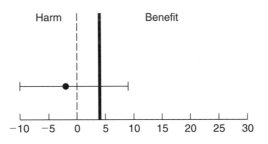

— FIGURE 8-6 —

no difference and also crosses the threshold above which we would actually recommend the therapy, we clearly would not be ready to use the treatment.

However, while such a trial fails to justify administering the treatment, we cannot be completely sure that a larger trial would not demonstrate a valuable benefit. In this case, we will certainly forgo recommending the treatment for now, but we will want to pay close attention to subsequent research, which could demonstrate a benefit.

EXAMPLE

If the Inspire™ study yielded results of ARR = −2% (95% CI −10 to 9), then while we certainly would not start using the medication, it may bear further study (Fig. 8-6).

Definitely Not Patient-important, Negative Results

If a study's results cross the no-difference line and the confidence interval does not cross our action threshold, then the study is definitively negative.

It is important to realize that researchers may have only looked at statistical significance and concluded that such a study was *not* definitive.

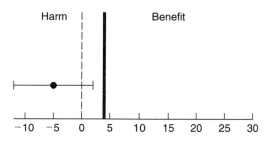

— FIGURE 8-7 —

This illustrates why confidence intervals, not *p*-values, best serve the needs of clinicians in evaluating the likely impact of random error.

EXAMPLE

If the Inspire™ study's results were ARR = −5% (95% CI −12 to 2), then we should not use the medication; this is a negative trial (Fig. 8-7).

Trends

Often, when reading studies, we will see the term *trend* used. What this refers to is a result that is not statistically significant, but which the researchers feel might have been if the sample size had been larger. From the discussion we have just had about confidence intervals, the evidence-informed reader can derive that the only trends we care about are those results with confidence intervals that cross our action threshold.

Down with *p*-values

Confidence intervals give far more information than *p*-values. It is for just this reason that many journals now request that treatment effects be reported with CIs as opposed to *p*-values. If a study does not provide confidence intervals, there are equations that allow us to calculate them ourselves.[39] Even easier to use are a number of websites, which do all of the calculations.

- For treatment studies: www.healthcare.ubc.ca/calc/clinsig.html
- For studies of diagnosis: www.healthcare.ubc.ca/calc/bayes.html

Study Power

One other term that we may come across in the methods section of a study is *power*. When planning a study, researchers need to calculate how many patients they will require to have their results achieve statistical significance. This calculation allows an estimation of the study's power to find a meaningful result. The power of a study is the likelihood of finding a predetermined outcome with a given sample size.[40] Although statisticians and researchers make much of this concept, it has little import to clinicians once a study has been performed and reported.

The determination of a sample size is based on:

- The accepted risk of making a type I error
- The accepted risk of making a type II error
- The number of placebo patients expected to respond
- The degree of desired relative difference between the two groups.

EXAMPLE

In a study of a new beta-blocker, researchers calculate a power of 90% (a 90% chance) to detect a decrease of 25 beats/min between the study drug and the placebo, given a sample size of 75 patients. This power calculation is based on a 5% chance of making a type I error and a 10% chance of making a type II error.

Power is important to researchers when planning a trial, but all that is truly important to us are the *confidence intervals of the results*. We mention the concept of study power only to familiarize you with the term.

PITFALLS IN THE ASSESSMENT OF STATISTICAL SIGNIFICANCE

A clinical trial is an enormous undertaking, requiring daunting investments of time and money. It is only logical that researchers like to see the trial yield useful information and positive results. In order to maximize the value of a study, many researchers use methods that increase the chances of a positive effect and broaden the results. Unfortunately, these methods also increase the risk of *random chance* causing apparently real results.

This is not to say that these strategies have no place, but as consumers of the literature we must be even more vigilant when using conclusions derived by these methods.

Secondary Endpoints

When planning a study, researchers determine how many patients they predict they will need to achieve statistical significance; we discussed this concept of *study power* in the previous section. This determination of required sample size is usually based on one, *primary outcome*; this is the outcome of most interest to the authors of the study. If two independent primary outcomes (or endpoints) are chosen, many more patients will need to be entered into the study to assure significance.

EXAMPLE

A colleague wishes to study the effects on mortality for a new drug when compared with a placebo. She estimates that she would need 400 patients to achieve adequate statistical significance. If, however, she wished to make both admission to the hospital for any reason and mortality the primary outcomes, she might need to enroll more patients to be equally certain that chance did not account for any discovered treatment effects.

The reasons why looking at multiple outcomes would increase the likelihood of random error may at first seem non-intuitive. We must remember that statistical significance is commonly determined using 95% confidence intervals (corresponding to a *p*-value of less than 0.05). This means there is always a 5% chance that the apparently positive results of a study could have occurred solely due to random error. If we look at 20 different independent outcomes, then chance alone creates a high likelihood that at least one of the outcomes will appear to be significant (falsely). If we look at two independent outcomes instead of just one, we double our chances of finding a positive effect by chance, unless we increase our sample size.

To avoid this need to enroll larger numbers of patients, when study designers wish to assess multiple outcomes, they often deem one of the endpoints to be primary and designate additional outcomes as secondary. These *secondary outcomes* are then not included in the estimate of the number of patients needed to power the study.

Even though these secondary outcomes are not included in the original power analysis of the study, they can still provide useful information if their effect sizes are sufficiently large and precise. While we cannot regard these secondary outcomes as strongly as primary outcomes, they can help us make decisions if two criteria are met:

Were the Secondary Outcomes Planned Prospectively?

If study designers plan ahead of time to analyze a small number of secondary outcomes, then their results are believable. If these secondary outcomes are chosen after the study results are available, there is a huge potential for chance to have caused the results.

Frequently, this latter situation occurs when researchers fail to find a statistically significant effect with their prospectively identified primary outcome. Rather than simply report the trial as negative, they can work through the data in an attempt to find an outcome they can report as positive. This approach is called *data dredging*; it refers to multiple analyses of accumulated study results (post hoc analysis) to find positive outcomes.

Retrospectively chosen secondary outcomes should never be regarded as anything more than interesting trends, suggesting the need for further research.*

Are the Secondary Outcomes Patient-oriented?

If a secondary outcome is patient-oriented evidence it is far more likely to provide useful information for our decisions. In many studies, the primary outcome is patient-oriented (mortality, need for intubation, etc.), but the chosen secondary outcomes are surrogate markers (such as FEV_1), which are correlated with clinically important outcomes.

These surrogate outcomes are often examples of disease-oriented evidence; they are not useful to help us decide how to treat our patients. This form of secondary outcome is often stressed in a study with a negative primary outcome. If we are to believe a secondary outcome, it must represent patient-important evidence.

Subgroup Analysis

Individual patient populations within the participants of a study can be analyzed separately; this method is called *subgroup analysis*. The resulting subgroups are comparable to a set of separate studies with many fewer patients than the original. The examination of subgroups within a study population can yield useful information and hone the applicability of a study.

At the same time, a subgroup analysis, when improperly performed or reported, has the potential to mislead. Both positive and negative results found by subgroup analysis can provide false evidence and lead us to bad decisions.[41]

If we are to believe the results of a subgroup analysis, it must be performed in a way that minimizes the potential of chance to create false effects. The following criteria can help us assess if we can derive useful information from a subgroup analysis:[41]

Have the Differences Been Supported by Other Studies?

It is extraordinarily rare that a subgroup effect can be accepted for clinical application when only a single study reports it. We should virtually never

---

*The CONSORT statement, the widely accepted standard for reporting trials, requires that primary and secondary outcomes be clearly identified prior to the start of the trial to allow us to assess for data dredging.

use an apparent effect in one subgroup from a single study as evidence for our decision-making. In most cases, we should consider evidence from a well done meta-analysis* to constitute the minimum strength of evidence supporting such an effect.

Were a Small Number of Subgroups Prospectively Declared?

Subgroup analyses performed on a large number of subgroups or those performed *after the results of the study are complete* can be dangerously misleading.[42] We have already mentioned data dredging in our discussion of secondary outcomes; the post hoc nature of this analysis makes it very likely that chance caused any observed subgroup effects. Prospectively declared analysis of only a small number of subgroups therefore has much greater weight as evidence.

EXAMPLE

A new drug turns out to have no benefit on mortality when compared to placebo. The frustrated researcher looks at the results and begins dividing the patient population into subgroups based on every criterion imaginable. He eventually discovers that green-eyed patients who are left-hand dominant had a 60% relative risk reduction.

Other Criteria

Oxman and Guyatt listed a number of additional criteria to assess the believability of a subgroup analysis.[43] One crucial element is that any subgroup effects should be assessed only in comparison to other subgroups in the *same study*. A subgroup from one study should not be compared to groups from another study, because we have no way of assessing for the presence of *confounders* (differences between the groups aside from the studied intervention).

The differences should be statistically significant, but as we have just discussed, this significance alone is not enough to allow us to trust the results of a subgroup analysis.

Any observed differences from a comparison between subgroups should make biological and clinical sense.

EXAMPLE

It is not immediately apparent why a subgroup of right-handed patients should have different clinical effects than the southpaws. On the other

---

*A meta-analysis is an integrative study, which systematically combines the results of multiple studies to yield believable estimates of effect. We will, shortly, discuss this form of literature in detail.

hand, if the subgroup analyzed in an asthma study was those patients with severe disease, then different clinical effects in this group are more believable.

Unless a subgroup analysis meets the above criteria, we should use the results only as indicators of possible qualitative trends and the impetus for further research.[42,44,45]

Composite Endpoints

Composite endpoints combine the possibility of multiple outcomes into a *single primary outcome*. For instance, a study's primary outcome may be mortality or myocardial infarction. The original purpose of composite endpoints was to avoid one outcome from falsely affecting the results of another outcome.[46]

EXAMPLE

A researcher wants to study the effects of a new drug on the 30-day incidence of myocardial infarction. As he is designing his study protocol, he realizes that if some of the patients die from a myocardial infarction during the 30 days, they may not actually be classified as myocardial infarctions. This is due to the fact that their death may precede the diagnosis of the heart attack. Unless post-mortem examinations were performed on all of these patients, some of the heart attacks may be missed. He decides to use the composite endpoint of myocardial infarction or death to avoid this problem.

Another use of composite endpoints, which has gained popularity, is to allow clinical trials to enroll *fewer patients* and still achieve a statistically significant treatment effect. This latter use can cause false study results if not performed properly.

Interpretation of studies using composite endpoints requires us to be diligent; a number of important criteria must be fulfilled in order for us to trust the results of a trial using composite endpoints. The treatment effect of the composite endpoint is assumed to be representative of all of its component outcomes. When used improperly, one of the components may falsely represent the effects of the entire component endpoint. In order to avoid error, we should evaluate the following points:[47]

Equal Meaning to the Patient

Each of the composite endpoints should be meaningful to our patient. This is perhaps the most important factor to keep in mind when analyzing composite endpoints. In order for a composite endpoint to be patient-important, all of its components must be of similar severity. If one of the components of the endpoint has much less significance than the others, it will be very difficult to apply the combined treatment effect to decision-making.

EXAMPLE

A study demonstrates 30% absolute reduction in death, stroke, myocardial infarction, or anginal chest pain. The presence of chest pain makes decisions regarding the use of this treatment difficult. Our patient may be willing to accept a higher cost and a larger risk profile to prevent the first three components of the outcome, than she would the reduction of anginal chest pain.

Individual Components of a Composite Endpoint

Authors often find it difficult to resist the temptation of reporting parts of a composite endpoint as *individual primary outcomes*, while downplaying the other components (especially if the composite endpoint showed no effect when analyzed together). Individual pieces of the composite endpoint should be reported as *secondary endpoints*; we can analyze and use this information as we have discussed in the secondary endpoint section above.[48] For the same reasons we have mentioned, when the reported component of a composite endpoint is a surrogate measure, which does not correlate with patient-important outcomes, it can be particularly misleading.

Reporting

We have just stated that all of the components of a composite endpoint should usually be interpreted together. However, if one of the parts of a composite endpoint had *little or no effect* on the combination, the authors should point this out. This is especially important when the outcome with little effect is the one that is most meaningful.

EXAMPLE

The composite endpoint used in a study is death, myocardial infarction, or stroke. At the end of the trial the authors note that, while the composite endpoint showed a 15% absolute risk reduction (ARR), there was no reduction in mortality at all. They should report the results as: "A composite endpoint of infarction, stroke, or death showed a 15% ARR; it should be noted that there was no observed effect on mortality."

Composite endpoints are becoming quite common, because they allow the enrollment of fewer patients. We must be vigilant in their interpretation if we are to use the results in practice.

Interim Results

Unless external factors intervene, a study should be allowed to continue for the duration planned before its inception. The temptation to examine data as they pour in from an ongoing study is large. Researchers should resist the temptation, as this examination dramatically increases the risk that chance can masquerade as actual effect.

Peeking Bias

In laboratory research, overeager scientists may check their experiments to see the interim results. If they terminate the study at a moment when the results are positive for the outcome they desire, then a huge bias has been introduced. Their experiment should have been allowed to continue to its predetermined endpoint; only then should the results be examined.[49] This bias is just as relevant in clinical studies as in laboratory research. If researchers had access to interim results during the course of the trial, then bias can be introduced. If a trial is terminated because of these interim results at a point when the researcher is pleased with the results, then the study cannot be trusted at all.

Ethical Considerations

When performing a therapeutic study of a new intervention, it is possible that the new treatment will be harmful. Even if evaluated on animals first, there is still a risk of any new medication or intervention. Ethically, we always seek to do no harm; especially with patients already vulnerable, because they are enrolled in a study. To counter this potential for harm, often treatment studies will have an interim examination of the data with a predetermined cutoff point for study discontinuation. In studies in which this is the case, a third party should perform the interim analysis; the results should be kept confidential from the researchers and any personnel involved in the study. The only information that should be relayed is that the study may continue or needs to cease.

Studies that are stopped because of apparent harm in the treatment group are quite believable. Studies stopped because of benefit in the treatment group should be regarded with skepticism if the interim analysis was not planned prior to starting the study.

Some studies are halted because a *third-party* interim analysis shows an unexpectedly large benefit in the treatment group. The study is stopped because it would be unethical to deny the control group the effective treatment. This can be a very unfortunate circumstance if the study's treatment effect has not yet achieved statistical significance.

Summary

All of the above forms of analyses can increase the likelihood of chance causing illusory study effects; they also can provide useful and essential information. We must be diligent in our assessments in order to make sure they provide good evidence, without allowing random error to sully the results.

CHAPTER 9

INTEGRATIVE LITERATURE

Integrative literature combines individual studies to form new pieces of evidence; their analysis combines the assessment tools we have already discussed for primary literature as well as new assessment methods specific to the forms.

SYSTEMATIC REVIEWS AND META-ANALYSES

The traditional form of review article seen in medical journals is the narrative or non-systematic review. These narrative reviews are also referred to as review articles, journalistic reviews, or overviews. The scope of most narrative reviews is quite broad with variable reporting of search strategies. The conclusions of narrative reviews may or may not be based on the latest evidence, but only rarely are the conclusions explicitly linked to the evidence.[50] We have to take the author's search and selection of studies on faith, as they are generally neither exhaustive nor disclosed. A good deal of opinion also guides the conclusions in a narrative review. Even worse, there is often no clear delineation of the recommendations that are based on evidence and those based only on opinion. We will further discuss the uses of narrative reviews in a later section.

Systematic reviews (SRs), in contrast to the above, attempt to answer a small number of questions based purely on the best available evidence. The search for, and evaluation of, the literature is exhaustive and explicit. While the authors' opinions may still infiltrate the discussion section, in a well-done SR, the summary of evidence will be objective and evidence-based. Many practitioners of evidence-based medicine consider a systemic review to be the highest level of evidence, as it minimizes the bias and chance treatment outcomes that can plague an individual study.

McKibbon outlines five reasons to create a systematic review:[51]

- To find a "bottom line" on a complex issue
- To increase the precision of estimates of treatment effect and side-effects
- To increase the numbers of patients in clinically important subgroups
- To resolve discrepancies that may exist between individual trials
- To plan new studies to address gaps in knowledge.

To create a *systematic review*, the authors first conceive a tight, focused clinical question and decide upon the criteria they will use to select studies for inclusion in their review. They then search for all of the available literature and research on their topic, using multiple databases.

They then evaluate the results of this search in a clear, predefined manner. If possible, they can go a step further and generate quantitative statistical results. If a systematic review includes these numeric conclusions, then it is termed a meta-analysis (MA).

Validity of Systematic Reviews and Meta-analyses

In order to assess the internal validity of a systematic review or meta-analysis, we ask the following questions.

What Question Will the SR Attempt to Answer?

A focused clinical question is the springboard for any systematic review. We discuss the way to formulate a question using the PICO format in Part III.* Using this method to formulate a clinical question allows the creation of a tight, usable query. This same PICO format will lead to a well-defined and answerable question for an SR. Broad questions lead to a greater amount of available evidence, but the resulting SR is rarely applicable to an individual patient.

Were There Clear Inclusion and Exclusion Criteria for the Literature?

Before performing the search for literature, the authors of a systematic review should create inclusion and exclusion criteria for which studies they will allow into the systematic review. These criteria should be clearly stated in the publication of the systematic review. Prospective creation of these criteria limits potential bias during the literature search.

---

*The PICO format divides a clinical question into the requisite components of Patients, Intervention, Comparison intervention, and Outcome measures. For more on this technique, see Part III.

Was There a Well-conducted Search of the Literature?

The acquisition of all available literature is the *sine qua non* of a systematic review. If an unstructured, inadequate search is used, then the results of the SR are biased.

The search strategy should be clearly outlined, so that readers of the SR can reproduce an identical search. A well-performed SR will include an extensive search of the following sources:

- MEDLINE, EMBASE*, and other large electronic databases
- Databases of systematic reviews and trials, such as the Cochrane Library
- Hand search of the references of all articles found thus far
- Relevant specialized databases, such as *Emergency Medical Abstracts* (see Part III)
  - Summaries of conference proceedings
  - Database registries of ongoing trials
  - Theses of researchers
  - Databases of pharmaceutical companies for unpublished trials
  - Consultations with experts in the field and authors of studies.

Unpublished data such as ongoing trials, theses, and conference proceedings are termed *gray literature*. The use of only published literature can lead to bias in a systematic review, because it may ignore conflicting evidence.

Inadequate Ascertainment of Evidence

When performing a systematic review, bias is introduced if there is not an adequate search for *all* of the available literature. Poor or cursory searches will result in systematic reviews based on less than complete evidence.

Publication and Positive Outcome Biases

Just because a study is performed does not necessarily mean it will be published in a journal. If studies are selectively published, a systematic review that searches only in the conventional literature will be biased. Positive studies are published far more frequently than negative studies.[52] An analysis of the emergency medicine literature revealed that negative results are also much less likely to be accepted to EM scientific assemblies and therefore will not appear in conference proceedings or published abstracts.[53,54]

---

*EMBASE is the European equivalent of MEDLINE. Articles will sometimes, but not always, be found in both databases.

The reasons for the lower rate of published studies with negative results are myriad. Editorial preference for impressive, positive results certainly plays a role. Study authors may also choose to shelve their work if they do not generate a positive result. This *file drawer bias* will affect a systematic review unless the researchers are specifically sought out and questioned by SR researchers.

A worrisome twist on the above is the practice of many authors to change the outcomes of their trial after completion to generate a positive result.

EXAMPLE

An author performs a trial on a medication to stop bleeding from peptic ulcer disease. Before the start of the trial, mortality is chosen as the primary outcome of the study. After the completion of the trial, the author finds that there is no change on mortality from the use of the medication; the trial is *negative*. However, the author finds, post hoc, that patients in the treatment group received fewer units of packed red blood cells. The author changes the *primary outcome* to number of units of blood and never mentions the fact that mortality was the original studied outcome. The trial is submitted and is published as a *positive* study.

While this form of manipulation can be used to deliberately mislead, sometimes it occurs simply due to the desire to publish positive results; what we do know is that it occurs frequently.[55] Obviously, this form of false reporting can add to publication bias in a systematic review.

Negative studies may be printed, but in less prominent journals. These journals may elude standard search strategies, as they are not indexed in the databases mentioned above. An inferior literature search may therefore skew the results of a systemic review.

Tower of Babel

Publications written only in foreign languages can also contribute to inadequate ascertainment of evidence. Frequently, positive studies, performed in non-English speaking countries, will be published in English in American or European journals. Negative studies may be only published in the native language, in the journals of the country of origin. If the SR researchers do not get these works translated, the SR may be biased. This source of error has been proven to influence the results of systematic reviews and meta-analyses. A well-performed search will attempt to avoid this potential error.[56]

Assurance of an Adequate Search

There are statistical methods to analyze a systemic review for the presence of publication and positive-outcome bias.[57,58] One such method, the funnel plot, utilizes a graphical representation to screen for publication bias (Fig. 9-1).[57]

Were the Inclusion/Exclusion Criteria Applied Appropriately to the Results of the Literature Search?

Once all of the studies have been located, the inclusion and exclusion criteria can be applied to the discovered literature. To avoid bias, more than one researcher should perform the weeding out of articles independently. At this point, the authors can decide if there is sufficient high-quality evidence to continue with the systematic review.

Were the Studies Critically Appraised?

Just as bias can invalidate the results of an individual study, it can poison a systematic review through the inclusion of biased trials. We discussed how to evaluate the validity of primary literature in the previous sections.

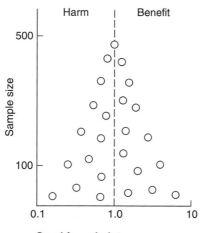

Good funnel plot:
plot should look like an upside down funnel

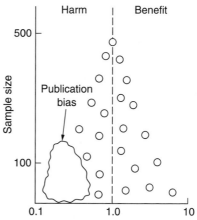

Possible publication bias:
smallest negative studies show largest effect; missing one side of the funnel. The studies that would fill out the funnel may have been performed, but not published or discovered.

— FIGURE 9-1 — *Funnel plots. The second plot indicates publication bias.*

Each individual trial needs to be evaluated using these criteria to determine its validity. In an attempt to decrease subjectivity, often trials are graded with quality scores. These scores assign points based on components of internal validity.

Quality Assessment

Each study must be examined to determine whether it was systematically free of bias, i.e. whether its results were believable. One means of performing this assessment is through the use of quality scoring. However, the main purpose of quality assessment in a systematic review is to allow the investigators and the readers to evaluate the effect of study quality on the observed results. This evaluation does not require the use of a scoring system.

Quality Scoring

These scoring systems can be used to determine inclusion, but often they are used to assign levels of evidence to each study. An example of a scoring system is the Jadad score,[59] which is used for evaluating randomized trials (Fig. 9-2).

There are many detractors to the use of these quality-scoring systems to assess study quality.[60,61] The argument against them is that neither the scoring systems (like Jadad), nor the criteria that go into them, have been shown to have a consistent impact upon the results of trials.[62]

The Cochrane collaboration is in the process of developing specific quality-assessment methods for each treatment subject area. These content-specific scoring methods may be a more powerful means to study quality assessment. Irrespective of what approach to quality assessment is used, the important thing is that a quality assessment is done. This allows the authors and readers to determine whether studies of different apparent quality observed different results.

The means of assessing each study included in a systematic review can change its conclusions.[63] Often, the complex methodology of an SR makes analyzing these study assessment methods difficult for the reader.

Garbage In, Garbage Out

The quality of a systematic review hinges directly on the quality of the literature on which it is based. Even highly skilled reviewers using pristine methodology cannot produce a useful systematic review from invalid articles. Unfortunately, this does not stop some authors from trying; hence, they create a review marred by poor literature support. This is why quality assessment of the studies is so vitally important.

The Jadad Score

This is not the same as being asked to review a paper. It should not take more than 10 minutes to score a report and there are no right or wrong answers.

Please read the article and try to answer the following questions (see attached instructions):
1. Was the study described as randomized (this includes the use of words such as randomly, random, and randomization)?
2. Was the study described as double blind?
3. Was there a description of withdrawals and dropouts?

Blind Assessment of the Quality of Trial Reports

Scoring the items:
Either give a score of 1 point for each "yes" or 0 points for each "no".
There are no in-between marks.

Give 1 additional point if:
For question 1, the method to generate the sequence of randomization was described and it was appropriate (table of random numbers, computer generated, etc.)

and/or:

If for question 2 the method of double blinding was described and it was appropriate (identical placebo, active placebo, dummy, etc.)

Deduct 1 point if:
For question 1, the method to generate the sequence of randomization was described and it was inappropriate (patients were allocated alternately, or according to date of birth, hospital number, etc.)

and/or

For question 2, the study was described as double blind but the method of blinding was inappropriate (e.g., comparison of tablet vs. injection with no double dummy)

— FIGURE 9-2 —   *The Jadad score.*[59]

Multiple Reviewers

At least two separate reviewers should appraise each of the articles. Their analysis of the quality and results of the included literature can be compared for agreement. Data extraction can be tedious, so it is subject to bias and error.[64] Having more than one reviewer analyze each article minimizes the possibility of error.

▓ Analysis

The analysis of a systematic review diverges into two types: *qualitative systematic reviews* and *meta-analyses*. If the researchers want to pool the results quantitatively, the result will be a meta-analysis. If, instead of a numeric outcome, the authors wish to derive answers to questions, we call the result a qualitative systematic review. The methodology is otherwise the same for both subtypes of systematic review.

Qualitative Systematic Reviews

When quantitative results are not desirable or feasible, an overall description of the combination of the studies is presented. The results of the trials should not contradict each other. If they do, then the researchers should attempt to explain this phenomenon. If certain studies did not obtain statistical significance, their trends should be consistent with the remainder of the trials.

EXAMPLE

In an SR performed on a pain medication, the qualitative results could be reported as: "Twelve trials of Thikskin™ were evaluated. Ten showed a clear reduction in visual analog pain scores. Two trials showed no benefit, but these trials used less than the conventional dosing regimen of the medication. One study showed much higher rates of the adverse events of nausea and vomiting; it is pertinent that this trial was performed exclusively on postoperative patients."

Discussion Sections

The job of qualitative systematic reviewers as investigators is completed when they report the results of the included studies. As with other research reports, SRs characteristically include a discussion section. We must be aware that discussion sections in systematic reviews are as subject to bias and spin as are the comparable sections in other types of studies. In all cases, you the reader must learn to take responsibility, on behalf of your patients, for drawing and implementing your own independent conclusions from even high-quality evidence.

Meta-analyses

The first thing to understand about meta-analysis is that all of the criteria we have just summarized must have been fulfilled for the meta-analysis to be valid. If a meta-analysis falls short, it is likely due to poorly defined criteria for study inclusion and/or an inadequate search, rather than due to inadequacies of statistical approach we are about to discuss.

The first step in a meta-analysis is to determine the degree of difference between the results of the included studies.

Heterogeneity of Studies

Heterogeneity is a measure of the variability of effect size between the trials included in the meta-analysis.[65] The *scatter* or *Forrest plot* included in most meta-analyses provides a crude representation of heterogeneity (Fig. 9-3).

Another graphical representation of heterogeneity and the contribution of each study to the meta-analysis is the L'Abbe plot (Fig. 9-4).

If any degree of heterogeneity is found, a search for an explanation can be elucidative. The causes for the observed variability can be different patient populations, different clinical settings, different assessment methods, dosages, etc. If heterogeneity is too great, either the studies may need to be pooled separately or the authors may decide to report only qualitative conclusions.

Analysis

The statistical machinations of meta-analysis can be even more complicated than those used for individual trials. They are far beyond the scope of this text; we refer readers to some of the recommended texts at the end of the book.

The essence of this portion of the meta-analysis is an analysis of the studies' data, adjusting for differences between studies and weighting based on study size. This *aggregate method* combines the conclusions of each study into a new combined effect parameter.

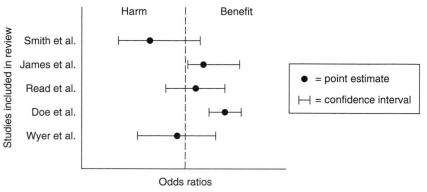

— FIGURE 9-3 — *Scatter plot.*

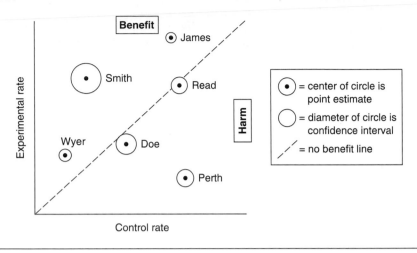

— FIGURE 9-4 —   *L'Abbe plot.*

Subgroup Analysis

Meta-analyses often include subgroup analysis of different patient groups. This is appropriate, as one of the advantages of meta-analyses is their ability to test the validity and significance of subgroup effects by considering and combining studies.

External Validity

Meta-analyses test the hypothesis of a constancy of effect. They have the ability to broaden the generalizability of a treatment or diagnostic method. This is why they are a legitimate form of research, and why they are so important. If there is a low enough degree of heterogeneity, then the risks and benefits represented are valid for a far greater number of patients than an individual study. The external validity of a meta-analysis is therefore greater than the individual studies it contains.

Reporting

The reporting method for the results of meta-analyses has been standardized in the QUOROM statement.[66] Similar to the CONSORT statement mentioned in the section on evaluation of treatment studies, the QUOROM statement gives a standardized template for the performance and publication of a meta-analysis.

Results

Meta-analyses of treatment will usually report treatment studies in *odds ratios* and *number needed to treat* (NNT). Diagnostic meta-analyses will provide *sensitivities/specificities* or *likelihood ratios*. These values can be utilized in the schema for diagnostic or treatment decisions described in Part I.

Summary

The systematic review and meta-analysis sit on the very top of the hierarchy of evidence. These literature types deserve their pedestal, but when poorly done they have vast potential to bias the decisions of clinicians. For an entertaining but frightening illustration of the dangers of meta-analyses, the reader is advised to examine the effects of rolling colored dice on stroke outcomes.[67]

LLSA AND NON-SYSTEMATIC REVIEWS

This section deals with *non-systematic* reviews. It is particularly pertinent in light of the recent changes in emergency medicine recertification.

In 2003, the paradigm of recertification shifted from intermittent testing to Emergency Medicine Continuous Certification (EMCC). The American Board of Emergency Medicine (ABEM) designed a program to allow continuous learning and testing throughout the course of an emergency physician's career. One component of this process is the Lifelong Learning and Self Assessment (LLSA) program.

LLSA

Each year, ABEM will choose 20 articles; the lists of articles for 2004 and 2005 are on ABEM's website.[68] All currently certified emergency physicians are required to read, analyze, and take an online test based on these 20 articles.

An excerpt from ABEM's website describes the purpose of the LLSA: "The primary goal of LLSA is to promote continuous learning by diplomates. ABEM facilitates this learning by identifying an annual set of LLSA readings to guide diplomates in self-study of recent EM literature. The readings are designed as study tools and should be read critically. They are not intended to be all-inclusive and are not meant to define the standard of care for the clinical practice of EM."[68]

Standard of Care

While the above description specifically states that the LLSA articles are not meant to define a standard of care, every emergency physician in the country is expected to read these articles. The conclusions and viewpoints in the articles have the imprimatur of our certifying organization. Since we will be tested on the information and recommendations of these studies, we cannot help but assume that ABEM believes they are representative of the way we should practice.

If we examine the articles chosen for 2005, we can classify the studies by literature type:

Prospective trial	Clinical prediction rule	Narrative review	Textbook chapter
┼┼┼┼	I	┼┼┼┼ ┼┼┼┼ II	II

We can thus see that narrative reviews and textbook chapters together make up the majority of the articles chosen for 2005. As we have mentioned in the section on systematic reviews, these non-systematic reviews present many obstacles to critical analysis.

Link to Page 207

Non-systematic Reviews

These reviews are excellent sources of answers to background questions. They can fill in the gaps in our knowledge base and provide the "whys" for our actions. They are less than ideal for providing the evidence to answer clinical foreground questions. There are various synonyms for narrative reviews (Fig. 9-5).

What Information Can Non-systematic Reviews Provide?

Non-systematic reviews can explain the underlying pathophysiology of a disease, the underpinnings of a treatment, and the recommendations of the author. This type of information does not merely satisfy our intellectual curiosity, but can help us make decisions. By building our illness scripts and treatment pathways, it can make our diagnostic and treatment choices more intuitive and therefore less prone to error.

Non-systematic reviews should *not* be used to answer specific questions that relate to the foreground of our practice unless they independently fulfill the criteria we previously summarized for evaluating systematic reviews.

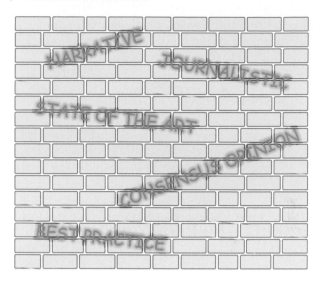

— FIGURE 9-5 — *Synonyms for non-systematic reviews.*

If they do not fulfill these criteria, they are not ideal to decide which medication to use or how well a test performs. When non-systematic reviews do not fulfill these criteria, they may still be useful stepping-stones to direct evidence on a question, if we understand that such evidence may itself be incomplete.

Surrogate Expert Opinion

In many clinical situations, the quality of available evidence falls short of that we would be inclined to trust as the basis of clinical decisions. At other times, we are just too busy to search for the best-available evidence during our shift. Ideally, we can rely on our consultants to provide evidence, but in some situations they may only offer opinions.

Non-systematic reviews invariably reflect the opinions of experts in the clinical area. The opinions expressed in a non-systematic review may be of superior quality to the opinions of consultants. What we must keep in mind is that this level of *evidence* is very different from the objective, verified evidence we have discussed previously.

Fodder for Illness and Treatment Scripts

While we may build the scripts we use to make rapid diagnostic and treatment decisions solely through our own clinical experience, non-systematic reviews also can provide a source to fill these mental databases.

By filling in the gaps of our understanding, non-systematic reviews give us a broader ability to make connections and insights during patient encounters.

A Quick Reference for Finding Primary Evidence

Frequently, non-systematic reviews constitute a source of citations to relevant primary research. We can take advantage of this, with the understanding that the references may reflect a biased and incomplete selection of published research on the question.

Mixed-type Reviews

Many reviews are now including trappings of systematic reviews, such as search strategies or tables of evidence. While these are nice additions, they do make the task of discerning which category a review article falls into more difficult.

One advantage of their presence is that, should an otherwise unstructured review fulfill *all of the criteria* we have outlined for a well-performed systematic review for one or two questions, it can be considered a source of definitive evidence for these questions.[69]

The JAMA Rational Clinical Exam series is an example of a mixed review type.[70] A meta-analysis is framed by a narrative type review that summarizes background information.

Shortcut Reviews

A new form of review found in the emergency medicine literature is the *shortcut review*. This evaluates the best evidence on an extremely focused clinical question. Conceptually, this is similar to a systematic review (SR); the difference is that a systematic review searches for all of the available literature ever written on a subject, while the shortcut review seeks out systematic reviews. If systematic reviews are not available, then carefully screened, well-done trials may be reviewed. The shortcut review attempts to answer a clinical question in the same manner informed emergency physicians might if they had the time and resources.

Examples of shortcut reviews in the emergency medicine literature include the Evidence-based Emergency Medicine (EBEM) section of the *Annals of Emergency Medicine*, as well as the Best Evidence Topic Reports (BETs) section of the *Emergency Medicine Journal*.[71]

A well-performed shortcut review will follow the precepts of a systematic review in spirit, though not in extent. Since shortcut reviews attempt to answer foreground questions, we must evaluate them far more carefully than a narrative review that provides background information.

Wyer described the questions that must be answered to trust a shortcut review.[72] We can ask these same questions about portions of narrative reviews, which are performed systematically:

- **Was there a well-formed clinical question?** The PICO format should be used to create a question for a shortcut review. Beyond formatting, the focus of the question should be narrow. These reviews are ideally suited to asking a question that comes up during a clinical shift, such as "Do antacids help in discriminating acute coronary syndromes from other non-emergent causes of chest pain?"[73] They are ill suited to questions in the vein of "What is the best treatment for hypertensive urgencies?"

- **Was there an explicit search methodology?** By their very nature, shortcut reviews will have inherent publication bias, since the less exhaustive search is limited to published systematic reviews or well executed trials. The inclusion and exclusion criteria for the trials of the shortcut review should be spelled out in the publication. The search strategy should also be described.

- **What was the quality of the included studies?** The authors of the shortcut review should assess the methodology of any trial that fulfills their predefined search strategy. Ideally, a systematic review or a large trial will be included. The authors should assess each study with the same rigor we discussed in the preceding sections.

- **What do we think of the included studies?** One of the true pleasures of a shortcut review is that it usually consists of a only a small number of articles, deemed to be the best evidence by trained reviewers. We can obtain and read these articles and see if we come to the same conclusions as the shortcut review authors.

CLINICAL PRACTICE GUIDELINES

Systematic reviews emerge only when there is sufficient evidence to be analyzed. If, instead, authors wish to describe the ideal care of a medical condition, they may choose to create a clinical practice guideline (CPG). Clinical practice guidelines make specific recommendations about a topic based on available evidence. When evidence is not available, *expert opinions* are often used. The fundamental difference between systematic reviews (SRs) and clinical practice guidelines is that, whereas SRs seek to identify and summarize the *best available evidence* on the questions they consider, CPGs seek to go beyond this by providing valid and

TABLE 9-1 COMPARISON OF SYSTEMATIC REVIEWS AND CLINICAL PRACTICE GUIDELINES

	SYSTEMATIC REVIEWS	CLINICAL PRACTICE GUIDELINES
Stem from...	Clinical uncertainty	Desire to improve patient care
Utilize...	Only the best evidence	Evidence and expert opinion
Yield...	Conclusions	Recommendations

convincing *healthcare recommendations* based not only upon the evidence, but also upon a consideration of patient values and the circumstances of care (Table 9-1).

The Institute of Medicine's definition of clinical practice guidelines is: systematically developed statements to assist practitioner and patient decisions about appropriate healthcare for specific clinical circumstances.[74]

Advantages of CPGs

- CPGs address care in situations with wide practice variation, where evidence exists for a better path.
- They attempt to intervene in clinical areas with substandard outcomes.
- They make literature more accessible to practitioners

Disadvantages of CPGs

- CPGs have the potential to limit physician autonomy and practice variation.
- They may not take into account the subjective views of the individual patient.
- They are difficult to implement.
- The are often considered a medico-legal standard of care, even if they are based on suboptimal evidence.
- It is difficult to resolve best care when multiple conflicting CPGs are published.

General Assessment of a CPG

The assessment of clinical practice guidelines can be broken into three parts. First, we ask general questions about the workings of the CPG. At this point, if we find the guideline to be flawed, we need not read any further. If it is acceptable, then we can assess the evidentiary and recommendations section for proper methodology.

Which Group Has Created the Guideline and From What Perspective?

Though occasionally created by individuals, most CPGs are created by groups or organizations. We certainly would have different feelings about a guideline created by the American College of Emergency Physicians (ACEP) compared to one created by a pharmaceutical company. We should always consider the motives and perspectives of the creating organization when analyzing a guideline.

Who Funded the Guideline?

Parties with a financial interest in the results often fund the development of a guideline. While this funding is frequently provided in the form of an *unrestricted educational grant*, it still creates conscious or unconscious *pecuniary bias*. A CPG created by a group funded entirely by sources without the potential for economic gain are more trustworthy.

Are the Guideline Authors Experts in the Subject Matter?

Guidelines written by acknowledged experts in the field automatically gain some degree of credence. This is not to say that guidelines should be ignored if we do not have immediate recognition of the authors.

Is there a Clearly Stated Target Patient Population?

In order for us to use guidelines in our clinical practice, we need to have clearly defined groups to which they are applicable. A guideline for pediatric emergency patients is probably not applicable to geriatric emergency patients.

Is the Guideline Usable in Our Practice Setting?

If a guideline is recommending tests or procedures, which we do not have available at our hospital, then it is of very little use in the care of our patients.

Is there an Expiration Date?

Authors should base guidelines on the best evidence available *at the time they are written*. Given the rapidly changing state of knowledge in medicine, there should be statement of when the data will be reassessed and any changes published. Sackett compares guidelines to cartons of milk: we need a clear date after which the product is no longer fresh.[1]

Were Interested Parties Allowed Input?

A more robust set of recommendations can be created if input from outside clinicians is solicited and utilized. A guideline vetted by acknowledged experts is stronger for their recommendations.

Was there Peer Review Prior to Publication?

This allows assessment by practitioners in a number of different practice settings. In addition, the guideline can be disseminated to the major emergency medicine organizations for commentary. If the subject of a guideline embraces other specialties of medicine, they should be involved as well.

Has the Impact of the Guideline Been Assessed?

The ultimate question for any guideline is: "Does it make a difference in patient care?" If a trial comparing the CPG recommendations to standard care has shown that the use of the guideline results in patient-oriented beneficial outcomes, then we can regard it as high-level evidence.

If the guideline passes the screening of the above criteria, we can divide further analysis into two parts: the summary of the evidence and the recommendations section.

Evidentiary Section

The evidentiary section of a clinical practice guideline is essentially a systematic review. We have discussed how to analyze this literature type in the previous section, but some of the key points are reconsidered here.

Just as with systematic reviews/meta-analyses, the performance of the evidentiary section of a CPG requires knowledge of research methodology and epidemiology beyond the level of the average clinician. While a non-research trained clinician naturally shies away from the creation of systematic reviews, the evidentiary section of a CPG may seem more approachable. However, this portion of the CPG should be held to the same rigor as a systematic review. Therefore, clinicians without this expertise should not perform this portion of a CPG alone.

Sackett advises that if asked to join the effort to produce a CPG, an emergency physician without advanced training in research methodology should stay clear of the evidentiary summary portion and utilize his or her skills in the recommendation section.[1] If *weekend warrior* physicians perform the search and classification of the evidence, they risk the creation of a flawed clinical practice guideline.

A poor search of the literature is the Achilles' heel of many CPGs (garbage in, garbage out). All available evidence should be sought, evaluated, and screened with clearly indicated inclusion and exclusion criteria.

Search for and Evaluation of the Evidence

Identification of the Target Questions Having Greatest Potential Impact on Outcome

Any search for evidence is only as strong as the clarity of the question that prompted it. If the authors of the CPG did not ask clear questions, it is unlikely that they will find strong answers.

Search Strategy

A structured search and selection of evidence should be performed for each target question. Authors should list the search methodology in the guideline so that we may evaluate for flawed ascertainment and publication bias. We have discussed these terms extensively in the systematic review section.

Link to Page 207

Classification of the Evidence

Each study included in the guideline should be assigned a class of evidence There are a large number of evidentiary classification systems. They almost uniformly follow the tenets of evidence-based medicine hierarchy discussed previously. The classification system utilized by the American College of Emergency Physicians is shown in Fig. 9-6.

Literature classification schema*

Design/ class	Therapy[†]	Diagnosis[‡]	Prognosis[§]
1	Randomized, controlled trial or meta-analyses of randomized trials	Prospective cohort using a criterion standard	Population prospective cohort
2	Nonrandomized trial	Retrospective observational	Retrospective cohort Case control
3	Case series Case report Other (e.g., consensus, review)	Case series Case report Other (e.g., consensus, review)	Case series Case report Other (e.g., consensus, review)

*Some designs (e.g. surveys) will not fit this schema and should be assessed individually.
[†]Objective is to measure therapeutic efficacy comparing ≥ 2 interventions.
[‡]Objective is to determine the sensitivity and specificity of diagnostic tests.
[§]Objective is to predict outcome including mortality and morbidity.

— FIGURE 9-6 — *The American College of Emergency Physicians' (ACEP) literature classification schema used in the organization's Clinical Policy Guidelines.*[119]

The importance of the classification of the studies used in the CPG is that the grade of each recommendation in the next section is directly dependent on the strength of the supporting literature.

Evidentiary Table

A citation of each study used in the guideline should be included with its evidentiary grade. Ideally, a table with a summary of the information each article provides is included as well. If journal space limitations do not allow the publication of such a table, a link to a companion website can be provided. This evidentiary table allows the reader to draw his or her own conclusions from the literature used for the guideline (Fig. 9-7).

Recommendations Section

In this section, the authors of the clinical guideline use the graded evidence to make specific recommendations. These recommendations should embrace possible variations in care, patient preference, and resources. We can evaluate this portion of the CPG by examining each recommendation.

Evidentiary Table

Article	Design	Patients	Outcome Measure	Findings	Limitations	Class of Evidence
Arienta, 1997	Retrospective	10,000 patients, 4 categories; α group: no LOC; β group: LOC/PTA, or vomiting, or subgleal hematoma	Deterioration	No patient in the group deteriorated; all 799 patients in the β group had skull radiographs performed; 73 (9%) had a fracture; 592 of 799 patients in the β group had CT scans performed; 21 (3.5%) results were positive; no patient with negative radiographic findings developed complications	Groups not well defined to allow for conclusions; follow-up not clearly defined	III
Ashkenazi, 1990	Case Series	6 patients; GCS score of 14-4; 2 patients had no LOC	Repeat CT scan showing epidural		All patients had a GCS score of <15	III/NA
Bell, 1971	Prospective Questionnaire	1,500 patients all ages/all types of injury	Fracture on radiograph	High-yield criteria were not sensitive for fracture	No CT correlation; no GCS	X

— FIGURE 9-7 — *An Excerpt of the Evidentiary Table from the ACEP Clinical Policy on Neuroimaging and Decisionmaking in Adult Mild Traumatic Brain Injury in the Acute Setting.*[119]

Level A recommendations. Generally accepted principles for patient management that reflect a high degree of clinical certainty (ie, based on "strength of evidence class I" or overwhelming evidence from "strength of evidence class II" studies that directly address all the issues).

Level B recommendations. Recommendations for patient management that may identify a particular strategy or range of management strategies that reflect moderate clinical certainty (ie, based on "strength of evidence class II" studies that directly address the issue, or strong consensus of "strength of evidence class III" studies).

Level C recommendations. Other strategies for patient management based on preliminary, inconclusive, or conflicting evidence, or, in the absence of any published literature, based on panel consensus.

— FIGURE 9-8 — *ACEP's Grading of Recommendations used in the organization's Clinical Policy Guidelines.*

Is Each Recommendation Properly Graded?

Every recommendation should be given a grade based on the evidence that supports it. If a recommendation is based solely on the opinion of the authors, this should clearly be indicated in the grading system.

Fig. 9-8 shows the grading system used by ACEP. The importance of this grading of evidence is that level C recommendations should be interpreted very differently from those at level A. The former are based on scant evidence or none at all, while the latter are based on solid evidence.

Is Each Recommendation Linked to its Supporting Literature?

When reading the guideline, we should know exactly which citations supported each recommendation. We can therefore evaluate for ourselves whether the evidence supports the recommendation.

Was there an Integration of Patient Values and Preferences?

There is no prototypical patient; if the guideline offers branch points to allow for the influence of patient values, then the applicability is infinitely higher. If patient values were not integrated in any way, the adoption of the guideline can cause dire consequences. The US Preventive Services Task Force uses a double grading system: one based solely on the evidence itself and the other for a the total recomendation incorporating patient-value considerations.

Reporting Format

Owing to the ubiquity and power of clinical practice guidelines, there has been a movement to standardize and improve the way in which they are conducted and reported. An international conference on clinical guideline formation yielded a number of recommendations on conducting this form of literature effectively.[75] The **GRADE** working group has also created consensus recommendations similar to the **CONSORT** initiative we discussed in the treatment section.[76,77]

Dissemination

One of the biggest problems with CPGs is that clinicians do not use them. Gallagher notes that the downfall of many CPGs is not the rigor of methodology, but instead poor dissemination and a lack of user-friendly design.[78] Even the most rigorous, meticulously designed guideline is useless unless emergency physicians receive and utilize them. Simply publishing the guideline or sending it by mass mailing has been shown to be ineffective.[78] What works best is small-group presentation of a new guideline, but this is often economically preposterous for large-scale dissemination. Computer-based decision aides incorporating the guideline probably have the most potential to alter care.

CLINICAL PREDICTION RULES

In the sections on diagnostic and prognostic decisions, we discussed the complex interplay between our history, exams, testing, and clinical impression, which culminates in a prediction or a decision. Clinical prediction rules (CPRs) attempt to standardize this process of decision-making into a validated, easily reproducible tool. They may augment making a diagnosis, the calculation of pre-test probability, and the determination of prognosis. Clinical prediction rules are alternatively referred to as "clinical decision rules." If designed to aid diagnosis, then we can call them "clinical diagnosis rules."

The following are examples of clinical prediction rules used in emergency medicine:

- Ottawa Ankle Rules (diagnosis)
- Ottawa Knee Rules (diagnosis)
- Canadian C-Spine Rule (diagnosis)

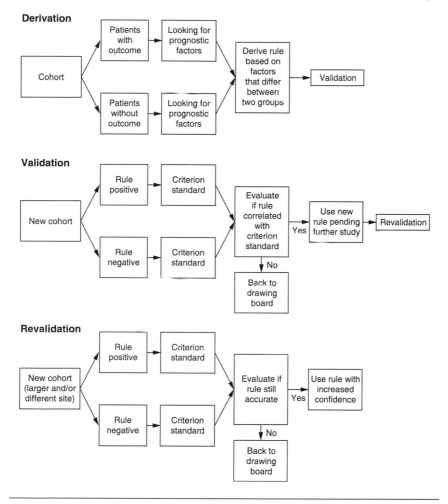

— FIGURE 9-9 — *The steps of the creation of a clinical prediction rule.*

- Nexus C-Spine Rule (diagnosis)
- PORT Pneumonia Score (prognosis)
- Well's Criteria for PE and DVT (risk stratification)

Clinical prediction rules are not established in a single study. It takes at least two and preferably more studies to assure that the rule is valid, impacts patient care, and is applicable to a wide range of practice settings (Fig. 9-9).

The first study used in the creation of a clinical prediction rule attempts to derive which variables predict a desired outcome.

The Derivation Study

The first step in the creation of a clinical prediction rule is to establish the outcome of interest. This outcome can be diagnostic (e.g., ankle fractures), prognostic (e.g., death from pneumonia), or the calculation of pre-test probability (e.g., risk stratification for pulmonary embolism).

Researchers postulate a wide array of variables from the history, clinical exam, and possibly from lab/imaging studies. A cohort of patients is then studied to see which ones have the outcome and which of the associated variables were present. The hope is that the authors will find a combination of these factors, which will accurately predict the outcome.

EXAMPLE

The Canadian C-spine Rule is a CPR that attempts to limit the number of cervical spine x-rays performed after trauma. The outcome studied was cervical spine injury. A long list of variables such as midline neck tenderness, ability to rotate neck, mechanism of trauma, etc. was assessed on each patient. They then either had radiographs or a follow-up protocol as their criterion standard for cervical spine injury.

After the completion of the derivation study, statistical analysis is performed on the variables to find the ones that are *independent predictors* of the outcome. There many different techniques used, but they are beyond the scope of this work; the reader is advised to examine the sources in the references section.[39,79] As this statistical analysis occurs post hoc, it can be thought of as a form of *data dredging*. This is entirely acceptable, because the authors of the derivation set should never advocate that this information is ready to be used in clinical practice. Only after the derived variables are prospectively validated do they have a place in our practice.

When evaluating a derivation study, we should assess the following points:[39]

- Were all relevant variables included?
- Were these variables present in the studied population in sufficient numbers?
- Was the number of patients adequate?
- Were the numbers of patients with the outcome sufficient?
- Was an adequate criterion standard used to determine the outcome?
- Were the assessors of the criterion standard blinded to the variables and vice versa?
- Does the rule make clinical sense in the setting of your practice?
- Is the rule easily remembered and applied?

It bears repeating one more time: it could be chance alone that caused the derived variables to appear to be sufficiently accurate. It can be extremely interesting to *hypothetically* apply the newly derived rule to see how it works with your standard care. This sort of "mini-validation" can test some of the external validity of the nascent rule. We should defer use of the rule to alter our care until after validation. We cannot emphasize this latter point enough; the use of a non-validated derivation set to make decisions (often spurred on by authors' spin) is a critical error.*

The Validation Study

The next phase of development for the CPR is validation in a second study. Ideally, the validation will be performed by clinicians in the course of their routine practice as opposed to being done by researchers. Validation should be performed on a different cohort of patients from the one used for the derivation. Though there are means of statistical legerdemain that allow for derivation and validation using just one set of patients, this method, sometimes called *split-sample validation*, is inherently less resistant to bias.[80]

Here are some questions to ask about a validation study:

- Did the patients chosen have a wide spectrum of disease?
- Was there a blinded assessment of the criterion standard?
- Was there 100% application of the criterion standard or follow-up?

External Validity: Revalidation

While a validated CPR is ready to be used by clinicians, an even more powerful proof of its accuracy is a third study to revalidate the rule. Revalidation is preferably performed at a different location and, perhaps, with a wider range of patients. It eliminates the potential for bias from the center the original validation was performed in, as well as assessing whether other clinicians will be able to apply the rule as effectively as the validating physicians. These latter reasons make revalidation especially helpful to ensure and broaden external validity.

Results

Impact Assessment

Many persuasive studies of new techniques for treatment and diagnosis do little to change patient outcome. If a CPR is evaluated for important

---

*It is important to recognize that the application of statistical techniques to test for random error and homogeneity within the original dataset do not themselves render it appropriate to use as a rule in clinical practice, even though authors frequently represent such analyses as a *validation* of the rule.

patient outcomes and proves to better, then the researchers have shown that their rule is not just accurate, but actually makes a difference.

EXAMPLE

The PORT score was a CPR developed to assess risk of mortality in patients with pneumonia.[81] To test the impact of this rule, we could do a prospective trial in which one group's decision to admit is based on standard care and the second is based on the PORT score. Using the outcome marker of 3-month mortality, we can see if the application of the PORT score has patient-oriented clinical utility.

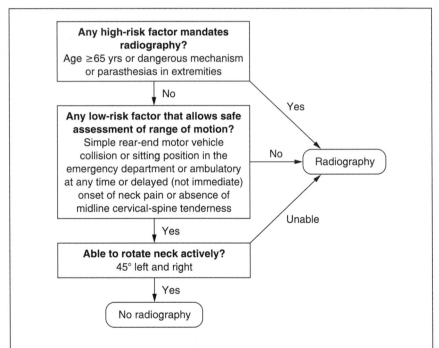

For patients with trauma who are alert (as indicated by a score of 15 on the Glasgow Coma Scale) and in stable condition and in whom cervical-spine injury is a concern, the determination of risk factors guides the use of cervical-spine radiography. A dangerous mechanism is considered to be a fall from an elevation 3 ft or 5 stairs; an axial load to the head (e.g., diving); a motor vehicle collision at high speed (>100 km/hr) or with rollover or ejection: a collision involving a motorized recreational vehicle; or a bicycle collision. A simple rear-end motor vehicle collision excludes being pushed into oncoming traffic, being hit by a bus or a large truck, a rollover, and being hit by a high-speed vehicle.

— FIGURE 9-10 —   *The Canadian C-spine rule.[7]*

Ease of Use

Even a meticulously designed CPR is fairly useless if it is too convoluted to be used clinically. Clinical prediction rules should be easily remembered or accompanied by a mnemonic device. Diagrams and flow charts also increase usability.

EXAMPLE

There are currently two CPRs used in emergency medicine to decrease the need for radiographs in patients with suspected cervical spine injuries. The NEXUS criteria are easily committed to memory:[6]

Cervical spine radiography is indicated for patients with trauma unless they meet all of the following criteria:

The Nexus Criteria[6]

Cervical Spine Radiography is indicated for patients with trauma unless they meet all of the following criteria:

- No posterior midline cervical-spine tenderness
- No painful, distracting injuries
- No focal neurologic deficit
- No evidence of intoxication

The Canadian C-Spine Rule is difficult to commit to memory, so a pocket card or wall chart is usually necessary to use this CPR (Fig. 9-10).[7]

MISCELLANEOUS STUDY TYPES

ECONOMIC ANALYSES

In earlier chapters we have outlined how to tell if a treatment or intervention actually benefits our patients. One factor we have not explored is whether the benefit is worth the cost; economic analyses broach this subject. For a number of reasons, this form of literature is difficult to assess. We include it here for the sake of completeness, but we offer the following only as an introduction. To avoid all of the pitfalls present in the evaluation of this literature type requires more extensive reading.[39,82]

There are a few "quick and dirty" criteria that can quickly be assessed to determine if an economic analysis has any validity.

Cost Calculations
Economic analyses would be simpler if all the authors had to calculate were out-of-pocket expenses. They would also be useless; cost must encompass far more than money spent for an intervention. Other factors must be taken into account, such as the benefit to a patient of getting out of the hospital earlier, additional quality of life, less tangible costs such as nursing and staff time, and projected future costs (e.g., the cost of increased antibiotic resistance from the use of a new drug). Many of these factors are not objective; the means by which they are assessed are subject to variability and possibly bias.

Underlying Literature
Ideally, the analysis should be based on the strongest available literature; in most cases this will be a meta-analysis or systematic review. If the underlying treatment studies are of poor quality, the economic analysis of these studies will also be flawed. This continues the concept of garbage in/garbage out that we discussed earlier.

Varying Perspectives

Any economic analysis must be viewed in the light of which group has performed or sponsored the study. A manufacturer of a new medication has a vested stake in showing that it is no more expensive than conventional therapy. It would be very unlikely that a chiropractor-authored economic analysis would reveal that manipulation for back pain is significantly more expensive than bed rest. In most cases, an analysis performed by authors with nothing to gain from the results is most trustworthy.

QUALITATIVE STUDIES

Qualitative studies provide information on things that cannot be reduced to numbers. The feelings, impressions, and desires of our patients provide the impetus for this form of research. Qualitative studies are usually easy to understand; the difficulty lies in assessing whether they represent the truth or merely the authors' opinions.

EXAMPLE

While patient satisfaction in the emergency department can be measured quantitatively using validated scales and rating systems, qualitative research may provide even more information.[83] Patients can be interviewed alone and in groups to gather information on problems and possible solutions encountered in the emergency department. Physicians and nurses can be asked for their perceptions on areas of patients' potential dissatisfaction. Families and friends of patients, who may have to wait for their loved ones, may also be approached for suggestions. A researcher may even place himself or herself into the role of a patient in order to experience first-hand the previously discovered complaints. This approach can provide the "whys" of patient satisfaction rather than merely quantifying its existence.

While typical studies demand a clearly defined research plan prior to gathering of data, qualitative studies often benefit from an ad-hoc plan which stems from immersion in the subject manner. This iterative approach allows the adaptation of the methodology as new information is gathered.[84] The danger of this approach is that the lack of firm structure can cause an erosion of strict research discipline.[85]

Critically appraising qualitative studies is made more difficult by the lack of a consistent methodology and the loose structure which governs this type of literature. Various sources have provided a starting point to evaluate qualitative research.[39,40] The following are some key points to evaluate.[39]

Study Population

While in quantitative studies we stressed the advantages of an entirely random selection of patients, in qualitative research we want to see just the opposite. The study population should be adapted as the researchers realize another valuable perspective can be provided by another group. An interview with a patient may lead to the realization that talking to the patient's family may be valuable as well. A large number of participants should be sampled to ensure that a broad representation of opinions is represented in the study.

Data Collection

Data for qualitative studies can stem from multiple sources. This form of research usually benefits from a multi-angular approach to better explore the many facets of an issue. Possible sources include:[40]

- **Documents:** recorded summaries of meetings or events.
- **Passive observation:** encounters in which the researcher is present, but separate from the events. This form of observation can also be obtained from video and audio recordings.
- **Participant or active observation:** encounters in which the researcher observes, but also takes a role in the events.
- **Interviews:** using discussion and questions with subjects to garner their thoughts and opinions.
- **Focus groups:** interviews with multiple subjects. Focus groups allow multiple inputs, but also add information from intra-group interaction.

Data Analysis

As the data are collected, researchers will have interim meetings to assure that the study is progressing appropriately. New approaches may be suggested and explored as the study progresses. Once the data collection is complete, the multiple sources must be synthesized into usable conclusions. These conclusions should be reached by multiple researchers, because if only a single author analyzes the data the danger is too great that opinion will etch the data.

Qualitative studies offer information that standard studies cannot provide. They are an essential counterpart to the research types we have discussed in earlier chapters.

CHAPTER 11

DELIBERATE MIS-REPRESENTATION

READING IS NOT BELIEVING

We have discussed the ways in which unintentional bias and imprecision can cause a study's results to diverge from the truth. Far more worrisome is when a piece of literature is designed to deliberately deceive its readers. The largest perpetrator of this practice is certainly the pharmaceutical industry, leading us to subtitle this section DRUG COMPANY "EVIL."

However, the pharmaceutical industry is not the sole culprit in the creation of deceptive evidence. Unfortunately, for reasons of academic advancement or other less tangible motives, even physicians with no industry relations may submit data that are misleading, or even false. We can divide deceptive literature into two categories: discoverables and undiscoverables.

Discoverables

Any of the biases and statistical manipulations we mentioned in earlier sections can be used to deliberately mislead. A careful appraisal of the literature will reveal these potential flaws, just as if they were unintentional. We can therefore refer to this form of misrepresentation as *discoverable*. If you have made it to this point in this text, you should have the tools necessary to find any discoverable deceptions when reading a study.

Undiscoverables

Fraud, direct lies, and hidden manipulations are much more difficult to detect simply by perusing a study. We refer to this class of misrepresentation as *undiscoverable*. Often it is only a significant period of time after publication that these forms of deception come to light. As you read this chapter, consider which types of deception may be identified by a careful and critical reader such as yourself.

Richard Smith, a former editor of the *British Medical Journal*, writes that one of the major problems in combating research misconduct is the lack of a clear definition. In one of his lectures on the subject, he presents a taxonomy of potential research wrongdoings (Table 11-1).[86]

Another way of conceptualizing this issue is to imagine you are a pharmaceutical company CEO (chief executive officer). If you temporarily abandon your moral restraint, how would you go about maximizing the sales of your product? When we think in this mode, we can quickly come up with many ways to deceive using the literature.

TABLE 11-1   TAXONOMY OF RESEARCH MISCONDUCT (from most to least serious)[86]

- Fabrication: invention of data or cases
- Falsification: wilful distortion of data
- Plagiarism: copying of ideas, data or words without attribution
- Failing to get consent from an ethics committee for research
- Not admitting that some data are missing
- Ignoring outliers without declaring it
- Not including data on side effects in a clinical trial
- Conducting research in humans without informed consent or without justifying why consent was not obtained from an ethics committee
- Publication of post hoc analyses without declaration that they were post hoc
- Gift authorship
- Not attributing other authors
- Redundant publication
- Not disclosing a conflict of interest
- Not attempting to publish completed research
- Failure to do an adequate search of existing research before beginning new research

DECEPTIVE AUTHORSHIP

When reading a journal, determining who actually wrote a study would seem an easy question to answer. Unfortunately, an examination of the authors listed at the top of the article may not reveal the whole truth. Authors' names may appear on the top of journal articles despite no actual contribution to the study. Conversely, the name of a true author may never appear on any part of the study.[87]

Ghost Authors

In recent years, a new industry has sprung up: medical writing agencies. These for-profit companies are hired by pharmaceutical and medical manufacturing companies to write journal articles and conduct studies of new drugs and products. A study authored by one of these agencies would not generate as much respect or regard as one written by a well-known physician expert in the field. These physician experts are known as *key opinion leaders* (KOLs).[88] If the pharmaceutical company offers KOLs a substantial honorarium, they might be convinced to submit the study as if they had designed and written it.

This chicanery is even more convincing if no connection to the medical writing agency remained attached to the journal article. The original study designers and article authors become *ghost authors*, with no mention of their contributions remaining.

Discovering whether the listed authors are the true authors of a study can be extremely difficult. Susanna Rees, a former employee of a medical writing agency, discusses the lengths that editors go to in order to eliminate any trace of the original authorship of these for-fee studies.[89] Alteration of word processor document properties to list the false author and exporting the file through numerous different computer programs to eliminate electronic traces were among the methods used. Identifying ghost authors can be nearly impossible after these machinations.

Honorary Authorship

In academia, often authorship will be given to physicians with no involvement in the actual research or writing of a study. This might occur because the honorary author has a high academic rank or greater standing in the field. The perception is that the addition of the guest author will improve the possibility of acceptance or the perceived value of a study. The granting of honorary authorship may be pressured; a higher ranking academic may demand authorship on any studies performed in his or her department.

These *gift authorships* are particularly dangerous when the non-contributing authors have not actually seen the study. Their names are now at the top of a piece of work which may be invalid or even fraudulent. The careers of eminent academicians have ended in just this manner.[90]

Undeclared Conflicts of Interest

It stands to reason that researchers being paid by the industry may be biased by their financial interests. We view with a certain justified skepticism studies authored by physicians with a financial conflict of interest. One way to avoid their works being viewed with a jaundiced eye is to never reveal these *conflicts of interest*. Many journals do not even ask authors to reveal potential conflicts of interest; the ones that do often have no means of enforcing their policy.[91]

These undeclared conflicts of interest become even more frightening when we learn how many of our scientists in the National Institutes for Health are supported by pharmaceutical companies.[92] Governmental physicians are expected to supply unbiased opinions for the good of the nation's health. Recommendations presented as "public policy" cannot be trusted when offered by doctors who have strong active connections to the pharmaceutical industry.

Possible Solutions

Obviously, the ideal solution would be a way to know exactly what each author contributed to a published study. Several journals now require authors to state their involvement as part of a study submission. The International Committee of Medical Journal Editors (ICMJE) has written guidelines for attributing authorship.[93] Their recommendations state that all three of the following criteria must be met for individuals to qualify for authorship:

- Substantial contribution to the conception and design of a study; or acquisition of data; or interpretation of data
- Drafting the study manuscript or critically revising it for important intellectual content
- Giving final approval of the version to be published.

Conflicts of interest must also be revealed. The Committee of Publication Ethics (COPE) guidelines demand the declaration of all relevant conflicts of interest for any published medical work.[94] Journal editors must attempt to enforce this policy, guaranteeing that the studies we read are trustworthy.

DECEPTIVE STUDY DESIGN

When we imagine the conception of a study for a new treatment, we hope that the researchers sit around a table and create methods that will minimize bias, lead to precision, and represent the truth. If instead, the study designers brainstorm the most effective way to prove what they wish, truth-be-damned, then many tactics are available to them.

Placebo Comparisons
A drug with even a modicum of efficacy should appear to be superior to a placebo in a study. However, even if the new treatment has only marginal benefit, or has no effectiveness at all, using the machinations below, a trial may be manipulated to make it appear useful.

Exclusion of Placebo Responders
We discussed the placebo effect in a previous section. Many participants in a study may improve simply because of the attention shown to them by a physician or caregiver. Pharmaceutical companies are now funding research to identify and eliminate these placebo responders from trials before their entry.[95] Techniques currently being explored include brain scans and DNA analysis. Drug researchers claim that screening for placebo responders will allow for smaller, less expensive trials. Of course, if the placebo responders were selectively eliminated only from the placebo group, the benefits to a dubious drug are obvious.

Equivalence Trials
Manufacturers of relatively useless drugs are petrified of a head-to-head trial with the standard, effective, cheap, existing therapy.[96] Ethics will sometimes preclude the use of a placebo, thereby forcing the hands of pharmaceutical manufacturers. When placed in this situation, the key is to maximize the potential of the new drug, while minimizing the effects of the standard therapy.

Straw-man Comparisons
False comparators are one of the primary reasons why industry-sponsored studies are almost uniformly positive.[97,98] Comparing a new treatment to an inferior regimen of an existing treatment is equivalent to setting up a *man of straw*, destroying him, and then claiming victory against a real, flesh-and-blood opponent (Fig. 11-1).[26] If *subtherapeutic* doses of effective medications are used as the comparison, the pharmaceutical company can claim their new drug is "just as good as standard therapy."

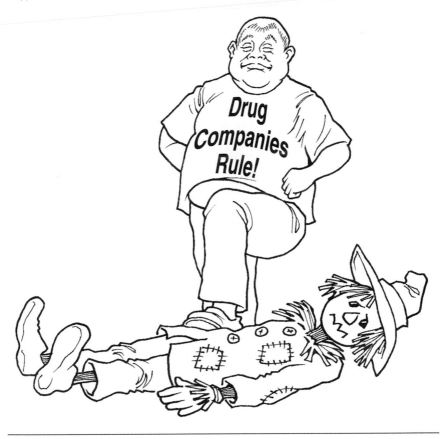

— FIGURE 11-1 —   *A victory over a straw man.*

EXAMPLE

A pharmaceutical company funds a study to establish the efficacy of their new COX-2 inhibitor. The COX-2 inhibitor, used at its maximally potent dose, is compared to ibuprofen in a randomized trial. However, the dose of ibuprofen used is 200 mg, far less than the 400–800 mg used by most emergency physicians. The COX-2 inhibitor and the ibuprofen groups have statistical equivalent reductions in the patients' visual analog scale representation of pain. The pharmaceutical company publishes in all of its advertisements for their new medication, "As efficacious as ibuprofen." The results may have been different if an adequate dose of ibuprofen was used rather than the straw-man amount.

At the same time a trivial dose of the standard therapy is tested, the new drug can be dosed at higher than recommended levels. Any additional side-effects from this supra-maximal dosing are handled by not assessing for them or not publishing the data if they are assessed.

Shifty Endpoints

As clinicians, we yearn for study endpoints that provide patient-oriented evidence. This type of evidence is the most useful and the hardest to obtain by deceptive means. As a result, many industry-sponsored studies avoid or de-emphasize the importance of such study endpoints in favor of the following.

Disease-oriented Endpoints

It is much easier to manipulate disease-oriented endpoints. Demonstrating a decrease in heart rate of two to four beats per minute can easily allow the claim that "our new drug is effective in controlling tachycardia." Proving that a new drug decreases mortality from myocardial infarction is much more difficult and therefore may be avoided by pharmaceutical manufacturers.

Surrogate Endpoints

The dodgy researchers frequently go even further and propose a direct connection between disease-oriented to patient-oriented outcomes. In this case the disease-oriented outcome is a "surrogate" for the patient-oriented outcome. Drug sponsors may promote their product on the basis of erroneous surrogates. For example, if a new drug is able to decrease heart rate (by even an inconsequential amount), the sponsors may make the logical leap that since beta-blockers reduce heart rate and beta-blockers decrease mortality in myocardial infarction, then their new drug also accomplishes both things.

Composite Endpoints

Composite endpoints also allow the extension of unimportant endpoints to apparently important ones. If the study authors make a combined endpoint of decrease in heart rate, reinfarction within 30 days, and all-cause mortality, then their new drug, which merely reduces heart rate, will seem far more vital.

Dubious Outcome Measures

Instead of validated scales, homegrown measures can be used to assess outcomes. For instance, a pain scale can be created that virtually guarantees equivalence with standard therapy. Validated scales and outcome measures are much more difficult to manipulate.

Unblinded Patient Assignment and Outcome Assessment

By unblinding patient assignment and outcome assessment, we allow bias to enter into the study. If physicians are being funded or paid by a pharmaceutical company, this bias will naturally lead to a more favorable assessment of the study drug.

Stacking the IRBs

The failsafe to all of the above deception is that an Institutional Review Board (IRB) must approve every study performed on patients. The IRB reviews the study design for validity and assurances that any participants are treated fairly and ethically. This of course assumes that members of the IRB are unbiased and free of conflicting interests. Unfortunately, statistics would lead us to believe that a substantial percentage of IRBs are not as unbiased as we would hope.[99]

DECEPTIVE DATA

There is no reason to stop at merely creating a study design that predisposes towards the desired results; the actual study data can be manipulated as well.

Falsification or Fabrication of Data

The easiest way to make a study say what you want is simply to make up the data. *Falsification* refers to the alteration of true data and *fabrication* is the creation of false data *de novo*. Both are devastating to the ethics of research and, what is worse, they are very difficult to detect. A study full of false data can still appear perfectly valid. There have been numerous episodes of fabricated and falsified data in the history of medical research.[100,101]

Interim analysis

We have discussed the necessity of researchers being blinded to any interim results, because of the bias that may result. Of course, if they are seeking to create deceptive results, such rules no longer apply. In a planned 6-month trial of a new medication, if the desired results occur at the 4-month mark, further study only has the potential to muck things up. Simply stopping the trial at this point by creating an explanation or never publishing the original 6-month planned duration, allows the publication of a positive trial. Conversely, if at the 6-month point the results they want are almost but not quite there, then there is no reason not to extend the trial for another few weeks until more data accumulate.

Slicing and Dicing the Dataset

If, at the end of a one-year trial, a drug is shown to be clearly inferior to the standard treatment, some might call this a negative trial. However, if the first 6-months' data show the new drug to be superior, then the solution is simple. The first 6-months' data can be published as if the second 6 months never existed. Authors can pretend that is all they planned to analyze in the first place. Some very well-known drugs published major trials using just this method.[102]

Outliers

Another deceptive means of cutting up the dataset is reflected in the way study authors deal with isolated data points, which differ from the trend. The proper method is to include all of the data, even if they do not fit neatly into the graph or calculations. The deceptive method is simply to strip out outliers; this *tidying-up* will certainly bias the study results, but that is the whole point.[103]

DECEPTIVE ANALYSIS AND REPORTING

How the information obtained from a study is analyzed and reported also offers much room for misleading the readership.

Post-hoc Secondary Endpoints

If the primary endpoint did not generate the desired results, then authors can simply choose another endpoint. If they can find one that is beneficial to their product, then they can emphasize it and downplay the primary endpoint. Furthermore, there is nothing to stop them from pretending that this secondary endpoint was the prospectively chosen primary endpoint. A surprisingly large number of trials have very different endpoints from the ones created when originally designing the study.[104,105]

Post-hoc Subgroup Analysis

Computers are truly wonderful inventions when it comes to the creation of deceptive literature. In the past, it may have taken weeks to retrospectively dredge a study's data, in order to find subgroups beneficial to a new drug. Now, all that is required is to enter the data into a statistical computer program; after this step, *data dredging* can be performed in minutes. If a drug shows a beneficial effect in redheaded males between the ages of 18 and $18\frac{3}{4}$, then there is no reason not to publish that fact.

Statistical Analysis

Faulty statistical analysis is one of the most difficult deceptions for non-statisticians to detect. If researchers choose the chi square over student's *t*-test, most of us are none the wiser. If one statistical method does not yield the desired results, researchers can keep trying others until they achieve the values they want.[40]

Suppress All Negative Information

If a study is designed to show the benefits of a new drug, why bother to report on side-effects? If harm from a new drug is discovered in a study, nothing aside from ethics and moral responsibilities obligate researchers to write about it. Recent allegations regarding Prozac™ and Vioxx™ make this point particularly apropos.

Blind Investigators and Researchers to the Data of the Study

We have previously discussed that it may increase the validity of a study to keep the researchers blinded to the data and results until the point at which they are ready to write-up the study. The pharmaceutical companies have taken this strategy one step further by never releasing the data to the study authors. By claiming the data is proprietary, they can hold on to the results of negative trials and not allow researchers to publish it. This is not merely a hypothetical situation; it is merely another deceptive practice which industry makes use of on a regular basis.[106]

Get the Spin Doctors

The Abstract and Discussion Section

Even if the results of a study show no benefit, it does not mean the abstract and the discussion section of the paper needs to state likewise. The negative can easily be made positive by simply adopting the right perspective.[3]

EXAMPLE

If a study to demonstrate equivalence of a new drug to an existing one shows your product is inferior, but this inferiority did not achieve statistical significance, then obviously the conclusion is: "There was no statistically significant difference between our new [expensive] drug and the cheap [effective] old drug."

Alternatively, if your new treatment shows a trend towards superiority which is not statistically significant, then you can say: "Our new drug showed a trend towards superiority compared to the treatment you have used for years."

Relative Risk

Often, relative risk looks far more impressive than absolute values. Nothing at all is keeping researchers from reporting relative risk and burying the absolute risk or not reporting it at all. A 50% reduction in relative risk is far more useful to drug sales than a 0.003% absolute risk reduction. Furthermore, why not simply say there was a 50% reduction in risk of death and never mention that the value is relative at all.[104]

Clinicians are not immune to this subterfuge, as is demonstrated by studies assessing the likelihood of physicians to change their practice when presented with absolute versus relative risk reductions.[39,107,108] Even though the actual change in risk was the same, physicians were much more likely to alter their practice when given the risk reduction in relative terms.

It is our responsibility to demand the proper reporting of treatment effect. Even prestigious journals often publish studies with only relative values reported.[109] The CONSORT statement, adopted by most major journals, addresses this issue.

DECEPTIVE PUBLICATION

"Journals have devolved into information laundering operations for the pharmaceutical industry." – Richard Horton[110]

This quote, written by the editor of *The Lancet*, evokes the oily connotations of mob money-laundering. It is an apt image; as journals are becoming less vehicles for the dissemination of the latest clinical advances and more repositories of industry propaganda. Without the revenue provided by drug company advertising and reprints, most journals would not be able to stay afloat.[96]

Publication Bias

Non-publication of Negative Trials

If a trial shows a product in a negative light and it is resistant to all of the techniques of data molding and spinning mentioned above, then the solution is simple: never publish it. Companies can simply pretend the study never took place and start a new trial; maybe the next time chance will allow a positive result. That is the true beauty of *p*-values of 0.05; if you keep trying, you have a one in 20 chance of making a completely ineffective drug look like a top seller.

Multiple Publications

Conversely, if researchers do manage to eke out a positive trial, then why waste that pot of gold on just a single study? First, they can publish the study in a prominent journal with some nice spin. Next, they can break out little pieces and subsets of the dataset and publish them as separate studies. If they publish enough times, people will begin to become convinced of the drug's efficacy by the power of *inundation*.[111] This strategy has been compared to matrushkas, the Russian dolls, which break open to reveal many smaller versions of the same doll (Fig. 11-2).[40]

Pooled Publications

By taking a few of these subset publications and pooling their results, still more studies can be generated. Two or three datasets can generate a dozen studies. It is difficult to see this much literature and still retain the belief that it is *all* flawed (Fig. 11-3).

If they can publish enough times, then the ultimate path of evidence-based deceit is available to the pharmaceutical company: the deceptive *systematic review* (SR). Of course, the SR should be performed by authors under the employ of the company. Since they are on the payroll, they certainly will not include any studies that cast the product in a negative light. After the creation of the systematic review, a *key opinion leader* can be found who will accept an honorarium in order to publish under his or her name.

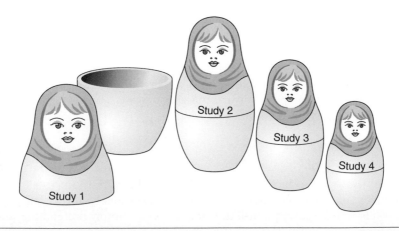

— FIGURE 11-2 — *Russian dolls.*

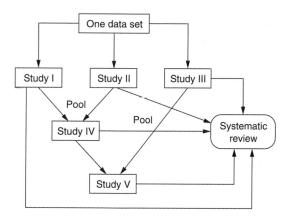

— FIGURE 11-3 —

Possible Solutions

The solution to many of the problems of deceptive publications is a registry of all clinical trials before they are executed. If a study is registered, then we will know of its existence, its pre-hoc methodology, and its primary endpoints. The data of all completed trials can also be placed in the registry, allowing independent analysis and conclusions. The World Health Organization (WHO) has offered its services as an international repository of clinical trials.[112] GlaxoSmithKline is the first pharmaceutical company to voluntarily adopt this principle. International pharmaceutical associations have recently agreed to follow suit.[113] As of this writing, many major journals are in the process of consolidating an agreement to refuse to publish randomized trials that were not prospectively registered prior to their outset. Such an agreement is expected to add an effective enforcement tool to this initiative.

DECEPTIVE MARKETING

The full range of techniques used by the pharmaceutical industry available to mislead through advertising can certainly fill whole books. Some of the techniques specific to medical literature are particularly apropos.

Advertising in Journals

The glossy advertisements in almost every medical journal, and now most mainstream magazines as well, are rarely peer-reviewed. Many of the claims in these advertisements are either misleading or blatantly false.[114,115] Evidence-literacy is the solution for practitioners of evidence-based medicine, but what of the public at large?

Panels of Experts

Large sponsorship fees allow pharmaceutical companies to create panels of experts. These panels can host conferences for hundreds of physicians. While the exclusive purpose of the conference is of course to promote a new drug, why not choose a title that makes it seem that impartial experts will recommend the ideal treatment for a disease? For instance, if you have a new antibiotic, sponsor a conference called "New Optimal Treatment for Community Acquired Pneumonia." In order to maximize this investment, the panel should produce a consensus paper of the conference proceedings to be published in a major journal.

Economic Analyses

A deceptive, falsely designed economic analysis showing that a company's new, ridiculously expensive drug actually works out to be cheaper than standard therapies is another extremely effective form of advertising. The use of multiple graphs and plots will make this effort appear even more valid.

Clinical Practice Guidelines

Companies can pay medical writing agencies or consultants to create practice guidelines, which are favorable to their product. The evidence-literate will discover that the conclusions are not supported by the evidence, but many physicians may still be swayed.

Reprints

If any favorable article is published in a major journal, then the manufacturer will pay millions to have reprints of the article made. The journal publishing the original article makes enormous revenue from these reprints, allowing further industry influence for future publications.

Supplements

Supplements are often attached to normal issues of prominent journals. Though they have the name of the respected journal on the cover, these supplements are not edited with the same rigor. Often, pharmaceutical companies pay for the production of these journal supplements and provide all of the articles. Key opinion leaders receive gift authorships in exchange for an honorarium. The pharmaceutical ghost authors are able to write about off-label uses of drugs, despite the fact that the FDA would ban the same off-label claims in normal advertising.[88]

SUMMARY

For a tongue-in-cheek discussion of the above issues, which nevertheless includes a wealth of information, we advise readers to peruse a copy of HARLOT plc's business proposal.[116]

Just as it is imperative to examine every study for validity and precision, we must also assess for deliberate misrepresentation. Unfortunately, as we have discussed, some forms of these devious practices are undiscoverable. We must therefore, as a profession, attempt to stamp out the impetus for deceptive practices in the literature. It is easy to characterize the drug companies as the villains and physicians as innocent victims.[96] The truth is that we aid and abet these misleading practices, either actively or passively; only a paradigm shift will limit the possibility of future abuses.

ONWARD

After the foregoing discussion of all that can go wrong with a study and its publication, it is easy to believe that the chances of finding the truth are slim. Hodgkin terms this sentiment of uncertainty as *medical credicide*: the death of belief.[117]

After initial training in evidence-based medicine and critical thinking, it may seem that every study is in some way flawed. The *nihilistic* desire to tear down imperfect literature can overwhelm the search for usable information.[1] Eventually, we must move out of this nihilistic phase and find what is valuable even in flawed literature.

The experienced clinician moves beyond methodological checklists and searches for usable evidence that can be applied to decision-making. We hope we have offered the tools to evaluate for validity, precision, and trustworthiness so that we may find the truth in the medical literature.

PART III
FINDING THE EVIDENCE

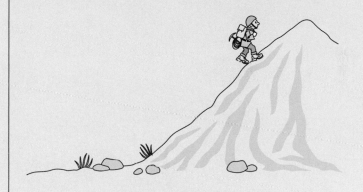

GOOD SEARCHES

CASE: THE BREATHING QUICKENS

A 49-year-old woman is brought to your emergency dpartment by a rescue squad because of acute shortness of breath and chest pain. A daughter tells you that the patient was well until 3 days ago when coughing and congestion worsened in the absence of fever. There was a sudden worsening early this morning with "tightness" in her chest and complaints that "she couldn't breath." The patient is now alert and responsive but in moderate respiratory distress. Obese, she has a respiratory rate of 30/min, a pulse of 120/min, a BP of 150/95 mmHg, and an oxygen saturation of 94% on room air. A medical student reports that jugular venous distention appears absent but is "difficult to judge," there is diffuse wheezing on chest auscultation, and no peripheral edema. This sedentary smoker takes no medications and denies any prior medical problems apart from mild untreated hypertension. You begin to evaluate the patient and to organize your thinking about the problems she presents. *To be continued . . .*

This part of the book is about asking questions and finding answers. In the past, students became doctors by emulating and accepting the mastery of clinical teachers. A search for answers was as easy as locating such a teacher or a colleague and asking our question.

The explosion of information and the advent of new technologies make this past method of learning by apprenticeship untenable. From the outset of our clinical training, modern emergency medicine now demands that we take responsibility for finding our own answers. We therefore must embrace a new skill set; along with learning patient care, we must master *evidence-literacy*. Evidence-literacy is the application of information literacy to the practice of medicine.[1] It contains the essential skills of integrating our need for evidence to make decisions and the ability to search for answers using a wide array of resources.

We discussed clinical reasoning in the first part of this book and dealt with integrating clinical evidence into our decision-making. In the second

Evidence/information-literacy in action

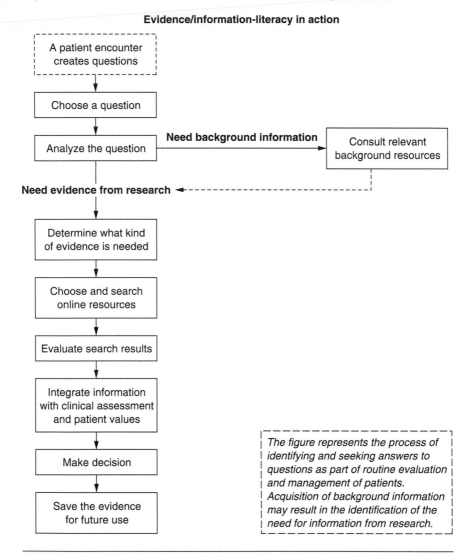

— FIGURE 12-1 —   *The process of answering clinical questions.*

part, we discussed the evaluation of evidence to determine if it is believable and important. In this third part, we address a deceptively simple skill set: finding the best and most relevant evidence pertinent to clinical decision-making.

We say "deceptively simple" advisedly. As medical students (and probably even before), we got pretty good at looking things up. Furthermore, we learned to routinely navigate the Internet in search of information with a facility that our clinically expert elders found dizzying. Despite this head start, finding the best and most relevant evidence to answer questions that arise in the course of our practice may be the last thing we will get good at in evidence-based medicine.

This does not mean that the content of this section is hard to learn. The skill-sets pertaining to finding evidence are easy to acquire; most physicians are undoubtedly already quite accomplished in many relevant areas. So why might this be the last thing we will get good at in the context of clinical decision-making? Simply because full evidence-literacy requires a mastery of the knowledge and skill sets that we have elaborated in the previous two parts of this volume. This is one reason that we have put *finding the evidence* as the third section of this book, rather than the first.

The process of finding relevant clinical evidence can be characterized as a stepwise process. It is important to acknowledge that even though application of clinical evidence to decision-making for individual patients is the fundamental precept of evidence-based clinical practice, in emergency medicine it is rare that we can carry a new inquiry through to a conclusion while an individual patient remains in the department. Therefore, while a search may be spurred by an encounter with one patient, the evidence we discover is often used for the next patient we see with a similar presentation (Fig. 12-1).

ASKING QUESTIONS

CHOOSING A QUESTION

We believe that one of the marks of a great emergency physician is a constant curiosity. In order to satisfy this urge for knowledge, we need to ask questions. Asking the *right* questions is the very first step in finding answers we can use for patient-important decision-making.

Questions can arise from a clinical encounter, questions from colleagues, in the course of our reading, or spontaneously while walking down the hall. Thousands of questions may present themselves on a daily basis. We can identify a few criteria that determine whether a question is likely to have patient-important impact on our practice and therefore whether we should pursue it further.

- *Is the question important to patient outcomes?* Some questions relate directly to patient care; they may impact on our application of tests, use of treatments, or quality of recommendations. These questions often demand a search for evidence, because we will directly use the answers with patients we see in the future.
- *Is the question important to our information needs?* Even if a question is not likely to directly impact upon patient outcome, it may be important if it corresponds to our own information needs. Such needs will ultimately benefit our care, if the information is essential to our ability to evaluate a patient and identify a reasonable course of action.
- *Am I likely to find an answer?* Although we may assume that all questions have answers, not all answers are known or knowable. Furthermore, we have some idea of what is known and knowable among possible questions as a result of our previous education and clinical practice. Such foreknowledge will vary with our experience of the particular disease entity and the context in which a problem presents.

At times, we may be inclined to pursue questions of a nature that do not satisfy these or other pragmatic considerations. We may then be called *curious* or *inquisitive*. If we do this kind of thing in a sufficiently obsessive way we may become known as *researchers*. As we aspire to such practice, we hope that there are sufficient numbers of the obsessively inquisitive within our ranks that our chances of finding answers to questions will continue to increase substantially over time.

For the duration of this part of the book we will be returning to the 49-year-old female with shortness of breath listed in the case at the beginning of this part of the book (page 257). Numerous questions may emerge from contact with this patient. Which questions occur to us will vary depending on our level of clinical experience and our practice environment. Clinicians taking a course in evidence-based medicine have frequently chosen the following questions in response to this scenario:

- How useful is jugular venous distension (JVD) in differentiating between previously undiagnosed cardiac heart failure and asthma in an obese patient?
- Does this patient have a pulmonary embolus?
- What does wheezing indicate is occurring in the lung?
- What are the possible causes of this patient's dyspnea?
- What are the mainstays of treatment for patients with chronic obstructive pulmonary disease (COPD)?
- Is it safe to administer albuterol in a patient with wheezing, tachycardia, and as of yet unexplained hypoxia?
- How sensitive and specific are B-natiuretic peptide (BNP) measurements for distinguishing between asthma and congestive heart failure?

ANALYZING THE QUESTION

Some questions have to do with augmenting our knowledge of a disease, a test, or a treatment in a general way. Others have to do with actions that will have direct impact on patient care.

Questions that pertain to our own requisite knowledge, are called *background questions*. Those having to do with specific choices, recommendations or expectations that you might present to a patient, are termed *foreground questions*.[2] One might say that background questions have to do with what we *know* and foreground questions with what we *say and do*.

- ***Background questions:*** The answers to background questions are readily found in sources that deal with disease-specific issues in relatively comprehensive terms. Textbook chapters and non-systematic reviews published in peer-reviewed journals are examples of such sources. In general, the information from these sources comes from both pathophysiological investigations and the personal experience of academic and clinical experts. Indeed, *consultants* in the relevant specialties may be as valuable a source of background information as are published sources. They are particularly important when the information is needed in the course of administering care to an acutely ill patient.

- *Foreground questions:* Answers to foreground questions are ideally found through clinical investigations. Sources of clinical evidence include primary research, systematic reviews and other systematic summaries. If you have ever conceived and designed a research project, you are aware that the question to be asked by a particular study is generally quite narrow. No doubt, if it did not start out that way it rapidly was made so through the interventions of your preceptor. Foreground questions are therefore narrower and more focused than are background questions. On the other hand, when well chosen, they go to the heart of the matter of what you are going to do or say to your patient in the course of an acute care encounter.

Whether we choose to ask a background or foreground question depends on our circumstances and our needs.

Clinical Experience

One factor has to do with the extent of our prior experience with the disease or circumstance in question. Figure 13-1 presents a useful construct for illustrating this principle.

As our experience with a particular condition increases from point A to point C on the horizontal axis, a greater percentage of the questions we are likely to ask fall into the foreground category. This is illustrated by the downward slope of the line separating the domain of foreground questions above from that of background questions below. At no point is the likelihood of asking background questions reduced to zero.

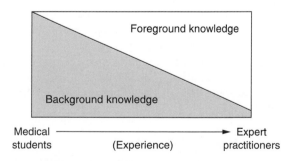

Foreground knowledge

Background knowledge

Medical students ———————————→ Expert practitioners
(Experience)

— FIGURE 13-1 — *The types of knowledge we need to answer our clinical questions changes as we progress in our careers.*

One might imagine the increase of experience with the condition of interest to correspond to the level of training of the practitioner. Indeed, medical students at the outset of their studies will tend to ask a very high proportion of background questions, irrespective of the nature of the condition at hand.

However, unfamiliar clinical conditions are commonplace in emergency medicine. When we encounter them, our background knowledge may be negligible, despite extensive clinical experience. In such situations, training in emergency assessment and resuscitation allows us to stabilize the patient. However, a basic orientation to the nature of the disease process soon becomes paramount and important background questions rapidly emerge.

Chaotic settings illustrate why background questions may be just as urgent in some situations as foreground questions, and why they need to be recognized as such and efficiently pursued. The answers to background questions provide the basis for identifying the relevant foreground questions (i.e., the questions whose answers shape the things we say and do). In general, therefore, it is our level of disease-specific experience, not our level of training, which best correlates with the likelihood that the important questions we will ask in relationship to a specific encounter are background or foreground.

Clinical Research

Answering a foreground question requires that research has been performed on the topic. Whether a particular question practically lends itself to a clinical research investigation is a potentially advanced topic. In the decade that has elapsed since evidence-based medicine (EBM) was first announced in the pages of *JAMA*,[3] additional clinical questions have been recognized by EBM authorities as potentially answerable by appropriate study types. Examples of the latter include studies on differential diagnosis and on clinical manifestations of disease.[4,5] Prior to this recognition, such clinical questions would have been referred to background information sources, even by experts in evidence-based medicine.

This process of blurring the boundaries separating background from foreground will doubtless continue. The assessment of whether a particular question can be answered through clinical research will therefore continue to involve a combination of knowledge and imagination.

Is a Clinical Study Conceivable?

One factor contributing to the likelihood of finding an answer from clinical research is whether such research is even conceivable. Rare diseases may be excluded from such studies because of the difficulty of assembling a sufficient number of patients. Some questions are relatively unanswerable for ethical reasons; for example, it will be unlikely that we will find clinical research on the advisability of administering blood transfusions to patients with exsanguinating hemorrhage. Questions pertaining to common disease entities may be relatively unapproachable via clinical research for particular patients due to an unusual complexity of concomitant disease. For example, patients on immunosuppressive medications may get appendicitis but are very unlikely to be included in a study on performance of peripheral white blood cell count as a diagnostic test in this context.

It is important to be clear on the *definition of clinical research*: it is research involving human subjects and measuring clinically important outcomes. Although animal studies contribute to our pathophysiological understanding and to the process of developing new interventions, it is misleading and even dangerous to base clinical decisions for human patients on such evidence. As an example, animal studies indicated the possible benefit of various pharmacological interventions for brain injury.[6] However, human trials have demonstrated no benefit and even harm from the same interventions.[7]

Likewise, as we emphasized in Part II, studies involving measurement of outcomes that are not directly important to patients, such as purely physiological evidence, are also subject to dangerous misinterpretation.[8] If only animal or physiological outcome studies are likely to have been performed on a question, it is best and most safely treated as a background question.

Has Clinical Research Been Done on This Question?

Having decided that a question *might* be answerable by means of a clinical study, we must still consider how likely it is that such a study has actually been done. If it is unlikely, the question might best be defined as a background question and referred to the sources appropriate to such an assessment.

EXAMPLE

In early 2003, a previously unknown infection with high mortality, the "severe adult respiratory syndrome" (SARS), was recognized in Asia and quickly spread to other parts of the world. There could be no clinical research on the entity in such a situation, and all decision-making had to be based upon *disease-oriented* considerations.

■ Our Case Scenario

If we return to the questions raised by our clinical scenario, we can classify two of them as background questions:

- ○ ***What does wheezing indicate is occurring in the lung?*** This question involves consideration of the pathophysiology associated with the clinical finding of wheezing and potentially pertains to the process of sizing up not only the differential diagnosis, but possibly the severity of the patient's condition.
- ○ ***What are the possible causes of this patient's dyspnea?*** This second question, under certain circumstances, might be referred to an appropriately designed study on differential diagnosis. However, in the setting of the scenario as we have defined it, and framed as it is in very general terms, we would be inclined to refer it to a relevant background source on clinical assessment of such patients.

BACKGROUND QUESTIONS

Answering background questions can be as easy as asking a colleague or may require a search for just the right monograph. The reader of this volume is likely already aware of many sources of background information and where to find them. Online information sources, such as UpToDate® and *eMedicine*,* are particularly popular among residents, because they provide rapid access to such information. For example, information pertaining to both of the background questions we identified above can be obtained from UpToDate® using the single words "wheezing" and "dyspnea" respectively in the search window that appears on the home page of the resource.

Sources of answers to background questions include:

- ○ Textbooks and monographs
- ○ UpToDate® and other online resources
- ○ Non-systematic review articles
- ○ Disease-oriented clinical research
- ○ Consultants and colleagues.

---

*These sources are online textbooks; we will discuss UpToDate® more extensively in the following pages.

Textbooks and Monographs

There is something extremely satisfying about the presence of large textbooks of emergency medicine sitting on our bookshelves. It is appealing to think that thousands of pages of information are just waiting for us to open to the right page. General textbooks of emergency medicine can answer many of our background questions at the beginning of our education. As we progress, we may get better information from disease or condition-specific monographs. One of the problems with learning from printed texts is that the nature of the publishing cycle dictates that these sources will be at least a few years out of date.

Online Resources

We have already mentioned UpToDate®, which is one of the most popular online resources to answer background questions. These sources are essentially textbooks on the web. There is a probability, but not a certainty, that these online sources will be updated more frequently than printed texts.

Non-systematic Reviews

Many journals publish articles of high quality and excellent readability that cover a broad range of disease-specific issues. Such articles do not follow the kind of structured format expected of research reports and are frequently referred to as *narrative reviews*. As long as we do not confuse these sources with foreground knowledge, we can garner the answer to many of our background queries through these articles. The search for non-systematic reviews can be performed using MEDLINE. We will discuss search strategies and databases in the next chapter.

Even in clinical studies, which can provide foreground knowledge, we may find answers to background questions. This is because the discussion sections of these studies often are narrative reviews in their own right and may be the most recent such review on the subject. These discussions may therefore provide useful *background knowledge*. We have discussed the relative merits of narrative and systematic reviews in an earlier chapter.

Disease-oriented Clinical Research

Research that is not patient-important, such as animal studies or studies of DOE, cannot help us answer foreground questions. It can provide further understanding of the underpinnings and pathophysiology of disease. These sources can therefore answer background questions.

Consultants and Colleagues

While we should not turn to expert opinion to answer foreground queries, asking questions of the physicians around us can serve as an excellent means of obtaining background information.

The remainder of this part of the book will deal with foreground questions.

REFINING FOREGROUND QUESTIONS

PICO: The Secret Acronym

Once a query is properly and fruitfully classified as a foreground question, we must proceed through additional analytical steps, if the process of seeking and evaluating an answer is to proceed efficiently. The most important of these is to break the question down into a number of smaller components, as a means of defining exactly the answers we are after. A widely used format for doing this is affectionately known as "PICO," an acronym standing for Patients, Interventions, Comparisons, and Outcomes."[2,9–11] PICO can be used for all of the types of foreground questions we may explore to aid our decisions.

- *P for Patients:* Under "P" we list the attributes of the patient population in question. We must define any factors that are likely to impact on the relevant patients' diagnosis or prognosis.
- *I for Interventions* (or exposures): "I" can be something we administer to a patient (intervention) or something that a patient is exposed to independently of medical treatment.
- *C for Comparisons:* "C" is used when the outcome involves a comparison, such as between two therapeutic effects, between the performances of two diagnostic tests, or of assessment instruments. While all foreground questions will contain P, I, and O, C will only be present when we are making these comparisons.
- *O for Outcomes:* "O" is a description of what results we would deem to be a relevant outcome for our question.

How Is PICO Used?

PICO is the tool that allows us to plot the entire course of inquiry, once a foreground question has been identified. It is to an inquiring clinician what a study protocol is to a researcher. Completing PICO for a question prepares us to answer the following questions:

- Does this question have to do with therapy, harm, diagnosis or prognosis?
- What kind of a study would best answer this question?
- What resource or database would provide me with the quickest path to finding such a study, if it exists?
- What terms should I use to search the resource I have selected?
- What criteria will I use to select the best and most relevant studies from my search?
- What criteria should I use to appraise the validity and importance of the studies I select?
- What considerations are going to guide my assessment of the applicability of such studies to my patients?

In our experience, physicians new to evidence-based medicine are initially tempted to reduce the use of PICO to identification of the search terms they will use. This is a mistake for several reasons. As we shall see, depending upon what kind of resource is chosen, only one or two search terms may be needed to find studies relevant to a question. In such a situation, completing a PICO grid goes far beyond what is needed to do a search. However, unless we think through PICO, or its equivalent, we may not have a sufficiently clear idea of what we are looking for to recognize or evaluate the best evidence when we find it. We may even choose an inappropriate resource for the search, rendering the choice of search terms moot.

PICO for Issues of Benefit or Risk of Treatments

Figure 13-2 illustrates the kind of information that might go into a PICO grid of a question pertaining to benefit or harm resulting from a therapeutic intervention. It is obvious that many more concept terms or "keywords" are called for here than would ever be needed for even the most challenging of electronic searches.

Let's try it out. One of the frequently asked questions (FAQs) listed earlier in connection with our 49-year-old dyspneic female was: "Is it safe to administer albuterol in a patient with wheezing, tachycardia, and as of yet undiagnosed hypoxia?" What information about our question would be important to have in mind prior to doing a literature search on this question and how would it fit into the PICO mold (Fig. 13-3)?

The information included within this PICO grid constitutes a guideline for limiting our search to studies that would be important and

Patients	Setting Disease Condition or injury Severity Age Time from onset of symptoms Comorbidities Important circumstances
Interventions	Range of drugs Range of doses Procedure specifications Ancillary care Other specific therapies
Comparisons	Placebo or alternative therapy Range of doses of comparison agents Ancillary care Other specific therapies
Outcomes	Relative likelihood of events Quality of life outcomes Process of care outcomes Minimum patient-important magnitude of effect for relevant outcomes

— FIGURE 13-2 — *Information potentially relevant to a foreground question on the benefit or harm caused by a medical or surgical intervention organized using the PICO format.*

applicable to our patients. We are not irreversibly bound to these predetermined limits. The choices we make in the course of selecting evidence to review may fall outside of them. Instead the guidelines serve as a starting point for seeking the type of evidence we require to make the right choices for our patients.

For example, the patients we treat are those who come to an emergency department, so we list this setting under Patient (P). However, if we find an otherwise well-done study that involved similar patients being treated by emergency services personnel in a pre-hospital care setting and that considered the outcomes we are interested in, we might well be willing to accept it as relevant and applicable.

Likewise, in the scenario, we were exclusively concerned with nebulized beta-agonists such as albuterol. However, we might find otherwise relevant research from a period in which subcutaneous sympathomimetics such as epinephrine were much more readily available and used in

P	Prehospital or emergency department setting, adults with moderately severe acute dyspnea of <24 hours duration and possibly due to bronchospasm or cardiac disease, patients without known cardiac disease and for whom an EKG and chest X-ray is not yet available.
I	Albuterol, or other sympathomimetic agents, administered by inhalation or subcutaneous injection in standard doses used for asthma in tandem with oxygen, absence of other agents with sympathomimetic effect such as aminophylline.
C	Placebo instead of sympathomimetic agents in tandem with oxygen, absence of other agents with sympathomimetic effect such as aminophylline.
O	>0.1% increase in cardiac arrest, >1% increase in life-threatening dysrhythmias, >5% increase in non-life threatening dysrhythmias requiring active intervention. Increased patient-important discomfort from palpitations or nervousness not requiring active intervention. All outcomes within 4 hours of administration.

— FIGURE 13-3 — *Information potentially relevant to the safety of albuterol administered to an adult patient with dyspnea and with yet undiagnosed hypoxia, wheezing, and tachycardia.*

pre-hospital emergency settings. Should we accept such research? If we believe that nebulized agents are not importantly *more* likely to cause the harmful outcomes we are interested in than are subcutaneous agents of the same general class, we may reasonably decide that the answer is "Yes." So as our Intervention (I), we list both nebulized and injectable sympathomimetic agents.

Where did the specific percentage increases of various harmful effects listed under the Outcome (O) category come from? Patients and practitioners certainly vary in terms of what constitutes an acceptable increase in events such as cardiac arrest or non-fatal dysrhythmias. Nonetheless, these thresholds are almost always greater than zero. Defining them qualitatively in advance forces us to address the issues of value and perspective that pertain to our question and prepares us to evaluate what we may find in the course of our search with greater objectivity. The exact choice of thresholds will, of course, vary from practitioner to practitioner and even from patient to patient.

There is far too much information in the PICO compartments of Fig. 13-3 to be reasonably put into a standard sentence. However, it is instructive to attempt an abbreviated reformatting of the original question drawing on the fruits of the PICO grid:

- BEFORE: *Is it safe to administer albuterol in a patient with wheezing, tachycardia, and as of yet undiagnosed hypoxia?*
- AFTER: *Do albuterol or other sympathomimetic agents administered to dyspneic adult patients with wheezing, hypoxia, or tachycardia, but without previously diagnosed cardiac disease in a pre-hospital or emergency department setting, increase above specified threshold levels the incidence of cardiac arrest, dysrhythmias, or discomfort compared to standard preliminary therapy without such agents?*

Comparing the new version of the question to the one we had at the moment that it first occurred to us, we can clearly see the effect and potential benefit of thinking it through in a *systematic* way.

In this example, our question has to do with a therapeutic intervention, specifically with the possibility of harmful effects of administration of the therapy in a particular clinical context. It is therefore a question about *harm*. No doubt we were already aware of this when we started to put it into PICO format. Later, we shall see that it is sometimes useful to suspend the final assessment of what kind of question is being asked until *after* PICO has been completed.

PICO for Diagnosis

Consider another question from our list of FAQs for the 49-year-old dyspneic female: "How sensitive and specific are BNP measurements for distinguishing between asthma and congestive heart failure?" This is a question about a diagnostic test; specifically, it is a question concerning the performance of the test in a particular clinical context. What kind of information is properly included in the compartments of the PICO grid for such a question?

Figure 13-4A makes it clear that the information pertaining to a question about performance of a diagnostic test is quite different from that pertaining to a question about therapy or harm:

- *Patients:* We no longer assume that we know whether the patient actually has the target disease or condition, but rather have only an estimate of how likely it is that he or she does.
- *Intervention:* The "intervention" is the diagnostic test in question.
- *Comparison:* The comparison is also no longer an alternative therapy or exposure, but rather a different test or an array of alternative tests, which we will accept as the criterion standard for the condition of interest.

A

P	Setting, clinical presentation, degree of clinical suspicion for a target disease or condition, severity, age, time from onset of symptoms, comorbidities, important circumstances.
I	Diagnostic test, including make and model if a device is involved and biochemical preparation if it is a laboratory test, specification of test results or range of test values, procedure specifications including category of expertise applied to interpretation.
C	Clinically acceptable criterion standard for comparison with results of index test, acceptable alternative criterion standards such as clinical observation over specified time period.
O	Sensitivity, specificity of dichotomous test results, likelihood ratios of results of interest, threshold values of post-test probability of the target disease or condition.

B

P	Emergency department, adult patient with moderately severe dyspnea, wheezing and mild hypoxia not previously diagnosed, intermediate pretest probability of congestive heart failure, <24 hours from onset of symptoms.
I	B-type natriuretic peptide test result greater than or less than recommended cutoff, or specified values or ranges of BNP.
C	Final discharge diagnosis for patients admitted to hospital, cardiologist opinion together with echocardiography result for patients discharged from emergency department.
O	Sensitivity, specificity, or likelihood ratios of BNP values above and below recommended cutoff value, or likelihood ratios for specific BNP values or ranges, such that the post test likelihood of CHF is either ≥70% or ≤15%.

— FIGURE 13-4 — *A Information potentially relevant to a foreground question on the performance of a diagnostic test, using the PICO format.* ***B*** *Information potentially relevant to a question on the performance of B-type natriuretic peptide as a test for congestive heart failure (CHF) in an adult dyspneic patient, using the PICO format.*

- *Outcomes:* Finally, the outcomes are now the measures of likelihood that the target disease or condition is present, given the result of the test of interest.

In our experience, learners frequently have a bit more trouble conceptualizing the use of the PICO format for analyzing questions of diagnosis as opposed to those pertaining to therapy. Their response is frequently to abandon the formatting process with the assertion that PICO does not *work* for questions of this sort. Our answer is that PICO in this setting works very well if its user understands the diagnostic decision-making process.

The stumbling blocks encountered by learners in this setting largely stem from an inadequate grasp of the basics of diagnostic clinical reasoning. Once the concepts of pre-test and post-test probability, action thresholds, and measures of test performance become clear, the means of using PICO for questions about the performance of a diagnostic test fall readily into place.

Let's see how PICO might work for the diagnosis question we have chosen from our scenario. As with Fig. 13-3 in the previous example, Fig. 13-4B reflects choices regarding the possible studies that would be accepted as valid and applicable to our practice.

The choice of attributes to be included under Patients, such as the length of time from onset of symptoms and severity criteria, pertain both to the patients' disease spectrum and to their similarity to the patients we are likely to see in our practice.

Under Interventions, we need to decide how precisely the diagnostic test in question needs to be specified. BNP is a relatively recent test and hence it is probably not necessary to define it more precisely. The opposite is true for a laboratory test such as d-dimer, for which several different techniques and preparations are available, each characterized by somewhat different test performance characteristics. In this case, we would need to specify exactly which d-dimer assay we wanted to analyze.

For Comparisons, we need to think carefully about the choice of criterion standard to be used to decide when 'positive' or 'negative' BNP values are *right* and when they are *wrong*. In clinical research, *definitive* criterion standards, such as autopsy or pathology reports, are rarely available. Nonetheless, the standards used in a study must be convincing. In our case, one would like to have a study that would include patients who are discharged from the emergency department. A different criterion standard may have to be used for this subgroup. Discharge diagnosis for patients admitted to hospital generally reflects a multitude of clinical and diagnostic inputs, including inferences from response to therapy. The same is generally not true for patients discharged from the emergency room. More stringent and objective criteria may therefore need to be specified for this latter subgroup.

The last category, Outcomes, reflects an important choice with respect to the way that the results of the test are approached. Investigators have proposed specific cutoff values for the BNP test, above which the test is considered "positive" and below which it is considered "negative" for congestive heart failure.[12,13] However, this approach to the results of diagnostic tests in which the result is a continuous measure has been challenged.[14,15] We may therefore choose to specify a range of values of BNP and seek to determine the likelihood ratios for those particular values from studies found in our search. If insufficient data are reported in these studies for the LRs to be calculated, we may find the studies to be inapplicable to our question. As in the case of questions of therapy, we may choose to define our outcome with reference to specific action thresholds. As we noted above, the choice of the thresholds will vary between practitioners and for individual patients and clinical situations.

Once again, the use of PICO makes it possible for us to think through many things that will equip us to assess the validity and relevance of the studies likely to come up in a search, as well as how we will use the results in decision-making, even before we find them. This is likely to limit confusion and multiple searches. It serves to set the stage for the subsequent steps of appraising and applying results to practice.

For the purposes of assessing the effect on the question as originally asked of the PICO analysis we have just performed, here is the before and after:

- BEFORE: *How sensitive and specific are BNP measurements for distinguishing between asthma and congestive heart failure?*

- AFTER: *In previously undiagnosed adult patients presenting to an emergency department with moderately severe dyspnea of less than 24 hours' duration and an intermediate likelihood of congestive heart failure, do the sensitivity and specificity of B-type natriuretic peptide, using recommended test value cutoffs for "positive" and "negative," yield likelihood ratios adequate to either increase the post-test probability of CHF to above 70% or to lower it to below 15% when either hospital discharge diagnosis or cardiology opinion aided by echocardiography are used as the criterion standard?*

Once more, we would not expect an "A" from our English grammar teacher as a reward for this rather preposterous construction. Nor do the specific choices we have made here for purposes of illustration constitute the "right" answer for this question. However, the revised version does reflect the effort we have put into analyzing our query. Furthermore, it is now in the form of a question whose answer we are directly prepared to act upon.

PICO for Other Questions

Therapy and diagnosis constitute the bread and butter of decision-making in emergency practice. To the extent that we are equipped to deal with the

P	Setting, disease, condition or injury, severity, age, time from onset of symptoms, comorbidities or specific characteristics, important circumstances.
I	Observation over specified time period.
C	(May not be applicable to this kind of question.)
O	Rate of clinically important events, such as death, stroke, myocardial infarction, or need for invasive therapy such as dialysis over observation period.

— FIGURE 13-5 — *Information potentially relevant to a foreground question regarding the prognosis of a patient with a specified disease, condition or injury using the PICO format.*

process of not only searching for, but also critically appraising and applying evidence pertaining to, other types of questions, we will find the PICO approach helpful.

Figures 13-5 to 13-7 provide examples of how the PICO format might apply to several other types of questions. Notice that for the simplest forms of prognosis or differential diagnosis questions, a "comparison" category is not necessary. In such cases, PICO becomes reduced to "PIO."

CHOOSING A CATEGORY OF EVIDENCE

Having parsed through our question using the powerful PICO tool, we are in a position to make a number of strategic assessments. While these assessments are interrelated and may ultimately be dealt with simultaneously by the clinician adept in evidence-based medicine, for the purposes of teaching it is best to deal with them separately.

We must first determine to which category of evidence our question pertains. There are four primary clinical categories of foreground questions:

- *Therapy:* Determining the relative effect of possible treatments on improving patient function or avoiding adverse events
- *Harm:* Ascertaining the relative effects of potentially harmful agents on patient function, morbidity, and mortality
- *Diagnosis:* Establishing the power of a diagnostic test to differentiate between those with and without a target condition or disease

P	Setting, clinical presentation consistent with a specific disease, condition or injury, severity, age, time from onset of symptoms, comorbidities or specific characteristics, important circumstances.
I	Structured application of a rule or scoring system based on presence or absence of elements of clinical evaluation and/or simple laboratory tests and images.
C	Results of an independent test or assessment.
O	Sensitivity, specificity or likelihood ratio of results of application of the prediction rule for predicting the results of the comparison test OR post-test probability of the target condition corresponding to the result of the application of the rule.

— FIGURE 13-6 — *Information potentially relevant to a foreground question regarding the performance of a clinical prediction rule using the PICO format.*

P	Setting, clinical presentation consistent with a number of specific diseases or conditions, severity, age, time from onset of symptoms, comorbidities or specific characteristics, important circumstances.
I	Structured multiphasic diagnostic workup applied systematically to consecutive patients.
C	(Not applicable to this kind of question.)
O	Percentage of patients having each of the target set of diseases or conditions.

— FIGURE 13-7 — *Information potentially relevant to a foreground question regarding the differential diagnosis of a patient presenting with a specific set of symptoms or findings, using the PICO format.*

- **Prognosis:** Estimating the likelihood of specific outcomes attributed to a patient's disease.

This level of categorization is familiar to all physicians. It is for this reason that we prefer to make the clinical categorization of questions primary and the determination of the various possible study designs secondary when teaching practitioners how to connect clinical questions to information from research.[16,17] The relationship of question type to study design is not linear. Nevertheless, this approach seems to provide clinical learners with the shortest path to understanding what can become fairly sophisticated relationships.

WHEN PICO CAUSES A REVISION OF THE QUESTION TYPE

For many, if not most, foreground questions we may ask in the course of caring for our patients, it is immediately evident whether a question has to do with therapy, harm, diagnosis, or prognosis. In this regard, subsequent PICO formatting only elaborates what is already obvious. However, occasionally the PICO format may cause us change the question type. Therefore, we have positioned this step *after* the PICO phase.

A concrete example illustrating the potential value of this subtlety might be drawn from the FAQ that we previously explored in relationship to our dyspneic patient: "Is it safe to administer albuterol in a patient with wheezing, tachycardia, and as of yet unexplained hypoxia?" After subjecting the question to the scrutiny of PICO, we arrived at: "Do albuterol or other sympathomimetic agents administered to dyspneic adult patients with wheezing, hypoxia, or tachycardia, but without previously diagnosed cardiac disease in a pre-hospital or emergency department setting, increase above specified threshold levels the incidence of cardiac arrest, dysrhythmias or discomfort compared to standard preliminary therapy without such agents?

In both cases, the question appeared to be a "slam-dunk" harm query. But let's take a step back and adjust the scenario to involve a patient with even more severe respiratory distress accompanied by more extreme elevation of the BP and heart rate. Let's furthermore confine the circumstances to a pre-hospital setting. The EMT-Intermediates call medical control and you answer the phone. From the information you receive, you determine that the situation is potentially life-threatening but does not yet call for an attempt at endotracheal intubation in the field. You consider that the patient is most likely experiencing an asthma attack but cannot rule out the possibility that she is in pulmonary edema. You are inclined to authorize administration of a beta-agonist and believe that it may buy important time for transport to the hospital emergency room, avoiding the dangers and pitfalls of a difficult field intubation under uncontrolled circumstances and perhaps indirectly saving the patient's life. However, you cannot exclude the possibility that the patient's apparent bronchospasm is a manifestation of pulmonary edema and that administration of a sympathomimetic agent could worsen underlying ischemia.

The issue at hand is still ostensibly a matter of harm caused by administration of intended therapy. However, it is now a matter of harm *in relationship to potentially life-saving benefit.* In other words, do the dangers of a dysrhythmia requiring cardioversion outweigh the likelihood of life-saving benefit? In the course of applying the PICO categories, you might well decide to call this a *therapy* question in which the need to weigh the benefits against the potential harms of an intervention is particularly pertinent. This in turn might affect your consideration of relevant study designs and your choice of online resources and databases to search for such a study.

This example also highlights the fact that, when considering the consequences of things that we administer to patients, benefit and risk ("therapy" and "harm") are flip sides of a single coin. Although our focus may at any point be more on the one side than the other, both sides are always present and decisions are always, implicitly, based on weighing the two sides against each other.

CHOOSING THE TYPE OF STUDY

The final step in understanding a foreground question well enough to find the best answer is to connect it to an appropriately designed study. This ultimately requires a basic knowledge of the types of study design that pertain to clinical research, and their relative strengths and weaknesses as sources of information. This is perhaps the biggest hurdle that clinicians face in coming to terms with evidence-based clinical practice.

Prior to providing a few pointers about navigating this hurdle, let us expose two commonly encountered misconceptions. The first, potentially lethal, misconception is that a lack of knowledge of statistics is the biggest obstacle to face in mastering EBM. Clinicians frequently fear that discomfort with, and lack of knowledge of, statistics will be their biggest obstacle in learning to practice evidence-based medicine. This misconception may result in early abandonment of efforts to absorb EBM methodology. In fact, the ready availability of online calculators makes it possible to practice "evidence-literate" medicine with virtually no knowledge of statistics. Further, no statistical knowledge is required to understand the important differences between the kinds of studies that pertain to different types of clinical question.

The second potentially lethal misconception is that randomized trials constitute the only acceptable study design for investigating clinical questions. We commonly encounter this misconception among learners attending their first course or workshop in evidence-based medicine. It mirrors a distortion that is frequently asserted by critics of evidence-based medicine.[18] These critics are generally very sophisticated types who should, and undoubtedly do, know better. Clinicians whose instincts tell them that the idea that the pursuit of all questions can be reduced to a quest for a single type of study is "too good to be true" may take comfort in the assurance that, indeed it *is*. An evidence-based practitioner needs to be prepared to search for a variety of different types of study to be able to maximize the potential value of clinical research to our patients.

These two misconceptions, i.e. that you have to be a statistical expert to be good at evidence-based medicine or that all you only need look for is a randomized trial on any question, constitute polar extremes. To harbor either of them is to undermine effectiveness in acquiring EBM skills. The truth lies somewhere in the middle ground that separates the "one size fits all" reductionist from the inscrutable obscurity of the mind of a statistician.

▪ The Four Primary Question Types

We have identified therapy, harm, diagnosis, and prognosis as the primary categories of question that suggest clinical investigation. Figure 13-8 identifies the types of study that are characteristically associated with such investigations. Things are not always so straightforward, and it is sometimes necessary to amplify Fig. 13-8 in important ways.

Let us look at the four primary question types in sequence, reviewing what we have already encountered and adding a few additional nuances.

Therapy

We have previously discussed the reasons why randomized trials are the preferred study design for determining the ability of therapies to improve patient outcomes.

Question type	Characteristic study design
Therapy	Randomized controlled trial
Harm	Population-based case control study
Diagnosis	Cross-sectional analytical study
Prognosis	Cohort study

— FIGURE 13-8 —   *The most characteristic study designs corresponding to the primary types of clinical questions.*

Such trials involve a control or comparison group which allows the calculation of measures of comparative outcome, such as relative risk reduction, absolute risk reduction, and number needed to treat. When many similar randomized trials have been performed on a question, a systematic review or meta-analysis becomes the preferred study type.

Harm

Issues of harm may involve exposures of a nature that would render it unethical for investigators to attempt to assign them to patients. These include addictive substances, environmental toxins, or drugs considered to be contraindicated in the clinical contexts in question. In these situations, randomized trials are categorically unfeasible.

Harm questions, by their nature, still require a comparison group, who did not receive the exposure, to be included as part of the study design. Various types of observational study can fulfill these requirements. A case–control study design is the common form for exposures that cannot be assigned to patients and in which the outcome of interest is rare.

Prospective observational studies, with control groups, are possible when the exposures and the outcomes are both relatively common, such as the use of addictive substances like tobacco. In the special case that the exposure is a medication that is legitimately administered to the target patients for therapeutic reasons and the adverse outcome is sufficiently common, then a randomized trial is feasible and should be sought for. If there are many such trials, a meta-analysis would be even more preferable.

Prognosis

Prognosis questions may seek estimates of simple outcome rates in patients presenting with defined conditions and clinical circumstances. However, they may also seek to determine the effect of specific patient characteristics (predictors) on increasing or decreasing those outcomes. In either case, prognosis studies characteristically involve a single study group.

When sufficiently large and continued for an adequate length of time, the control arm of a randomized trial may be taken as the basis for a study on prognosis. In this circumstance, the randomization plays no role in the analysis of the prognosis study aside from creating a group to follow. Systematic reviews of observational prognosis studies may be performed, but this form of literature is controversial.[19]

Diagnosis

We have saved diagnosis for the end, because it causes the most confusion on the part of learners. There are several kinds of questions that we ask about diagnosis and diagnostic tests; very different study designs are used to answer them.

Early efforts aimed at equipping clinicians to bring information from clinical research to bear on the diagnostic process focused on studies of diagnostic test performance, as measured by parameters such as sensitivity/specificity, predictive values, and more recently, likelihood ratios.[20,21]

However, the diagnostic process encompasses a multiplicity of phases, of which interpretation of diagnostic test results is only one.[22] Information from clinical research can be brought to bear on many phases of this process, including recognizing a disease by its clinical manifestations, and forming a differential diagnosis.[4,5]

Furthermore, even when the focus of a diagnosis question is on a diagnostic test, measures of *performance* of the test may not constitute the desired outcome. Rather, the clinician may seek information on whether performing the test results in measurable benefit to the patient. In this case, the question is said to pertain to the *utility*, not to the *performance*, of the test, and the outcomes are measured in ways otherwise associated with studies of effectiveness of therapy.[23,24]

For a diagnosis question pertaining to the accuracy of a diagnostic test in distinguishing between patients with and without a target condition, a study that subjects patients with a common clinical presentation to both the test in question and to an appropriate criterion standard is preferred. This is conventionally termed an *analytical cross-sectional study*; it may be done prospectively or retrospectively. Attempts to demonstrate the former to be superior to the latter have been unsuccessful.[25]

When the diagnosis question pertains to the utility of using a test in improving patient-important outcomes, a randomized trial is the ideal study design. This may, in fact, constitute the highest level of evidence supporting the systematic use of a diagnostic test in the relevant clinical circumstances.[26] However, we must understand that the results of a randomized trial will not provide us with the information needed to estimate the post-test probability of the condition when a particular test result is obtained.

Systematic reviews and meta-analyses may be performed on studies of diagnostic test accuracy and of diagnostic test utility, when such studies are sufficiently numerous and similar.

The use of our old friend, the PICO tool, can be of considerable help in sorting out what kind of a diagnosis question we are asking. Figure 13-9 addresses the application of PICO to issues of the accuracy and utility of a diagnostic test.

Returning to the second *lethal misconception* above, although we see that randomized trials potentially play an important role with respect to questions in all four categories of clinical evidence, they are frequently

Diagnostic test question type (study design)	Accuracy (cross-sectional analytical study)	Utility (randomized trial)
Patients	Emergency, diagnostic uncertainty present	Emergency, diagnostic uncertainty present
Interventions	Proposed diagnostic test	Proposed diagnostic test
Comparisons	Criterion standard for diagnosis	Alternative test or no test
Outcomes	Sensitivity, specificity, likelihood ratios	Relative risk of morbidity, comparative length of stay

— FIGURE 13-9 — *Comparison of two types of questions clinicians may ask about a diagnostic test, using the PICO scheme. Questions about accuracy are answered via cross sectional studies using measures of performance of the test compared to a criterion standard. Questions about utility are answered via randomized trials using measures of relative benefit to patients.*

unfeasible and sometimes undesirable. We must accustom ourselves to routinely asking and analyzing a variety of different kinds of questions arising in the course of our practice. We should become increasingly comfortable with matching questions to the study design most likely to provide the best and most pertinent information. The PICO tool can be extremely helpful in this process.

WHEN THE IDEAL STUDY IS NOT AVAILABLE

What should we do when a study of the preferred design has not been performed, or at least is not readily located in the course of a litera-ture search? This is perhaps the ultimate test of our *sure-footedness* in traversing the nooks and crannies of study design in relationship to clinical questions. We have discussed the concept of hierarchies of evidence in the context of evaluating with clinical recommendations as characteristically found in evidence-based practice guidelines.

Link to Page 221

The very same approach pertains when the ideal study design (i.e., the "highest level of evidence") is not available. We move down the hierarchy and consider the appropriateness of other types of study. There are several generic principles that pertain to this process.

- *Correct categorization:* First one needs to be sure that one has correctly categorized the question itself. For example, if a question regarding a diagnostic test pertains to its accuracy, a randomized trial will not provide the sought for information (see discussion above). It will be to no avail to move down the hierarchy of evidence that would pertain to questions of effectiveness of therapy. Such subsequent endeavors will have no greater chance of success than did the initial one.
- *Different hierarchies:* The hierarchy of study designs will be different for each type of clinical question.

Figure 13-10 demonstrates an appropriate and characteristic hierarchy for therapy questions. There are many variants of this hierarchy in the literature, some of them very elaborate; our version is consistent with most of them.

The hierarchy will implicitly be different for other types of question. Furthermore, there is more variability in how such hierarchies will be defined in different contexts. Figure 13-11 demonstrates possible hierarchical schemes for the four primary types of clinical question that is consistent with the foregoing discussion. There is substantially less consensus in the literature regarding the hierarchies corresponding to categories other than therapy.

Hierarchy of study design for questions of therapeutic effectiveness
Meta-analysis of randomized trials
Single randomized trial
Observational study
Retrospective case control study
Consecutive case series

— FIGURE 13-10 — *Standard hierarchy of study design pertaining to questions regarding the effectiveness of therapeutic interventions. The possible study types are listed in descending order of preference.*

Question type	Likely study designs
Therapy	Meta-analysis of randomized trials Randomized controlled trial Observational studies
Harm	Meta-analysis of randomized trials (for therapeutic interventions) Randomized trial (for therapeutic interventions) Prospective observational study with control group Population-based case control study
Diagnosis	Meta-analysis of cross-sectional analytic studies Cross-sectional analytic study Case-control study
Prognosis	Cohort study, prospective or retrospective Case control study

— FIGURE 13-11 — *An abbreviated hierarchy of study designs corresponding to the primary types of clinical questions. The "diagnosis" category assumes a question regarding accuracy of a diagnostic test. The hierarchy listed under "therapy" would also pertain to questions regarding the utility of a diagnostic test.*

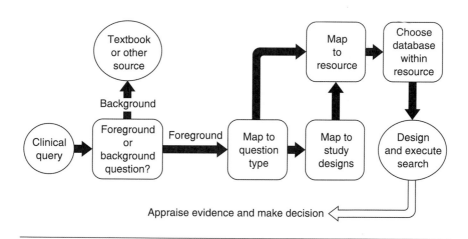

— FIGURE 13-12 — *A systematic approach to sorting and seeking clinical evidence about clinical questions. This figure should be compared to the one presented at the outset of the chapter; it may be seen as an expansion of the central portion of that figure.*[52]

SUMMARY

Armed with the concepts and tools outlined above, we are at the crossroads of our journey. We understand our foreground question and are ready to select a resource and do a search for the best clinical evidence pertaining to it. Figure 13-12 summarizes the process we have described in this chapter, including the initial distinction between background and foreground questions and extending through the issues to be discussed in the next section. For some questions, we can immediately select a resource that reflects selection, appraisal, and summary of the highest level studies for a question. For others we will need to think more carefully about our question and the preferred or likely study design before proceeding.

In the next chapter we discuss how different types of resources relate to different types of question and study design. This is an additional step that requires knowledge and experience. It is, however, all downhill from here. Heretofore we have had to deal with concepts and principles. The rest is just a matter of knowledge and learning; as doctors, we are quite used to accumulating this!

CHAPTER 14

SEARCHING FOR ANSWERS

PREFILTERED RESOURCES

We have selected a foreground question, put it into the PICO format, and identified the outcomes most important to our patients. We have determined whether the question has to do with therapy, harm, diagnosis, or prognosis, and we have decided on the kind of study that would be likely to constitute the *best-available evidence*. We are now ready to select a target resource and to plan our search.

Our first task is to decide whether a small, filtered, database is likely to contain the evidence we are seeking. If so, we may avoid the challenge of searching a huge database such as the 12 million or so citations of MEDLINE. Depending on the resource in question, we may be able to take advantage of a professionally performed critical appraisal of the evidence, further expediting the use of the evidence for our decisions. To be able to exercise such options effectively, we need to understand how the resources are created and which ones are most relevant to the questions that arise in our practice.

Some concepts and definitions are necessary to the understanding of resource options and of how to select them.

Concepts and Definitions

What is a Resource?
A *resource* is any source we turn to for information. This could be a friend, a consultant, a book, or notes from a course we took. In this section, we will use the term to specifically signify *an online source of any kind that we would consider using in the course of looking for clinical evidence on a foreground question.*

What is a Database?

A database can be conceived of as a searchable repository of items conforming to a predetermined rule of inclusion. This rule may be very broad and inclusive, such as:

- All of the articles published in the ~4000 biomedical journals indexed in MEDLINE.

It can be very narrow and selective, such as:

- Systematic reviews of randomized trials of effectiveness of therapeutic interventions performed under the auspices of the Cochrane Collaboration.

The latter rule defines the contents of the Cochrane Database of Systematic Reviews (CDSR).

A database is, by our definition, a resource. However a resource may encompass more than one database or may not include a database at all. The Cochrane Library, the periodic electronic publication of the Cochrane Collaboration, comprises a number of independent databases, of which the CDSR is only one.[27] Furthermore, some resources of potential utility in the answering of foreground questions neither are nor contain databases. *Clinical Evidence* is an example of such a resource.[28]

What is a Filter?

A filter is most clearly thought of as a rule of inclusion for defining a database. Strictly, the term might be considered to refer to a rule for systematically extracting citations otherwise included in a larger, parent database, into a smaller, subsidiary database. However, "filtered" databases are frequently generated independently of the creation of larger databases, even though the latter may independently include all of the same citations. The rule underlying the "filter" may pertain to clinical question type, study design, specialty area, or subspecialty area (Fig. 14-1).

The possible types of filtering are independent of each other. A resource may be largely restricted to issues of therapy but not strictly to study design. *Clinical Evidence* and UpToDate® are examples of such resources; they consider study types other than randomized trials. A database may be filtered by study design but not by question type. The Cochrane Controlled Trials Registry (CCTR) is an example. Although most randomized trials pertain to effectiveness of therapy, they may also be designed to test comparative utility of diagnostic tests, including screening tests, or the clinical impact of using a prediction rule. Hence the CCTR includes randomized trials that are relevant to questions other than therapy. Resources may be filtered for relevance to a particular specialty but not systematically for

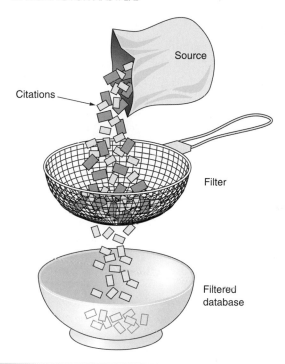

— FIGURE 14-1 — *A filter used to build a database. Bibliolographical citations originating from a well-defined source, which may itself be a database or simply a target set of biomedical journals, are passed through a set of rules for inclusion (filtered). The result is a subset of citations that fulfill the requirements of the rule, now organized into a structured database to facilitate and streamline retrieval.*

quality. *Emergency Medical Abstracts* is an example. The user of such a resource needs to know that the critical appraisal of the included articles remains to be performed.

Finally, resources evolve over time. *Clinical Evidence* is considering, and UpToDate® is already actively including, diagnostic questions within their summaries.

To summarize, the advantage of small, filtered, databases is that their use obviates the need for specialized searching skills. Their disadvantage is that the user needs to understand how the particular database is generated and to what kinds of questions and study designs it applies if time is not to be wasted in futile searches. When a resource contains multiple databases, the user needs to understand them individually in these ways to be able to maximize their value.

Now let's throw one final monkey wrench into the works.

Pre-appraised Resources

When a resource not only contains citations but also reflects the application of methodological standards for the included studies, it may be said to be *pre-appraised*. The appraisal may be performed at any of several stages.

The authors of *Clinical Evidence* perform the equivalent of a systematic review, without pooling of data, on the therapy questions they consider. They routinely search for systematic reviews as well as randomized trials on those questions and provide an estimate of the quality of the studies they find. Hence this resource offers a quality filter, critical appraisal, *and* summary of the evidence on their target questions.

ACP Journal Club publishes minimum standards required for studies of diagnosis, therapy, prognosis, systematic reviews, and other publication types to be included in their index. In addition, a subset of articles, selected as reflecting high clinical impact, undergoes a second, even more intensive quality review. For these, a critical appraisal and summary of the study, written by ACP Journal Club editors, is accompanied by a clinical commentary in the main body of the journal.

Well-performed systematic reviews also reflect an appraisal process. Only studies conforming to predetermined study designs, such as randomized trials, are included. The high-quality reviews done by the Cochrane Collaboration subject the included trials to an explicit set of methodological appraisal criteria and report the results of studies meeting those criteria separately.[29] As a result, readers can judge for themselves whether study quality affected the results.

Pre-appraised resources save time for the busy clinicians by relieving them of the burden of having to appraise the methodological quality of individual studies "from scratch."[30] Use of clinical evidence at the bedside is maximized when both the need for searching and for appraisal skills are minimized. The clinician can then maintain his or her concentration where it ultimately belongs: on the individual patient and on issues of the applicability of the evidence from research to the decisions at hand.

Why Filtered Resources?

Some readers' instincts may now be telling them that it should be easier just to use MEDLINE, or even Google, than to grapple with the complexity of smaller databases. We urge them to bear with us. The actual complexity is not that of the databases and resources; it stems from the challenges posed by the questions themselves. If you have accurately thought through what kind of question you are asking and what kind of study is likely to answer it, getting to know a few readily available databases will not add much more to the burden.

Searching Pre-appraised/Filtered Databases

A relatively small number of primary filtered databases are relevant to the foreground questions most commonly encountered by emergency physicians. Although we are not aware of a rigorous survey of the distribution of such questions in an actual practice setting, our experience in practicing and teaching emergency evidence-based medicine leads us to a few, challengeable conclusions:

- As emergency physicians, we seem to be primarily involved with matters of diagnosis and therapy, and to a lesser extent with prognosis questions.
- We are involved with harm issues largely as downsides of the therapeutic interventions we offer to our patients.
- We are particularly interested in clinical prediction rules.
- Our practice overlaps that of every other specialty, albeit in different degrees. However, our context and priorities are unique.

Few electronic resources and databases have been developed specifically to meet the needs of emergency physicians. This is a frontier development area for our specialty. As a result, we are forced into the role of *scavengers*. In other areas of our practice, such as emergency airway management and ultrasound skills, we have *parasitized* and adapted resources and technologies developed within the cultures of other specialties. The use of online resources to inform emergency practice follows the same principle. We ultimately need to develop our own specialized resources; until then we must adapt resources developed for use in overlapping specialties for our own use. The following is a summary of the most relevant resource options for emergency physicians in search of evidence.[28]

ACP Journal Club

ACP Journal Club began in 1991 as a supplement to the *Annals of Internal Medicine* and is currently published independently on a bimonthly basis. It is available by subscription from the American College of Physicians. A closely related journal, *Evidence-Based Medicine*, was initiated in 1995 and is currently published by *BMJ*. Both journals are available electronically, and much of the content of the two journals is issued as a compendium on CD-ROM called *Best Evidence*. Approximately half of the entries in *ACP Journal Club* are common to the two journals. *ACP Journal Club* largely reflects an internal medicine perspective, while *Evidence-Based Medicine* maintains a somewhat broader clinical focus. Analogous "meta-journals" exist in other specialty areas under the auspices of various publishers and include *Evidence-Based*

Cardiovascular Medicine, *Evidence-Based Mental Health*, and *Evidence-Based Nursing*.

ACP Journal Club may be considered the prototype of a pre-appraised source of clinical evidence. One hundred and twenty-five target journals are regularly hand searched. Primary research reports and systematic reviews conforming to specific types of clinical questions, and which meet a predefined set of minimum quality criteria, are selected for inclusion. Articles of high clinical impact are provided with critical abstracts and commentaries by *ACP Journal Club* editors and consultants.

The criteria used for selection and appraisal of articles included in *ACP Journal Club* are very similar to those to be found in the *Users' Guides to the Medical Literature* for the respective study types.[31] However, clinical impact plays an important role in determining whether an article that meets the quality standards makes it into the front of the journal with abstract and commentary. The other eligible articles are included as non-abstracted citations in the database. Studies published prior to 1991 will not be found in *ACP Journal Club*.

While we can be fairly confident that *ACP Journal Club* will provide quality-screened evidence on topics of high clinical impact to *internists*, we need to be mindful of its specialty focus and of certain other limitations. The methodological standards for inclusion of some study types of key significance to emergency physicians, such as studies of performance of diagnostic tests, may be so high as to exclude studies of clinical importance to our specialty. Nonetheless, when we are seeking evidence on therapy questions that overlap internal medicine and emergency medicine practice, we will frequently find *ACP Journal Club* useful. Further, the online summaries are of sufficient quality to obviate the need to consult the full text of the original articles.

Clinical Evidence

Clinical Evidence is useful for issues of therapy that intersect with the practice of internal medicine. It is available online by subscription through the *BMJ* publishers. It presents systematically assembled, qualitative syntheses of evidence pertaining to specific clinical questions within defined topic areas. Over 1200 questions are addressed in over 19 sections, organized by organ system. Although currently limited to questions of therapy, as of this writing, *Clinical Evidence* is in the process of developing a protocol for dealing with diagnosis questions as well.

The syntheses in *Clinical Evidence* stop short of rigorous systematic reviews and meta-analyses. However, the methodology used by the authors is structured, explicit, and involves a systematic search for randomized trials and systematic reviews in multiple databases as well as a methodological appraisal of the included studies. Many advisors and contributors are also involved with the Cochrane Collaboration. The resource is organized around foreground questions within the clinical topic areas; this lends a further appeal to the busy clinician.

Clinical Evidence may be particularly useful to emergency physicians in connection with questions involving therapy or harm in areas related to internal medicine practice when multiple studies render impractical a primary critical appraisal at the point of care. In such situations, an unsuccessful search of the Cochrane Database of Systematic Reviews might be followed by a search of *Clinical Evidence*.

UpToDate®

UpToDate® is an online textbook with some features characteristic of an evidence-based resource. It is particularly liked by residents because it is a very quick source of background information in a user-friendly format. Specific recommendations are linked to abstracts of primary studies via citations. Like *Clinical Evidence*, UpToDate® reflects an internal medicine orientation. The focus is largely on therapy questions, but recently it has begun to address diagnosis issues as well. A full-time staff of methodologically trained editors contributes to the quality of this resource. However, although efficient and easy to use for background questions, UpToDate® is substantially less explicit than *Clinical Evidence* in identifying the relevant foreground questions and the evidence pertaining to them.

The Cochrane Library

As mentioned previously, the Cochrane Library is made up of multiple databases, three of which are particularly useful to emergency physicians.[27]

The Library is available by subscription, either via CD-ROM or online, to individuals and to institutions. It is a useful source of systematic reviews and randomized trials on issues of therapy and prevention.

CDSR

As of Issue 3, 2005 of the Cochrane Library, the Cochrane Database of Systematic Reviews (CDSR) included over 2400 reviews, constituting rigorous syntheses of evidence on questions of therapy and prevention. Protocols of an additional 1600 reviews are posted for completion within the next 2–3 years. Abstracts, but not the full texts, of the reviews included in the CDSR are available via free access. A survey published in 2002 found that 18% of reviews included in the CDSR were directly or indirectly relevant to emergency practice.[32]

DARE

The Database of Abstracts of Reviews of Effectiveness (DARE) is another database within the Cochrane Library. It is made up of over 5300 structured summaries and appraisals of systematic reviews published in standard biomedical journals. The resource is available for free access independently of the Cochrane Library at www.york.ac.uk/inst/crd/darehp.htm. The critical abstracts obviate the need for the user to consult the full text of the parent review. The resource is, in this respect, analogous to *ACP Journal Club*.

CCTR

The Cochrane Controlled Trials Register (CCTR) currently includes 450,000 citations and is the largest such registry in existence. A quick search of the CCTR is the fastest single way of determining whether a question has been studied by means of a randomized trial. This, together with the CDSR and the DARE database, make the Cochrane Library a reasonable first choice for the emergency clinician seeking evidence regarding a question pertaining to therapy, prevention, or to any issue for which a randomized trial would constitute a preferred and likely study design.

Emergency Medical Abstracts

Emergency Medical Abstracts (EMA) is a product developed and marketed by subscription for use by both emergency clinicians and academics for the purpose of keeping up to date with literature in our specialty. *EMA* is available both on a CD-ROM version and online. The search engines of the two versions differ and users must become familiar with the idiosyncrasies of their own preferred mode of access.

As of 2005, EMA comprised two databases totalling over 160,000 citations extending back to 1977. The resource is drawn from the English language journals indexed in *Current Contents* (www.isinet.com/products/cap/ccc/), corresponding to a target set of up to 1120 peer-reviewed medical journals. *Current Contents* allows the titles of all abstracts of this journal set to be periodically screened. Citations of articles perceived to be relevant to emergency medicine are identified and included in the EMA database.

Forty articles per month are selected from the parent set and are included in a separate database of abstracted citations. The two databases overlap substantially, with the non-abstracted database of *EMA* encompassing most of the total resource. In practice, an effective search of *EMA* for articles relevant to a particular topic or question may require separate searches of both the abstracted and non-abstracted databases.

Although filtered for relevance to emergency medicine, the citations included in *Emergency Medical Abstracts* have not been systematically screened for study design, nor have they been critically appraised. Users must therefore be prepared to undertake a critical appraisal of the results of a search on their own.

Emergency Medical Abstracts is a particularly suitable choice when the user is searching for evidence on a question relevant to emergency medicine not involving an issue of therapy or prevention. For example, as mentioned above, *ACP Journal Club* imposes a relatively high quality standard for inclusion of studies of diagnostic test performance and clinical decision rules. Failure to find a relevant study pertaining to such questions in *ACP Journal Club*, even if relevant to both emergency medicine and internal medicine, should prompt a search of *EMA* prior to diving into the huge MEDLINE database or to giving up the effort. Weak evidence also supports the use of *EMA* as a first-line resource for all emergency medicine questions.[9]

Cumulative Index to Nursing & Allied Health Literature

CINAHL is an independent database of citations related to nursing and other allied health practice areas. It is not, strictly speaking, a "filtered" database. However, it is of potential usefulness to emergency physicians seeking answers to questions pertaining to out-of-hospital care and quality issues in emergency medicine. The contents date from 1982 and are not formally restricted by question type, study design, or specialty. It is not a pre-appraised resource.

PubMed's Clinical Queries

Clinical Queries is an evidence-based search program that is an included feature of the PubMed access to the large MEDLINE database. We will describe it below when we address approaches to searching large databases.

Link to Page 306

Choosing a Suitable Filtered Resource

Having summarized the characteristics of the most important filtered resources of use to emergency physicians, Fig. 14-1 summarizes their relationship to specific types of questions and study designs. Figure 14-2 summarizes the characteristics of the resources we have reviewed.

From Figs 14-1 and 14-2 we can derive rules of thumb that might guide our efforts to locate evidence on clinical questions in a quick and efficient manner. A few such rules are summarized below.

A Therapy Question

- Check the Cochrane Library unless you are quite sure that no controlled trial has been done on the question.
- If you think a lot of trials have been performed, check the CDSR and DARE first. Otherwise check the CCTR.

A

Question type	Best feasible study designs	Suitable filtered databases
Therapy	RCT* or systematic review of RCT's	ACP journal club, clinical evidence, up-to-date, Cochrane library, emergency medical abstracts, clinical queries[†]
Diagnosis[‡]	Cross-sectional analytic study comparing test results to a criterion standard in symptomatic patients	ACP journal club, up-to-date, emergency medical abstracts, clinical queries[†]
Harm	RCT, cohort study, population-based case control study	ACP journal club, Cochrane library, clinical evidence, up-to-date, emergency medical abstracts, clinical queries[†]
Prognosis	Cohort study, placebo arm of RCT	ACP journal club, emergency medical abstracts, clinical queries[†]

B

Resource	Quality filtered	Pre-synthesized	Question types	Specialty orientation
Cochrane library -CDSR -DARE -CCTR	✓ ✓	✓ ✓	Therapy[+]	All
ACP journal club (1991-present)	✓		All	Internal medicine, some pediatrics
Clinical evidence	✓		Therapy	Internal medicine
Up-to-date			Therapy, some diagnosis	Internal medicine
Emergency medical abstracts (1977-present)			All	Emergency medicine
PubMed clinical queries	✓		All	All

— FIGURE 14-2 — *A Grid demonstrating the study designs associated with the common types of clinical question and the filtered resources most likely to yield relevant clinical evidence.*
*RCT = randomized controlled trial
†PubMed's Clinical Queries
‡"Diagnosis questions" refers here to questions regarding the performance of diagnostic tests as measured by sensitivity, specificity, or likelihood ratios.
B Characteristics of specific databases in a fashion that facilitates their use by emergency physicians. Resources limited to evidence published more recently than 1966 are identified by the relevant dates of inclusion in parentheses under the first column. Systematic reviews of studies of diagnostic test performance are included in the DARE database and randomized trials investigating the utility of diagnostic test are included in CCTR.

- If you think that no controlled trial has been done and the question overlaps internal medicine and is fairly important, try UpToDate® or *Clinical Evidence*, otherwise turn to *Emergency Medical Abstracts*.

A Diagnosis Question

If you are asking a question about the performance of a diagnostic test:

- Consider *ACP Journal Club* if it overlaps internal medicine practice and is high profile (like d-dimer for venous thromboembolism).
- Otherwise try *Emergency Medical Abstracts* or PubMed's *Clinical Queries*.
- If you think there are a lot of relevant studies, search DARE within the Cochrane Library. This database, but not the CDSR, includes systematic reviews of studies of diagnostic test performance.

If you are asking a question about the effect of using a diagnostic test on the process of care, or on patient-important outcomes,[33] then treat the question as if it were a therapy question. Look in:

- The full Cochrane Library
- *ACP Journal Club* if it is a high-profile internal medicine issue
- *Emergency Medical Abstracts* if it is not.

A quick review of Figure 13-9 may solidify your grasp of the different kinds of diagnosis questions.

A Harm Question

This is perhaps the most challenging category to match to a resource as different kinds of harm questions can be approached with very different kinds of studies. Let's consider two cases.

We are concerned about a harmful effect of a therapeutic intervention   If we think there are large trials that went on for a reasonable length of time and the effect is not very rare, a randomized trial might give us the answer we are looking for. In this case the Cochrane Library would be a good choice. If these conditions are not met, we need to look for an observational study.

- If it is an internal medicine question, consider *ACP Journal Club*, *Clinical Evidence* or UpToDate®.
- If it is not a question of interest to internists, *Emergency Medical Abstracts* or PubMed's *Clinical Queries* are our best choices.

We are concerned about a harmful effect of a non-therapeutic exposure   In this case, a randomized trial is pretty much ruled-out and the Cochrane Library will not help us. Since the question is also not related to a therapy question, *Clinical Evidence* and UpToDate® will not be useful. *ACP Journal Club, Emergency Medical Abstracts* or PubMed's *Clinical Queries* are our best bets, depending on the specialty area and the level of clinical impact.

A Prognosis Question

Once more, we need to decide what kind of study design is most likely. Most prognosis studies are observational. Occasionally a randomized trial may go on long enough for the placebo arm to serve as the equivalent of such a study. In emergency medicine, we are frequently concerned with very short-term outcomes. For us, therefore, the placebo arm of a randomized trial may provide the answer to many prognosis questions.

For all other prognosis questions, *ACP Journal Club, Emergency Medical Abstracts* or PubMed's *Clinical Queries* are the best targets, once again depending on the specialty orientation and impact.

Summary

If we have accurately thought through our question and have decided on the appropriate study type most likely to have been performed, the above rules of thumb should rapidly guide us to appropriate clinical evidence, assuming it exists. If this approach fails, and we are still determined to seek such evidence, or if we do not have access to the appropriate filtered resource, we have no choice but to plunge into the world of large biomedical databases.

MEDLINE AND OTHER LARGE DATABASES

Large databases such as MEDLINE have been the mainstay of electronic literature searching since the dawn of the cyber age. The advantages of such sources are their inclusiveness and established familiarity. They are what our librarian will turn to, should we request professional help with a search. We propose only the selective use of large databases, restricting their use to the questions for which they are uniquely suited. We anticipate that, as time goes on, clinicians will turn to them for fewer and fewer queries.

MEDLINE

MEDLINE is familiar, comprehensive and accessible. It became available on the Internet almost 20 years before the Internet itself became available to most individuals via the World Wide Web. It constitutes an electronic form of what prior to 1966 existed only as a paper resource called *Index Medicus*. It encompasses over 4000 biomedical journals on an issue by issue basis and currently includes over 12 million citations.

There is a greater than 50% chance that a study relevant to your question, if it has been published anywhere in the world since 1966, is in the MEDLINE database. Finally, MEDLINE is available freely without a subscription anywhere in the world via PubMed.

While also an asset, the principal disadvantage of large databases is their size. Imagine looking through 12 million items for anything at all. Even an elephant might be hard to find among 12 million rabbits. Now consider having to use not your eyes or ears but rather words and names. The richness of the English language, with its density of synonyms, works against us when we have to guess the name that someone else may have used in the title or abstract of an article.

MeSH Headings

The MEDLINE database, located at the National Library of Medicine (NLM), is structured using an elaborate indexing framework, referred to as the Medical Subject Heading (MeSH) system. This system helps eliminate much of the guesswork otherwise inherent in medical nomenclature by linking a broad array of synonyms to standardized MeSH terms within a searchable hierarchy of topics. Indexers at the NLM scan each journal article before it is entered into the database in order to assign the MeSH terms most appropriate to the topic, study design, and other aspects of the article. This allows a search program to connect many of the synonyms we might enter into the search line to the common standardized MeSH term.

However, even when sophisticated indexing is combined with expert training and experience, the challenge of finding a given article in MEDLINE may be formidable. A study performed in 1990, in which expert librarians performed searches aimed at finding articles included within a target set, found that the highest percentage of target citations found by any two of them was 33%.[34] Although search technologies have become more sophisticated in the last 15 years, the size of the MEDLINE database itself has nearly doubled in that period of time (Fig. 14-3). Hence, even in the best hands, non-exhaustive searches of MEDLINE still have a high likelihood of missing relevant articles.

Busy clinicians in search of clinical evidence are concerned not only with finding the best relevant evidence but also with avoiding the need to sift through large numbers of irrelevant citations in the process of answering questions. Borrowing terminology familiar to us from our discussions of diagnostic test performance, we may consider the "sensitivity" of a search

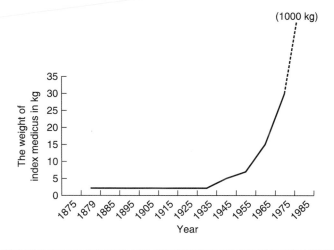

— FIGURE 14-3 —   *The weight of the Index Medicus (the printed forerunner of MEDLINE) through the years.*[53]

strategy to constitute the proportion of relevant articles in the target database that it identifies. We may then consider its "specificity" to constitute the proportion of irrelevant articles in the target database that are excluded by the same search. Low search specificity therefore means a lot of irrelevant articles amongst our hits.

When librarians or researchers use exhaustive protocols to search MEDLINE, their results can have high sensitivity. Such searches are done in the context of preparing original research projects or systematic reviews. Characteristically, an investigator doing a systematic review or other original study is prepared to sort through several thousand citations emerging from a MEDLINE search, to assure they do not miss even one important and relevant prior study. In other words, such a user must be prepared to accept a very low "specificity" in exchange for high "sensitivity" when a large database is used as the target resource.

How well can MEDLINE perform in the context of the kind of searches that busy clinicians do in the course of pursuing focused clinical questions? Haynes et al. used a structured protocol similar to that used by researchers developing a diagnostic test, to develop and validate MEDLINE search strategies for locating high-quality evidence pertaining to the primary question types (therapy, diagnosis, prognosis and harm).[35] They identified a criterion set of articles from a predetermined target set of journals and measured the sensitivity and specificity of various search strategies. They achieved a maximum sensitivity of 99% in locating articles on therapy, and 80–90% sensitivity for studies pertaining to the other question types. Specificities ranged from 72% for harm to 98% for therapy.

These results are impressive and the strategies developed by Haynes et al. have since been incorporated into several MEDLINE search programs, including PubMed's *Clinical Queries*. However, it is important to realize that the high performance on therapy questions may still fall short of that achievable through use of the Cochrane Controlled Trial Registry (CCTR) for locating randomized trials on a question. Furthermore, a "specificity" of 72% may correspond to hundreds of irrelevant citations when the full MEDLINE database of 12 million citations is searched.

For these reasons, we advise that MEDLINE be considered primarily for situations in which the clinician is very intent on finding an answer to a question, is quite sure that a study is likely to exist, and has failed to locate relevant studies through the use of available filtered resources.

EXAMPLE

As an example, let us return to the foreground questions that emerged from our original scenario regarding our patient with dyspnea. The first and last questions point to diagnosis questions for which filtered resources would be appropriate. The fourth question pertains to a harm issue which, because it is wedded to issues of therapy, would also invite the use of filtered resources. This leaves the second and third questions:

Does this patient have a pulmonary embolus? To an evidence-literate clinician, this question suggests a quest for a clinical prediction rule that could identify this patient's likelihood of pulmonary embolus, given the findings resulting from clinical evaluation. Such an instrument exists.[36] Although prediction rules are included in *ACP Journal Club* and in *Emergency Medical Abstracts*, rather than wasting time in searching limited databases that may not contain the studies we are after, we may turn to MEDLINE for this question.

What are the possible causes of this patient's dyspnea? One could consult a textbook or a non-structured review for a summary of possible causes of dyspnea; but there may actually be foreground evidence pertaining to this question.[5] If we suspect the latter possibility and are therefore inclined to define it as a foreground question, we are again faced with important uncertainty regarding the likelihood of relevant evidence being included in our preferred filtered databases. Again we may reasonably be inclined to choose MEDLINE as our resource.

■ EMBASE

EMBASE is a European database corresponding to *Excerpta Medica* indexes. These indexes are independent of the *Index Medicus* upon which MEDLINE is based. EMBASE currently contains upwards of 9 million citations, making it comparable in size to MEDLINE.[37] There is about 30% overlap between the 3800 journals indexed in EMBASE and those indexed in MEDLINE.

EMBASE, unlike MEDLINE, is not available for free access, but it will usually be accessible to clinicians through the libraries of their medical centers. For this reason it is less useful for the purpose of rapid searching for clinical evidence. Clinicians need to be aware of it as an option when they are doing comprehensive searches for specific projects such as development of clinical pathways for their hospitals. They will then almost certainly be engaging the services of a research librarian.

■ Original Search Strategies for Large Databases

The MEDLINE indexing system developed under the auspices of the National Library of Medicine is as complex and sophisticated as the database itself is large. To master it fully is far beyond what can reasonably expected of a busy clinician. A few basic concepts can allow us to undertake straightforward searches with a fair degree of surety. We present these here and refer the reader to other sources for a description of the more sophisticated aspects of the total resource.[10,37,38]

Choosing the Search Terms

Which search terms should we select when using a large database? This depends on how much research has been done in connection with the disease entity in question. When we are dealing with a relatively uncommon condition, the *name of the disease* itself may be a reasonable choice; this may hold for common conditions as well.

A search of MEDLINE 1966 to January 2005 with the OVID interface using the single term "burns" and limited to randomized trials yields a total of 467 hits. Restricting the search using the term "acute" reduces the yield to a grand total of 47 citations. When a lot of research has been done on the clinical entity in question (e.g., asthma), and the intervention is quite specific to that entity (e.g., ipratropium), then the intervention is a better choice of search term.

MeSH Terms versus Text Terms

The system of medical subject headings (MeSH) was developed by the NLM as a way of streamlining searching of the large database. The user needs to understand that a MeSH term is *assigned* to an article at the time that it is entered into the index. The term itself may not appear in either the title or abstract of an article to which it is assigned. However, the user is relieved of the task of guessing which of the many possible synonyms the author chose to use in a study.

Text terms are terms that actually appear in either the title or abstract of relevant articles. Searching for text words bypasses the indexing process. This may be efficient when we are very sure that a particular word is likely to occur in the abstracts of the relevant studies.

EXAMPLE

We have a question concerning a patient with right upper-quadrant pain, for which studies focusing on either biliary colic or cholecystitis may be relevant. There are many possible terms that might be chosen by authors of relevant studies, including "biliary colic," "cholecystitis," cholelithiasis," "gallstones," "cholecystolithiasis," and "choledoco-lithiasis." Even if we could be sure of anticipating all of these possible terms, including them all would render the resulting search strategy formidably complex. By using the MeSH system, we can quickly determine that most (but not all) of these terms can be encompassed by a single term, "biliary tract diseases" (see "Exploding and Focusing MeSH Terms" below).

Use of either MeSH or text terms involves guesswork. In either case we have to guess which term, among many possible terms, someone else might have used to refer to a common entity or concept. The MeSH term "biliary tract diseases" does not include the term "gallstones"; the latter is an independent term within the MeSH system.

MeSH coding can also be idiosyncratic. An article on predicting outcome in patients presenting to emergency departments in pulmonary edema was originally coded under the MeSH term "edema."[39] This made it almost impossible to find using the MeSH system. The author's idiosyncratic use of the term "triage" in their title made it difficult to find it using text terms without an inordinately broad strategy that would have yielded thousands of hits.

To be sure of not missing important articles, we advise users of MEDLINE to consider use of both broad MeSH terms and also text terms that authors would find hard to avoid using in the abstracts of their articles.

Exploding and Focusing MeSH Terms

MeSH terms are organized into an extensive tree. Figure 14-4 illustrates a small excerpt of the tree pertaining to our example.

By selecting a MeSH heading and including all subsidiary headings, we can search for articles that have been indexed under all those headers at the time of entry into the database. This is called *exploding* the original term.

Virtually all MEDLINE search programs provide for the ability to explode MeSH terms. We can, at the same time, choose to *focus* the search to the exploded MeSH term. This instructs the search program to select only those articles for which any of the relevant MeSH terms have been identified by the indexers as of *central importance* to the subject of the article. Using these functions, we can therefore maximize both the sensitivity and specificity of MeSH terms for finding articles relevant to our question.

Natural Language Searching

It is important to be aware of an emerging search technology that may ultimately surpass the framework of MeSH and text search terms. This is most commonly referred to as *natural language search technology* It was originally developed by Aries Knowledge Finder (www.kfinder.com/newweb). Natural language searching allows the entry of phrases or entire questions in a form that we would conventionally use, without consideration of MEDLINE indexing techniques. Variations of the natural language approach have been adopted by some other MEDLINE programs including PubMed and are under development by commercial MEDLINE vendors such as OVID.

```
┌─────────────────────────────────────┐
│  All MeSH categories                 │
│     - - - - - - - - - - - - - - -    │
│       - - - - - - - - - - - - - - -  │
│     Diseases category                │
│       - - - - - - - - - - - - - - -  │
│         - - - - - - - - - - - - - - -│
│        Digestive system diseases     │
│        Biliary tract diseases        │
│        Gallbladder diseases          │
│        Cholecystitis                 │
│        Cholelithiasis                │
└─────────────────────────────────────┘
```

— FIGURE 14-4 — *An excerpt from the Medical Subject Heading (MeSH) tree structure. The tree encompasses "Cholecystitis" under "Digestive System Diseases."*

Limiting and Narrowing a Search

To avoid having to wade through hundreds, or even thousands, of articles in the course of a search, busy clinicians need to know how to restrict it to the citations most likely to be relevant. There are two ways of doing this. We can add more search terms or we can impose direct limits. The first option entails knowledge of *operators*.

Using Boolean Operators

Don't be intimidated by the fancy terms *operator* and *Boolean*. The latter comes from set theory and corresponds to a very simple principle. If we take a look at Fig. 14-5, we can see why connecting two search terms by the operator "AND" limits the search to include only articles identified by both of them. Conversely, when we connect them by the operator "OR," it expands the search to include articles identified by either of the terms.

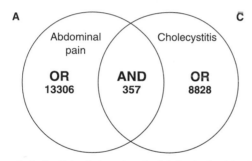

'A' = set of all articles indexed under 'abdominal pain' = 13306 + 357   = 13663 citations
'C' = set of all articles indexed under 'cholecystitis' = 8828 + 357   = 9185 citations
Total hits using 'OR'   = 13306 + 357 + 8828 = 22491 citations
Total hits using 'AND'   = 357 citations

— FIGURE 14-5 — *Illustrating the effect of 'operator' terms 'AND' and 'OR' using a Boolean diagram. Circles 'A' and 'C' are sets including all the citations in the MEDLINE database indexed under 2 different terms. Set A includes 13663 articles indexed under the exploded MeSH term 'Abdominal Pain' and set C includes 9185 articles indexed under the exploded MeSH term 'Cholecystitis'. The area of intersection of the 2 sets includes 357 articles identified by both MeSH terms. Connecting the 2 MeSH terms by the 'operator' AND restricts the search to this area at the intersection of the circles. The area of the 2 sets lying outside the area of intersection corresponds to articles identified by one or the other, but not both, of the MeSH terms. A search connecting the 2 MeSH terms by the 'operator' 'OR' will identify 22491 citations, including those lying outside the area of intersection and those lying within it. The search of MEDLINE used exploded forms of the 2 terms over all citations from 1966–2004.*

Operator terms are universal to the search programs connected to most online databases; some programs may require that they be capitalized.

The use of AND and OR pertains to all categories of search terms, including MeSH terms and text terms. Hence, by adding new search terms to a search, we can effectively expand or contract the number of citations we find, depending upon which operator term we choose to connect them. If we have too many hits, then we can add a new term and connect it using AND; if we have too few, we can connect the new term using OR.

Built-in Limits

The second way of limiting a search is to use direct *limits* built into the search program. Available limits include age ranges of the patients, year and language of publication, journal subsets, and elements of study design. We will almost certainly want to employ some of these limits (particularly year of publication) in most of our searches for relevant and up to date clinical evidence.

Medline Quality Filters

A special type of limit has to do with study design. We can create our own *quality filter* in the course of a search for evidence on a therapy question, by restricting our search to the publication type "randomized controlled trial."

Even more powerful are the quality filters developed by Haynes et al.[35] and described above. They are available as *single-click* search strategies on a number of MEDLINE programs, including PubMed and OVID. If one of these is available and applicable, we only need to plug in a few terms specific to our question, decide on how far back in time we wish to go, and use the quality filter to have a reasonable chance of finding relevant evidence, if it exists.[38] If using the PubMed program, a truly appealing option exists in the form of *Clinical Queries*.

PubMed's *Clinical Queries*

The *Clinical Queries* program within the free-access MEDLINE package of the National Library of Medicine deserves special mention. It is based upon the validated quality filters developed for questions regarding therapy, harm, diagnosis, and prognosis.[35] The user selects the question type and also indicates whether "sensitivity" (minimizing missing important articles) or "specificity" (minimizing irrelevant articles) is to be prioritized. The user can also select "systematic reviews" as the preferred publication type under any of the clinical question categories.

Clinical Queries frequently rivals the performance of filtered databases such as *ACP Journal Club* in accuracy and efficiency. Analogous applications have been adopted by other MEDLINE search packages, including that of OVID.

Summary of Tips for Searching Large Databases

Transferring Strategies

If we have access to more than one large database, such as EMBASE, we need to be aware that search terms and strategies may perform somewhat differently from how they perform on MEDLINE. Guidelines for EMBASE and other databases may be found in McKibbon et al.[37]

"Sensitivity" versus "Specificity"

When beginning to do searches, busy clinicians are most concerned with efficiency and may perceive even as few as 50 or so hits to be more than they have time to peruse in order to find an answer. As clinicians gain experience, particularly with the challenges posed by MEDLINE, they frequently come to the conclusion that it is better to spend a little extra time looking through a few more citations than it is to waste *all* of the time, and come to a false conclusion that there is no good evidence, as a result of an overly narrow search. Our inclination is therefore to start out with a fairly broad strategy and to narrow the search judiciously until 100 citations or fewer are left to scan. We also find that we get better at the rapid screening of citations for relevance as time goes on.

Start with a Few Maximized Terms

You should pick a small number of strategic terms that go to the heart of the question. You can then maximize them, using both exploded MeSH terms, if they exist, and text terms. By adding strategic qualifying terms such as "acute" or the MeSH term "Emergency Service, Hospital," you increase your chances of finding applicable studies. Finally, restrict your search by applying quality filters and limiting to an appropriate range of publication dates and patient ages.

If you used PICO to format your question, you will no doubt wind up with a large array of potential search terms. Do *not* expect to use very many of these in your actual search; that is not the main point of PICO.

Consider the Likelihood of Relevant Studies

Consider the likelihood of relevant studies. If there is a small likelihood that many studies exist, use a very broad search. Frequently, a single clinical identifier combined with "randomized controlled trial" will yield only a handful of studies. Sometimes, it pays to start only with the clinical term, even in MEDLINE, if primary research is unlikely.

Scan before narrowing

If your first search yields a large number of citations, take a quick look to see if they are at all relevant before narrowing. If they are very distant from what you are looking for, revise the search using different terms, rather than attempting to narrow what you have. If you find one article that is related among many that are not, many programs will provide an option to "find similar articles to this one." It is worth trying.

Access Packages to Large Databases

A common point of confusion on the part of clinicians learning to search electronic databases is the distinction between a *target database* itself and the *program* used to access and search it. For example, as we already mentioned, MEDLINE constitutes a database comprised of all citations included in *Index Medicus*. The latter source was first converted into an electronic resource in the mid 1970s; 1966 was arbitrarily established as the earliest date of publication accepted into it.*

Many programs and software packages have been developed over the years as means of accessing and searching the MEDLINE database. One of these, PubMed, was developed under the auspices of the custodian of the database itself, the National Library of Medicine, and is available free, online, to anyone who has Internet access. Other access packages are available only by subscription. The OVID package is priced out of the range of individual subscription and is only marketed to institutions.

If one imagines a database to be the electronic equivalent of a large warehouse, then the different access packages and search programs used to find things in the warehouse are like different forklifts used to retrieve the warehouse's contents (Fig. 14-6A).

The user needs to understand that, by switching from one resource product such as PubMed to a different one such as OVID, we are simply using different forklifts to bring the contents to us (Fig. 14-6B).

Beginners frequently misconstrue such a switch to constitute the equivalent of looking into a new warehouse. One would need to switch to a different database, such as EMBASE, for this to be true.

This distinction is made slightly more complex by the fact that a single product may in fact provide access to multiple different databases. OVID, for example, can provide access not only to MEDLINE but also to EMBASE, the Cochrane Library, *Clinical Evidence*, *ACP Journal Club* and other databases (Fig. 14-7). OVID can provide full text access to a large number of biomedical journals. The health science library of your institution

---

*Since then, efforts have begun to extend MEDLINE backwards in time. *Old* MEDLINE currently includes sporadic citations dating back as far as 1958.

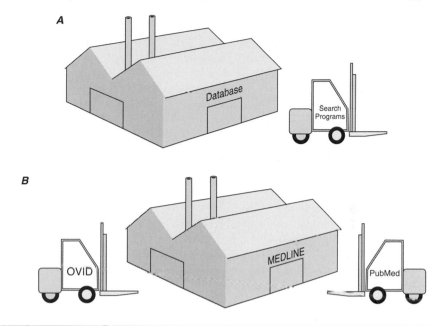

— FIGURE 14-6 — *A We can think of databases as warehouses and search programs as forklifts.* **B** *Both the OVID forklift and the PubMed forklift access the same MEDLINE warehouse.*

may subscribe to all or to only some of these options within the OVID package.

The search engines provided by different access programs perform differently even when applied to the same database, and it is important to know some of the differences. Some MEDLINE access programs automatically connect terms entered into the search to relevant MeSH terms. Some treat such terms as text terms and require a separate application to connect to the MeSH system. Terms entered into a MEDLINE search on OVID are automatically linked to a selection of possible MeSH terms which can, in turn, be selected, exploded and/or focused by the user. The same menu also lists the terms entered by the user as "keywords." It is important for the user to know that the keyword will treat the term as both a MeSH term and as a text term. Hence the broadest use of a single term using OVID will be achieved using the "keyword" option, not the exploded MeSH terms. On other programs, "keyword" may designate text terms only.

Another thing to be aware of when using packages such as OVID is that your institution's version may include only selected components of the resources offered. For example, although OVID offers three databases

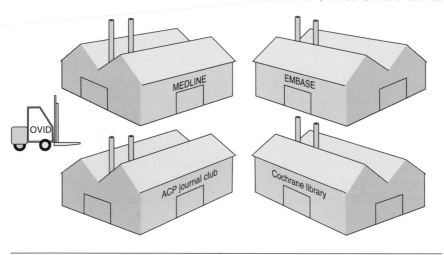

— FIGURE 14-7 —   *The OVID forklift can also access many different warehouses, in addition to MEDLINE.*

from the Cochrane Library, the Cochrane Library also includes databases pertaining to methodology and health technology that are not included in OVID. Similarly, of the full *ACP Journal Club* database, OVID offers only the high-clinical-impact articles for which *ACP Journal Club* publishes abstracts and commentaries, not the larger database of *all* articles from the target journals that pass the initial quality filter.

Full Text Access

Beginners are also commonly confused by the fact that some packages that include MEDLINE also include full text access to many articles. The MEDLINE database itself includes only the citations and the abstracts (when they exist) of indexed articles. When more than this is available through a MEDLINE access program, it has been added by the proprietor. Some biomedical journals are themselves available online via free access and are not restricted to subscribers. PubMed takes advantage of this and provides links from MEDLINE citations to the full text when it is available by free access. OVID offers full text access to a substantial number of journals with which it has contracted. Health science libraries that subscribe to OVID may or may not choose to purchase OVID's full text access package. Such libraries may also purchase online access directly from journals or from other online vendors. In no case is full text access a part of MEDLINE per se.

Additional Summary Points

- Get good at one or two MEDLINE programs: We advise clinicians to learn what they need to know about MEDLINE searching in connection with one, or at most two access programs. These might best be the one that your own institution's health sciences library offers, and PubMed for use when the former is not available.
- Be prepared for surprises: Access programs will perform differently, even when supplied by the same vendor. A good example is *Emergency Medical Abstracts*. This resource is supplied in offline, CD-ROM, and online Internet versions; the search programs for these versions perform differently. If we elect to use both routes of access, we need to be prepared for surprises that will occur when the same search term performs differently on the two versions.
- Full text access is an add-on: Get to know what journals your health sciences library or hospital has available online, to save time and trees.

INTERNET RESOURCES

If clinical evidence is to be used in clinical decision-making at the bedside, speed of access is paramount. Sackett found that evidence was used most frequently during ward rounds when its sources could be located within *eleven seconds* of asking the question, and that uptake decreased significantly when access time increased to 90 seconds.[40]

Internet Search Engines

Residents and attendings are well aware of this when they turn to quick-access resources such as UpToDate®, which provide comprehensive information while requiring virtually no search skills. More and more, they are turning directly to the Internet and to search engines such as Google (www.Google.com).

How good are search engines at finding good evidence? The quick answer is that nobody knows for sure. A rigorous trial comparing the performance of Google to that of conventional biomedical resources in finding a target set of high-quality evidence pertaining to a variety of predetermined clinical questions has not been published as of our writing. It is easy to convince ourselves that Google allows us to find something pertaining to almost any question that we might have, in not much more than 11 seconds. Google searches commonly link to abstracts and to full texts of articles via PubMed, without our having to know or use the few streamlined search skills we have summarized earlier in this chapter. Google is particularly impressive when we want to find a *hot topic* article in a high-impact journal, which has recently received newspaper or media attention.

Google, as of this writing, is enhancing its portfolio of Internet search packages to appeal particularly to a professional and scientific audience. A subsidiary package, Google Scholar (http://scholar.google.com) has been announced as a resource that can customized for the needs of academics. So why not just use Google or Google Scholar?

CLINICAL SCENARIO

You are at work in the emergency department and are attending to a 45-year-old male patient who recently seized. The patient is now fully alert and is free of evidence of trauma, except for a superficial tongue abrasion. The patient tells you that he has been on phenytoin, but ran out a few days ago. His story is consistent with his phenytoin level, which the lab reports as $<0.5 \, mg/L$. You would like to provide the patient with the protection of a therapeutic, or near-therapeutic anticonvulsant level prior to discharging him from the hospital, to minimize the risk of a recurrent seizure in the next one or two days prior to his reevaluation by his regular neurologist.

You ask the nurse to hang up an appropriate weight-based dose of phenytoin for intravenous infusion. The nurse responds: "We aren't using phenytoin anymore, we have switched to fosphenytoin, because it is so much faster and safer." You go along with the nurse's revision of your order to avoid a prolonged standoff at your patient's expense.

You are skeptical, however, and although tired after a busy shift, you decide to do a quick search. You are interested in stable patients such as the one you have just treated, in the emergency care setting and using the comparison of loading regimens of phenytoin to fosphenytoin. Your outcomes of interest include effectiveness in preventing seizures, adverse effects, and cost-effectiveness. You decide to use the new Google Scholar program for your search.

Your instincts, combined with fatigue, have steered you in the direction of a quick approach to a comprehensive resource. Using the "advanced search" option on Google Scholar, you enter "fosphenytoin" and "phenytoin" and immediately are led to a total of over 400 hits. The seventh hit is a cost-effectiveness analysis sponsored by the maker of Cerebryx (fosphenytoin's brand name) and published in 1996 for which a full text link is available.[41] The conclusions of the analysis are highly favorable to fosphenytoin. You find analyses published between 2000 and 2002, and coming to conclusions unfavorable to fosphenytoin, as citations 53 and 76, respectively.[42,43] The most recent analysis, also unfavorable to fosphenytoin, is found as citation number 96.[44] Depending upon whether you change the hits per page default on the Google Scholar program, it might take you 10 panels to locate the most recent relevant analysis.

Is there a pro-industry bias to Google? Not necessarily. Doing the same search using Google, as opposed to Google Scholar, you first find one of the unfavorable analyses as number 17.[45] The industry-sponsored analysis is not found among the first 100 hits; however, neither is the most recent analysis.

Database Searches

By comparison, an indexed search of the abstracted database of *Emergency Medical Abstracts* from 1977 to 2004, using the single search term "fosphenytoin," yields a grand total of 146 hits, of which the most recent analyses are included among the first ten, and the industry-sponsored analysis is number 18. A search of the NHS Economic Evaluation Database of the Cochrane Library, Issue 4 for 2004, using the single search term "fosphenytoin," yields three critically appraised economic evaluations, including two of those found in the other searches. Important flaws and limitations in all three are identified in the critically appraised abstracts.

What about MEDLINE for this question? A search of MEDLINE on OVID, using the terms "fosphenytoin" and "phenytoin" as keywords and limited to the years 1990–2005, yields a total of 143 citations, of which the most recent analysis is number seven and another recent one is number 20. When the search is further limited using the MeSH term "cost–benefit analysis," the number of hits is reduced to seven, of which the most recent analysis is number three.

PubMed's *Clinical Queries* performs with comparable efficiency. Setting the program to "therapy" and using only the terms "fosphenytoin" and "phenytoin," the specific search yields only 12 citations between 1966 and the present, and includes most of the important articles, including the most recent analysis. Changing the setting to maximize sensitivity yields a grand total of 122 citations from 1966 to the present and identifies the additional two economic analyses included in the Cochrane registry among the first 54 citations.

The foregoing example illustrates why primary use of the Internet as a resource for finding quick answers to clinical questions can be *problematical.* The selection of hits may be arbitrary and idiosyncratic. Furthermore, no quality or specialty filter is guaranteed when a free Internet search is done. Such a search may therefore turn out to be the fastest route to the *wrong* answer.

The Internet is also a source of other free access online resources of relevance to clinical practice. Many of these fall into the general classification of online *CAT Banks*. We will further describe what CATs (critically appraised topics) are and how they are useful later in the book. In the context under discussion, CATs are loosely structured summaries of evidence performed outside of the auspices of formal peer review. There may or may not be a defined oversight process and disclosure of methods. However, such oversight and disclosure generally falls far below that of peer-reviewed, published systematic reviews.

BestBETs

A website of relevance to emergency practice is BestBETs (www. bestbets.org), an online collection of shortcut reviews. The BETs is short for Best Evidence Topics. They are focused clinical questions maintained by the Emergency Department of the Manchester Royal Infirmary in the UK. The site is free access, easy to find and, when a question has been considered, the corresponding summary can be found relatively quickly on the site. When a relevant "BET" is found, the information within it may be useful. However, there is no guarantee that it reflects a comprehensive review of relevant evidence, nor that it is current.

Returning to our fosphenytoin scenario, a relevant BET is located on the Google search: (www.bestbets.org/cgi-bin/bets.pl?record=00303). Although it pertains to a slightly different question from that in our scenario (i.e., fosphenytoin versus phenytoin in patients arriving in the emergency department in status epilepticus), the biggest limitation of the BET review is that although updated in April 2005, it is based on only one study from 2002[43] and does not include the more recent cost effectiveness analyses.

We will not attempt here to provide a comprehensive summary or catalogue of potentially relevant Internet resources. We believe that such a summary would be the very first thing in this book to become hopelessly out of date. One umbrella site that is worth knowing about is the "Netting the Evidence" site: www.shef.ac.uk/scharr/ir/netting, developed and maintained as part of the website of the School of Health and Related Research of the University of Sheffield, UK. One can obtain links through this site to just about all websites and resources relevant to evidence-based medicine.

RATING RESOURCES

At the outset of the chapter we introduced the concept of *information literacy* as a precedent for many of the concepts we have introduced.[1] *Evidence-literacy* entails the necessity of appraising the validity and relevance of clinical evidence to be considered for application to patient care, and of the sources used to locate it. What criteria should be used to assess the quality of electronic sources of clinical evidence? Various concerns and criteria have been offered over the years.[46] We suggest that these should be closely related to the criteria that are used to assess the quality of systematic reviews.

Link to Page 221

Are the Sources Explicit and Well-defined, or Was the Search Comprehensive and Well-defined?

MEDLINE fulfills this criterion. All articles, except for explicit and consistent exclusions, such as obituaries, from an expanding target set of biomedical journals, starting from the year 1966, are indexed in the database and authors' abstracts are reproduced when available. A well-reported systematic review, such as characteristically found in the Cochrane Database of Systematic Reviews, fulfills this criterion in a different way, as does *Emergency Medical Abstracts*.

Resources such as UpToDate™, Clinical Evidence and BestBETS fall short of meeting this criterion. Although the editors describe their general approach to finding the evidence used to inform their summaries, it is not clear to the user how this was done for a particular question.

Are the Criteria Used to Appraise the Quality of the Evidence Explicitly Identified?

Many resources, such as large databases, make no claim to having screened or assessed for quality in the process of compiling their contents, nor do such resources themselves present or imply health recommendations. When resources present syntheses of evidence and other related information, they need to be judged by the standards of systematic reviews. *ACP Journal Club* may be considered to constitute the criterion standard for pre-appraised resources in this regard. UpToDate™ must be considered to be largely opaque with respect to its quality assessment, and *Clinical Evidence* again falls in between.

Are the Outcomes Well-defined and Explicitly Reported?

This is an expected feature of systematic reviews which is shared by resources such as MEDLINE and EMBASE, insofar as the authors' abstracts are included. *ACP Journal Club* also presents the specific quantitative results of included studies in a standardized format. Resources such as UpToDate™ and *BestBETs* commonly present results in only qualitative and generalized form, making it impossible for the user to assess their clinical importance.

When resources do not meet the above criteria, we must treat them only as stepping stones to finding relevant clinical evidence; we must be prepared to independently appraise the original studies prior to drawing conclusions.

Is the Resource Up to Date?

It is important to know whether and how reliably the resource you are using is updated. If updating is not a built-in feature of the resource, it should be explicitly stated when the last update occurred. How do standard evidence-based medicine resources measure up in this regard?

The MEDLINE indexers at the National Library of Medicine require up to a month to get all citations from the target journal set into the full database. However, users who are intent upon finding articles that may have just appeared may be able to access PreMEDLINE, the set of very recent citations that have been preliminarily entered into the database but that are still awaiting MeSH indexing. Through this means, we should be able to find a new study within days of its publication.

Emergency Medical Abstracts is updated monthly but is characterized by a 6-month lag between an article's appearance in the database and its original publication. Users therefore need to be aware that they will not find an article in this source if it has appeared within the last 6 months.

Systematic reviews published in the Cochrane Library may or may not be up to date. However, the date of the most recent update is included at the top of each review, and users can also review a catalogue of articles awaiting evaluation for potential incorporation into the analysis.

Similarly, *Clinical Evidence* may be several years behind in updating summaries of evidence in relationship to specific questions. However, the date of the most recent search is routinely provided under each topic header.

The CAT bank of the Oxford Centre for Evidence Based Medicine (www.minervation.com/cebm2/cats/allcats.html) includes summaries that are characteristically 8–10 years out of date. They are to be viewed for demonstration purposes only.

SEARCH RESULTS

DID WE FIND WHAT WE NEED?

When a search yields high-quality, pre-appraised, and synthesized evidence that exactly fits our question and is applicable to our patients, we are home free. More often, our searches are likely to yield results that are less satisfying. What should we do when this happens? This is a complex question, but we can offer a few, non-exhaustive suggestions.

There are two possible ways that a busy clinician may be unsatisfied with the results of a search: we found too little or we found too much.

Paucity of Results

What should you do if you find less than you hoped for? In patient care, when a patient is not responding to our therapy, we take a step back and systematically run through the possible sources of error. In the same way, by thinking through the elements of our question using the PICO categories, with particular attention to the link between intervention/ exposure and outcome of interest, we can improve our search.

Have You Correctly Linked Your Question to the Preferred Study Design?

For example, are you looking for the measures of accuracy of a diagnostic test compared to a criterion standard? If so, you should *not* be searching for a randomized trial.

Have You Chosen an Appropriate Resource?

If you have a question regarding the treatment of a trauma patient, resources like *Clinical Evidence* or *ACP Journal Club*, even though oriented to therapy questions, are unlikely to include relevant evidence. Internists are not routinely treating the victims of trauma.

Have You Used Too Many Search Terms?

If you are using a filtered database, you should not need more than two or three search terms to find what you are after. If you use more, you are only increasing your chances of missing relevant evidence.

Are You Being Overly Demanding on the Applicability of Studies?

For example, you may be asking a question about a 45-year-old male with diabetes and a hip replacement. However, if you reject a study as irrelevant, because it only included 47-year-old females with diabetes and knee replacements, you are making unreasonable demands on the exactitude of the match between a study and your patient.

The Solution

Depending upon the above and on how convinced we are that clinical research relevant to the question exists, we may choose from various options. We may revise our strategy by looking for a study that enrolled a broader range of patients or for a different or less ideal study design. If we were limiting ourselves to prefiltered databases, we may switch to a more comprehensive resource such as MEDLINE. We may need to search for indirect links to evidence, such as narrative reviews, relevant practice guidelines, or consultants. If relevant clinical research does not exist, we will have to rely on disease-oriented evidence or expert opinion.

Plethora of Results

What if you have found too many citations to look through in the time available? Again there are several possibilities, depending upon the relevance of the articles you have identified.

Are There Many Relevant Citations?

If this is the case, it means that this is perceived to be an important research area and a systematic review is likely. You can try the Cochrane Library or a PubMed *Clinical Queries* search focused on systematic reviews.

Are There Many Irrelevant Citations?

How far off the mark are the articles you have found? If, after looking through the first 30 or 40, you are finding nothing even close to your question, you are doing something wrong. If you are using a small database, is it the right one for your question? If it is, you can try several synonyms for the search term you have chosen and see if relevance improves.

If we are using a large database, we must broaden our search by adding different exploded MeSH terms connected by "OR." If we find even one related article, we can take a quick look at the full abstract and citation to see which MeSH terms were designated as the most important and retry our search using these terms.

If we are finding both relevant and irrelevant articles, the judicious narrowing of our search, by adding another MeSH term connected by "AND" and eliminating all but the most recent articles, will narrow our search.

Our approach to unsatisfying search results tests our knowledge of everything that has been covered in this chapter and a lot of the content of the previous chapters as well. As in clinical medicine, expertise develops over time. Shortcuts which bypass elements of searching such as formal PICO analysis and search strategies become more justified as we refine our skills. Beginners are advised to be *systematic* and *thorough* in analyzing their questions and planning their searches.

SOURCES OF ERROR

When we first begin to routinely perform searches for clinical evidence in response to questions arising from patient care, we may perceive the activity to be methodical and maybe even burdensome; this is because initially, it is a *knowledge-based* behavior. If we force ourselves to engage in the process routinely, it soon becomes *rules-based*, allowing rapid searches with little conscious thought. Errors are therefore likely and particularly important to become aware of during the initial, knowledge-based, phase of acquiring searching expertise.

We have seen that there are useful analogies between the ways we traditionally measure the performance of diagnostic tests (i.e., "sensitivity" and "specificity") and the use of search strategies for finding evidence. There are comparable analogies between the common cognitive errors in forming a differential diagnosis and the most frequent mistakes made in the process of choosing, formulating, and researching questions.

Considering, among all possible questions raised by a clinical scenario, the subset that potentially warrant a search for external evidence is analogous to considering the list of possible diagnoses that need to be actively considered. To help strengthen this analogy, we have included both practice and teaching scenarios among the following examples.

Errors in Choosing Questions

- *Availability bias:* When considering a patient problem under the time pressure of emergency practice, it is tempting to give priority to questions relating to subjects for which we already have a strong knowledge base. We may already know where to find additional information and how to search for it in these subject areas. As a result of this bias, we may overlook important questions for which relevant clinical evidence also is likely to exist. These latter questions may be even more important to our practice, because of our lack of familiarity.
- *Prior extensive work-ups:* Some questions come up again and again in the course of practicing and teaching; we may well have searched for relevant clinical evidence on multiple occasions. It is a mistake to dismiss the possibility of new evidence or of evidence missed in the course of less than exhaustive previous searches. We must put *expiration dates* on our conclusions for all clinical questions to account for new evidence, which is constantly emerging.

Errors in Choosing Resources

If we gain skill with one evidence resource or one mode of searching, we may be biased towards using it in every situation. Residents frequently prefer and confine themselves to resources such as UpToDate, because they yield answers very quickly to most questions and because of their ease of use. Habituation to one or two target resources due to ease of use alone is likely to result in missing many important and relevant studies, particularly in the broad practice context of emergency medicine.

Errors in the Performance of a Search

- *Search satisficing:* When the emergency department is busy and we are pressed for time, it is a great temptation to stop the search at the first article that fulfills our criteria of relevance and importance. Other studies or systematic reviews may exist that might lead to different conclusions. We should continue our searches until we are reasonably sure we have found the *best-available evidence.*
- *Entrapment:* A poor search strategy may yield thousands of irrelevant results. If we continue parsing through these countless citations, rather than choosing a new search strategy, we may waste time and never find answers.

- *Confirmation bias:* We must be cognizant of our existing beliefs when we perform a search for evidence. Our search can be biased, if in the course of researching a question we stop at the first article that seems to *confirm* our preconceptions. We must put our prior beliefs aside when performing the search and evaluation of new evidence.

CHAPTER 16

SAVING THE EVIDENCE

We have just discussed the essential skills of finding clinical evidence relevant to our questions. We can then use the methods discussed in Part II to determine the strength of this evidence. Once we have made that determination, to allow this discovered evidence to be truly useful for decision-making, we need some way of saving it, so that it is readily available for patient care.

This chapter discusses "CATs" and "NEEDLEs." CATs are a way of documenting our search for, evaluation of, and results from a study or piece of evidence. NEEDLEs are the purest distillation of a piece of evidence to only the essentials needed for bedside decision-making. We can use these related methods of saving literature in tandem as well.

CRITICALLY APPRAISED TOPICS (CATS)

By building our own collection of electronic resources, using clinical evidence that we have screened and evaluated, we can bypass the need to search online resources *de novo* each time a clinical question arises. One such resource constitutes an adaptation of something known as the *critically appraised topic* (CAT).

What Are CATs?

Critically appraised topics predate the advent of ready public access to the Internet. They were invented as a teaching aide by David Sackett at McMaster University.[47] Fellows in clinical epidemiology, in the course of their training, were encouraged to compose one- or two-page summaries of their appraisals of evidence in relationship to focused clinical questions. The summaries included the citations of the articles they selected, outcomes in the form of NNTs and likelihood ratios, and a few comments pertaining to the quality of the studies and their applicability to patient care. At that time, search options were limited to a MS DOS version of Grateful Med, a MEDLINE package produced by the National Library of Medicine. As a result, the fellows did not include information regarding the searches they did to gather the evidence in their CAT summaries.

The original CATs were done on paper. Subsequently they were assembled on a floppy disk, which could be installed on computers in relevant locations such as ward lounges. They were developed for use within the teaching hospital where they originated, as a special kind of mnemonic for use in teaching and standardizing practice. Much later, many of these CATs were posted, without update or revision, on a free-access website developed by the Oxford Centre of Evidence Based Medicine. Following this development, a plethora of CAT sites and CAT banks flourished on the Internet. Recently, a Google search using the phrase "critically appraised topics" yielded over 21,000 hits. An Internet CAT crawler, a search engine exclusively for CATS, has also been announced.[48]

Do-It-Yourself

The best way of guaranteeing access to something that you may need in a hurry is to put it in your pocket. The advent of hand-held personal digital assistants (PDAs) has enabled the technology-savvy individual to increase the size of his or her pocket to far beyond anything conceivable even 10 years ago. It is currently within the grasp of anyone so inclined to create their own CAT bank (or CATalog) of evidence summaries for instantaneous use during clinical practice and teaching.

When should we create a CAT?
In principle, a CAT is appropriate any and every time we do a search on a question and come up with relevant information. In practice, time constraints will probably force us to be selective. If our goal is to maximize the proportion of our own care and teaching that encompasses an evidence-literate approach, we will be best advised to choose and document inquiries on questions that arise most often in practice and teaching and for which relatively high-quality evidence is available.

What should we put in a CAT?
The best answer to this is "whatever you need to fulfill the purpose of the retrievable record." A more formal answer lists the elements that go into a search and appraisal of a focused clinical question.[49] You may or may not find that all of these elements are required for a particular situation.

These are possible elements of a CAT:

- The clinical question that inspired the search
- The search strategy

- The best evidence discovered
- Evaluation of this evidence
- Summary of results and applicability
- Expiration date.

Elements that are always important to include are a precise documentation of the search we performed, including the resources and strategies used, and, of course, the full citations of the articles selected. This allows us to reproduce the search at such time that we choose to update our summary. The date of the original summary can serve as a useful reminder regarding when such an update is appropriate. The amount of detail we include with respect to the other relevant elements will depend upon many factors, including whether we plan to use the summary as a vehicle for clinical teaching, for communicating with peers and consultants, or simply for our own use.

Unlike a systematic review on a particular well-defined question, the content of CATs done by different individuals for different uses and circumstances, but on the very same question, *should* be highly variable (Fig. 16-1).

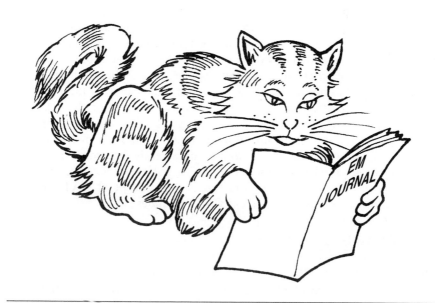

— FIGURE 16-1 —

▦ Are CATs born free?

There are a few potential misconceptions that arise with the posting and publishing of CATs for others to use. The profusion of CATs on the Internet raises the question: "What happens when a CAT, a species born and bred in a confined domestic setting, is released to the wild of cyberspace?"

- ○ Should we let the CAT out of the bag?
- ○ Are CATs born free?
- ○ Do they belong in the wild?

A likely consequence of free access posting of CATs is that they will be misconstrued as reflecting a more rigorous search and appraisal of evidence than is actually justified. If online CATs are to be regarded as reviews, they must answer to the standards that we require of published summaries of evidence.[50] These standards reflect the methodology of rigorous systematic reviews and meta-analyses.

> ### *Link to Page 221*

However, they apply as well to any *shortcut reviews*; i.e., any reviews that seek to identify the best and most relevant evidence bearing on focused clinical questions and to incorporate it into decision-making.[51]

It is not surprising that most CAT banks on the Internet fall far short of these standards. Such sites are to be criticized for inconsistency with respect to warning potential users of their methodological shortcomings. However, to the extent that we are evidence-literate practitioners, we need not throw out the kitten with the litter. Rather, we may heed the wisdom of the original CAT-maker, David Sackett, communicated in the course of a phone conversation some years ago. Sackett's concept of the CAT was of something quite downstream of the process of collecting and appraising the evidence. He saw them not as reviews, but rather as instruments of evidence-uptake or examples of what are currently becoming known as *translational aides*. They are means of getting the evidence, once identified and appraised, to the bedside. And this is the concept of CATs that we recommend to you the reader: Treat CATs as mules.

▦ CATs on a Leash

The concept of the CAT-on-a-leash is embodied in a free-access, password-protected CAT site available to emergency physicians at www.EBEM.org. This Journal Club Bank is an online vehicle which allows users to enter information pertaining to questions they have researched for purposes of immediate retrieval at the point of care. Password protection is used to prevent the contents of the Journal Club Bank from being misconstrued as systematic reviews, designed for the acceptance and use of practitioners other than those who created them. Online posting has one advantage over hand-held devices: the summaries may be used by others within the same department or facility.

NEEDLES

CATs contain evidence-based answers to clinical questions. They are a brief summary of the search, evaluation, and uses of evidence. As we discussed in Part I, NEEDLEs distill this information even further to only the absolutely essential information for bedside decision-making:

- Necessary
- Evidence for
- Emergency
- Decisions:
- Listed and
- Evaluated

NEEDLEs contain only:

- The results and downsides from a study
- Information to assess applicability
- Citation for the evidence
- Brief (1–2 sentences) description of validity and precision.

NEEDLEs are sufficiently small to be kept in our memory, ready to be used for clinical decisions or bedside teaching. As we accumulate a greater number of NEEDLEs, the cognitive load for all but the eidetic becomes unwieldy, causing us to yearn for a means of recording them.

NEEDLEs can be placed on paper (or when sufficiently distilled, even the back of a matchbook). Just as with CATs, they become more powerful when recorded on a PDA or online. As we will discuss shortly, perhaps the most utile form of NEEDLEs are when they are a part of or derived directly from a larger CAT.

NEEDLE for Diagnosis

A diagnostic NEEDLE should contain:

Benefits and Downsides

- The characteristics of the diagnostic test, preferably already turned into likelihood ratios (LRs)

- Any risks of performing the test, such as the possibility of headache with a lumbar puncture
- Any prohibitive cost.

Applicability Information

- Patient data, such as inclusion/exclusion and the external validity we assessed when evaluating the study
- Specialized interpretation
- Setting where the study was performed.

Citation
Brief Notes on Validity and Precision
Figure 16-2 shows an example of a diagnostic NEEDLE for one of the d-dimer tests for pulmonary embolism.

Diagnostic Evidence: Elisa d-dimer for Pulmonary Embolism

Benefits/Downsides

- LR + 1.73, LR − 0.11

- No risks, cost minimal

Applicability

- Adult patients in outpatient setting

- Performed in normal hospital laboratories; interpreted by laboratory staff

- Specificity lower in patients >70; sensitivity and specificity lower if symptoms >3 days

Brown MD et al. Annals Emerg Med 2002;40(2):133-144
-Valid meta-analysis. (Sens 95% CI 0.88-0.97) (Spec 95% CI 0.36-0.55)

— FIGURE 16-2 —   *An example of a diagnostic NEEDLE.*

NEEDLE for Treatment

A treatment **NEEDLE** should contain:

Benefits and Downsides

- The benefit parameters of a treatment
- Any risks of using the intervention
- Any prohibitive cost.

Applicability Information

- Patient data, such as inclusion/exclusion and the external validity we assessed when evaluating the study
- Setting information that may affect its use
- Specialized training necessary to perform the intervention.

Citation
Brief Notes on Validity and Precision
Figure 16-3 shows an example of a treatment **NEEDLE** for the use of tPA for acute ischemic stroke.

NEEDLE for Prognosis

A prognostic **NEEDLE** should contain:

Results and Prognostic Factors

- The results of primary outcome
- Any prognostic factors which define higher risk groups.

Applicability Information

- Length of follow-up
- Patient demographics
- Setting where the study was performed.

Citation
Brief Notes on Validity and Precision
Figure 16-4 shows an example of a prognostic **NEEDLE** for patients sent home after a transient ischemic attack.

    These examples should serve as templates for your own **NEEDLEs**; they are not set in stone. Whatever pieces of information you deem

Treatment NEEDLE:
tPA for acute ischemic stroke

Benefits/Downsides

- 0.9 mg/kg (10% as bolus, 90% as infusion over 60 minutes)
- ABI 13%, RBI 50% compared to placebo for minimal/no dysfunction at 3 months
- ARI 5.8%, RRI 900% compared to placebo for symptomatic intracerebral hemorrhage at 36 hours
- 90% probability of cost savings due to decreased hospitalization and rehabilitation costs

Applicability

- NIH Stroke Scale 5-21
- CT without signs of bleed or early infarct; read by neuroradiologists
- BP <185/105; may give labetolol × 2 doses if BP <220/140. If BP still >185/105 patient is not a lysis candidate
- Standard tPA contraindications

Original Study: *N Engl J Med.* 1995; 333:1581.
Cost Data: *Neurology.* 1988 Apr; 50(4):883-90.
–Valid RCT (ABI 95% CI 8.9-23.7)

— FIGURE 16-3 —   *An example of a treatment NEEDLE.*

important for decision-making can be included. If you understand the concept of NEEDLEs, you can easily create them for other forms of evidence, such as clinical practice guidelines, qualitative studies, etc.

*Maisel AS, Krishnaswamy P, Nowak RM et al. for the Breathing Not Properly Multinational Study Investigators. Rapid measurement of B-type natriuretic peptide in the emergency diagnosis of heart failure. N Engl J Med 2002;347:161–167. McCullogh PA, Nowak RM, McCord J et al. B-type natriuretic peptide and clinical judgment in emergency diagnosis of heart failure: analysis from Breathing Not Properly (BNP) multinational study. Circulation 2002;106:416–422.
Lader E. BNP levels had high sensitivity but moderate specificity for detecting congestive heart failure in the emergency department. ACP Journal Club 2003;138:23. Hohl CM, Mitelman BV, Wyer P, Lang E. Should emergency physicians use B-type natriuretic peptide testing in patieints with unexplained dyspnea? CJEM 2003;5:162–165. Schwam E. B-type natriuretic peptide for diagnosis of heart failure in emergency department patients: a critical appraisal. Acad Emerg Med 2004;11:686–691.

Prognosis Evidence:
Prognosis of patients sent home from ED after TIA

Results

● Patients with TIA discharged from ED: 10.5% had a stroke in following 90 days, half of these within two days of discharge

Prognosis worse if:

● Age >60 years
● Diabetes mellitus
● Longer duration of TIA
● Signs or symptoms of weakness, speech impairment, or gait disturbance
● Patients with symptoms still present upon arrival to the Emergency Department

Applicability

● Adult patients (~80% >60 y/o), many with comorbidities
● HMO patients, hospital use discouraged may represent sicker population
● Academic Emergency Department
● Ninety day follow-up important, 2 day data especially relevant

Brown MD et al. Annals Emerg Med 2002;40(2):133-144
-Valid Prospective Cohort Study, (Risk of stroke at 90 days 95% CI 9-12%)

— FIGURE 16-4 — *An example of a prognosis NEEDLE.*

Impaled CATs

If you create a CAT, a NEEDLE can be integrated into it, ready to be used for teaching and decision-making. This is perhaps the most versatile tool for bedside teaching, as all of the information of search, evaluation, and results are immediately available. NEEDLE information can be in a separate area of the CAT or simply derived "on the fly" from the CAT summary (Fig. 16-5).

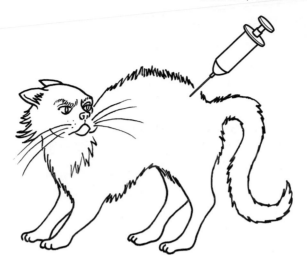

— FIGURE 16-5 —   *A NEEDLE embedded in a CAT.*

EXAMPLE:

The following illustrates the application of these concepts, starting with a clinical scenario.

CLINICAL SCENARIO

You are the senior emergency medicine resident on call when a 53-year-old female is brought in by the paramedics as a "difficulty breathing" notification. They assessed her as having an asthma attack and began administration of albuterol by continuous nebulization. They now report that she is "a little better" since they initiated therapy.

   She is a slightly obese female whose vital signs are heart rate of 108/min, blood pressure 160/100 mmHg, respiratory rate 30/min, and an O_2 saturation of 97% with oxygen powered nebulization in process. She is in moderate respiratory distress, with some use of accessory muscles, but able to interact verbally and to answer questions. She has a history of hypertension, an "enlarged" heart, and asthma, going back to childhood, for which she has been admitted to hospital twice as an adult. When asked whether her current symptoms are consistent with previous asthma exacerbations, she replies in the affirmative. On the other hand, she mentions that she ran out of her blood pressure medications about a month ago and has not had time to refill them.

CAT summary
BNP for the Diagnosis of Congestive Heart Failure

Question:
What is the power of BNP to distinguish between CHF and other causes of acute dyspnea in emergency patients whose clinical evaluations and chest X-rays are unable to distinguish between CHF and COPD/Hyperactive Airway Disease?

Search:
OVID MEDLINE with links to ACP Journal Club 1995-March 2005. 'Natriuretic', 'congestive heart failure' using keywords and relevant exploded MeSH terms and limited using the clinical query diagnosis (sensitive) yielded 107 citations including entries from ACP Journal Club citing both original studies and critically appraised commentaries.

Citations:
Lader E. BNP levels had high sensitivity but moderate specificity for detecting congestive heart failure in the emergency department. ACP Journal Club 2003;138:23.

Hohl CM, Mitelman BV, Wyer P, Lang E. Should emergency physicians use B-type natriuretic peptide testing in patients with unexplained dyspnea? CJEM. 2003;5:162-165.

Schwam E. B-type natriuretic peptide for diagnosis of heart failure in emergency department patients: a critical appraisal. Acad Emerg Med. 2004;11:686-691.

Study Summary and Critical Appraisal:
The parent study, published in the New England Journal of Medicine, Circulation and elsewhere, was large, international, multicenter and ED based.

The principle methodological weakness was a failure to restrict, or at least focus, the analysis on patients for whom clinicians harbored important clinical uncertainty. Even though such patients were identified as part of the study protocol, they constituted less than a third of the total population. BNP values are likely to be very high in patients for whom CHF is clinically unequivocal and very low in patients judged clinically to have a low likelihood of CHF. BNP values are likely to be in the middle range for clinically ambiguous patients and to perform much less accurately in identifying patients with CHF. Sensitivity and specificity of BNP using the cutoff recommended by the authors (100 pg/cc) were only 79% and 71% respectively for the uncertain group, much lower than for the total population, verifying the presence of spectrum bias in the parent study.

Results:
LR's for interval ranges of BNP reported by Hohl and amplified by Schwam for patients who are clinically indeterminate for the diagnosis of CHF:

BNP range (pg/cc)	Likelihood ratio (95% CI)
<100	0.3 (0.2-0.4)
401-1000	5.0 (3.3-7.9)
>1000	16 (10-26)

Interpretation:
The interval LR analysis suggests that BNP values have to be either <100 pg/cc or >1000 to have a significant impact on clinically assessed pre-test probability of CHF. These estimates do not take into account the effect of spectrum bias noted above. Hence, the useful BNP threshold values pertaining to clinically equivocal patients may, in reality, be even more extreme than one would expect from the above table.

Date of Creation:
December 15, 2004

— FIGURE 16-6 — *Your newly created CAT.*

Diagnostic Evidence: BNP for the Diagnosis of CHF

Benefits/Downsides

BNP (pg/cc)	LR
<100	0.3
>1000	16

No risks, cost minimal
At least 40% of the time, the test results will be inconclusive

Applicability

● Adult patients in outpatient setting who are
  clinically indeterminate as to the diagnosis of CHF

● Performed in normal hospital laboratories; interpreted by
  laboratory staff

Original studies: N Engl J Med. 2002;347:161-167, Circulation. 2002;106:416-22.
Reanalysis: Acad Emerg Med 2004;11, (6):686-691, CJEM 2003;5(3):162-165.
–Prospective Diagnostic Cohort with Possible Spectrum Bias.
(LR <100 95% CI 0.88-0.97), (LR >1000 95% CI 0.36-0.55)

— FIGURE 16-7 —   *From the CAT, you can create a NEEDLE.*

Physical exam reveals bilateral rhonchi and occasional expiratory wheezes. You find mild lower extremity edema, which the patient says her doctor told here was due to her amlodipine. The electrocardiogram is unremarkable and a chest radiograph reveals cardiomegaly and increased vascular markings, but no clear pulmonary edema.

You present this case to your attending with the question: "Should we treat her for asthma or for congestive heart failure?" Your attending suggests that you continue to treat with albuterol, give her a little furosemide, and order a B-natiuretic peptide (BNP) assay. He comments: "If the BNP is over 120, we will treat her for CHF."

The patient continues to improve; meanwhile, the BNP result comes back 95 pg/mL. You and your attending are satisfied that the issue has been adequately addressed *for this patient*. However, you have heard that the use of BNP to distinguish between CHF and other causes of acute dyspnea is controversial and decide to do your own literature review.

A search of your library's integrated OVID package leads you to two publications on a study of the diagnostic performance of BNP in this setting,[54] as well as several published critical appraisals of that study.[55] Because the results of this study were scattered over a series of parallel publications, and because of the complexity of some of the statistical issues, you elect to rely on the latter references for your assessment. After reviewing them, you find some disagreement between their assessments and conclusions. You therefore decide to draft your own CAT summary and to post it on your department's resident teaching website for quick reference when this issue comes up in the future (Fig. 16-6).

From this CAT, you can derive a NEEDLE that contains only the minimum amount of information necessary for bedside decisions. You place a copy of this NEEDLE on your personal website and attach it to the original CAT (Fig. 16-7).

CATs stuck with NEEDLEs may be the most powerful means of saving our searches and evaluations of evidence. This combined form is useful for bedside teaching and decision-making. In this way, the NEEDLE provides the information necessary for evidence-based teaching or practice scripts. Having pre-appraised information immediately available in the emergency department can allow us to make unbiased decisions and teach with literature support, rather than just opinion.

CONCLUSION

Questions of various types arise in the course of practice. Depending upon the circumstances and our degree of familiarity with a condition, the questions may pertain to background information or to information from clinical research. Online resources sometimes even make it possible to bring information of both types to bear on clinical decision-making in the same time-frame as patient care itself.

To accomplish a search for evidence efficiently and accurately, a practitioner needs a selective knowledge of study design, outcome measures, and the criteria that determine the quality of information stemming from such sources. Categorizing this selective knowledge by modes of action and decision-making (i.e., diagnosis, therapy, harm, and prognosis) allows it to be understood in terms that pertain to clinical reasoning: *what doctors do and say*.

This same conceptual scheme, the categorization of these components of knowledge as pertaining to the four types of medical questions, allows an evidence-literate clinician to connect questions to the fastest online sources of answers. As is true of all clinical skill, expertise results from practice. The tools and concepts we have presented here, such as PICO and goal-directed searching, are aimed to facilitate your acquisition of expertise in a fashion that avoids the most common pitfalls. We anticipate that, over time, the development of even more sophisticated evidence-based resources, within and without emergency medicine, will make the challenges even easier to overcome.

PART IV
ENDMATTER

EPILOGUE

We hope you have enjoyed the journey as much as we have enjoyed being your guides. As the cartoon suggests, while this book ends upon a summit of knowledge, there are still many more peaks to climb.

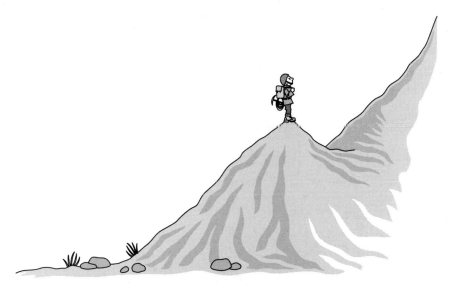

Evidence-based Medicine

This book introduces many of the concepts of evidence-based medicine, but there are innumerable areas that would reward further study. At the end of the book we list some of the sources to delve further into this vital subject area.

Research

Part III of this book discussed asking questions and searching for answers. Sometimes, you cannot find an answer to an important question, because the evidence does not yet exist. This might spur you to invest the time and energy into answering the question yourself. We hope that this book offers you a good perspective on what the consumers of the literature will need from your study.

Teaching

If you have taken the time to integrate the precepts of this book into your clinical practice, please teach them to your residents, students, and colleagues.

Visit Us at http://critdecisions.com

Please go to our website to find additional information, updates, and our contact information. We would love to hear from you.

SELECTED ONLINE RESOURCES

- *ACP Journal Club*: www.acpjc.org
- *Annals of Emergency Medicine* EBEM: http://journals.elsevierhealth.com/periodicals/ymem/content/ebemresources
- Aries Knowledge Finder: www.kfinder.com/newweb
- BestBETs: www.bestbets.org
- Centre for Evidence Based Medicine: www.minervation.com/cebm2/cats/allcats.html
- Cinahl: www.cinahl.com
- *Clinical Evidence*: www.clinicalevidence.com
- The Cochrane Library: www.thecochranelibrary.com
- *Emergency Medical Abstracts*: http://ccme.org
- Evidence Based Emergency Medicine (The "Journal Club Bank"): www.EBEM.org
- Google: www.Google.com
- Google Scholar: http://scholar.google.com
- National Guideline Clearinghouse: www.guideline.gov
- OVID Technologies: www.ovid.com
- PubMed: www.ncbi.nlm.nih.gov/entrez/query.fcgi
- The ScHARR Centre ("Netting the Evidence"): www.shef.ac.uk/scharr/ir/netting
- UpToDate®: www.utdol.com

ADDITIONAL READING

Evidence-based Medicine

- Guyatt G, Rennie D. *Users' Guides to the Medical Literature.* American Medical Association, 2001. This text is the next step if you want to study the EBM concepts we have just presented in greater depth.
- Sackett DL, Straus SE, Richardson WS et al. *Evidence-based Medicine: How to Practice and Teach EBM,* 2nd edn. Churchill Livingstone, 2000. This book established the very beginning of the EBM movement by one of its founding fathers.
- Jenicek, M. *Foundations of Evidence-based Medicine.* Parthenon, 2003. This monograph offers an exploration of the epistemology, philosophy, and cognitive basis of EBM. It is not a book for beginners.

Cognitive Errors

- Reason, J. *Human Error.* Cambridge University Press, 1990. Reason's work offers an eminently readable description of the underpinnings of cognitive error. While not a book specifically about medical error, the theories presented are directly applicable.
- Schwartz S, Griffin, T. *Medical Thinking: The Psychology of Medical Judgment and Decision Making.* Springer-Verlag, 1986. This volume provides perhaps the most in-depth analysis of the cognitive psychology of medical errors.
- Skrabanek P, McCormick J. *Follies & Fallacies in Medicine.* Prometheus Books, 1990. A list of biases and cognitive pitfalls, this book is written for general practitioners, but is useful for emergency physicians as well.

Deliberate Deceptions in Medical Literature

- Angell, M. *The Truth About the Drug Companies*. Random House, 2004. Dr Angell discusses not only the manipulation of the literature by the pharmaceutical industry, but the way they have used every facet of commercialism to advance their bottom line. It is chilling but necessary reading for every practitioner.
- Montori VM, Jaeschke R et al. Users' guide to detecting misleading claims in clinical research reports. *Br Med J* 2004;329:1093–1096. This article serves as an addition to the *Users' Guides* text; it addresses many of the topics we discussed under the deliberate misrepresentation section of Part II.
- *British Medical Journal*, 31 May 2003. The BMJ devoted an entire issue to the crucial problems of the interaction of the pharmaceutical industry and medicine.

REFERENCES

PART I

1. Elshove-Bolk J et al. A description of emergency department-related malpractice claims in the Netherlands: closed claims study 1993–2001. *Eur J Emerg Med* 2004;11:247–250.
2. Kuhn GF. Diagnostic errors. *Acad Emerg Med* 2002;7:740–750.
3. Macartney FJ. Dziagnostic logic. *Br Med J* 1987;295:1325–1331.
4. Jenicek, M. *Foundations of Evidence-Based Medicine.* Parthenon, 2002.
5. Kyriacou DN. Evidence-based medical decision making: deductive versus inductive logical thinking. *Acad Emerg Med* 2004;11:670–671.
6. Schmidt HG et al. A cognitive perspective on medical expertise: theory and implications. *Acad Med* 1990;65:611–621.
7. Croskerry P. Achieving quality in clinical decision making: cognitive strategies and detection of bias. *Acad Emerg Med* 2002;9.1184–1203.
8. Kassirer JP. Diagnostic reasoning. *Ann Intern Med* 1989;110:893–900.
9. Charlin B et al. Scripts and medical diagnostic knowledge: theory and applications for clinical reasoning instruction and research. *Acad Med* 2000;75:182–190.
10. Pauker SG et al. Towards the simulation of clinical cognition: taking a present illness by computer. *Am J Med* 1976;60:981–996.
11. Barrows H, Feltovich P. The clinical reasoning process. *Med Educ* 1987; 21:86–91.
12. Barrows H et al. The clinical reasoning of randomly selected physicians in general medical practice. *Clin Invest Med* 1984;5(1):49–55.
13. Jones AE et al. Randomized, controlled trial of immediate versus delayed goal-directed ultrasound to identify the cause of nontraumatic hypotension in emergency department patients. *Crit Care Med* 2004;32:1703–1708.
14. Norman GR, Brooks LR, Colle CK, Hatala RM. The benefit of diagnostic hypotheses in clinical reasoning: an experimental study of an instructional intervention for forward and backward reasoning. *Cognit Inst* 1999;17:433–448.
15. LeBlance VR, Brooks LR, Norman GR. Believing is seeing: the influence of a diagnostic hypothesis on the interpretation of clinical features. *Acad Med* 2002;77:S67–S69.
16. Reicher GM. Perceptual recognition as a function of meaningfulness of stimulus material. *J Exp Psychol* 1969;81:274–280.
17. Klein G. *Sources of Power: How People Make Decisions.* MIT Press, 1999.
18. Guyatt G, Rennie D. *Users' Guides to the Medical Literature. JAMA and Archives Journals* 2002:449–459.

19. Schaider J, Hayden SR et al. *Rosen & Barkin's 5-Minute Emergency Medicine Consult*. Lippincott, 2003.
20. Richardson WS, Wilson M, Lijmer J, Guyatt G, Cook D. Differential diagnosis. In: Guyatt G, Rennie D (eds) *Users' Guides to the Medical Literature: A Manual for Evidence-based Clinical Practice*. AMA Press, 2002:109–119.
21. Reagen RT et al. Quantitative meanings of verbal probability expressions. *J Appl Psych* 1989;74:433–442.
22. Bryant GD. Expressions of probability words and numbers. *N Engl J Med* 1980;302:411.
23. Cecil RL. Acute intermittent porphyria. In: *Cecil's Textbook of Medicine*. WB Saunders, 2000.
24. Richardson WS, Polashenski WA, Robbins BW. Could our pretest probabilities become evidence based? *J Gen Intern Med* 2003;18:203–208.
25. Morgenstern LB. Worst headache and subarachnoid hemorrhage: prospective, modern computed tomography and spinal fluid analysis. *Ann Emerg Med* 1998;32:297–304.
26. Kapoor WN, Karpf M, Wieand S et al. A prospective evaluation and follow-up of patients with syncope. *N Engl J Med* 1983;309:197–204.
27. Kaupacis A, Sekar N, Stiell IG. Clinical prediction rules: a review and suggested modifications of methodological standards. *JAMA* 1997; 277:488–494.
28. Kline J. *Use of Pretest Probability to Reduce Unnecessary Test Ordering in the Emergency Department*. www.studymaker.com, accessed 5 July 2004.
29. Shields GP, Turnipseed S, Panacek EA, Melnikoff N, Gosselin R, White RH. Validation of the Canadian clinical probability model for acute venous thrombosis. *Acad Emerg Med* 2002;9:561–566.
30. Phelps MA, Levitt MA. Pretest probability estimates: a pitfall to the clinical utility of evidence-based medicine? *Acad Emerg Med* 2004;11:692–694.
31. Hunt KJ. The utility of pretest probability assessment in patients with clinically suspected venous thromboembolism. *J Thromb Haemost* 2003;1:1888–1896.
32. American College of Emergency Physicians Clinical Policies Committee; Clinical Policies Committee Subcommittee on Suspected Pulmonary Embolism. Clinical policy: critical issues in the evaluation and management of adult patients presenting with suspected pulmonary embolism. *Ann Emerg Med* 2003;41:257–270.
33. Brown MD, Vance SJ, Kline JA. An emergency department guideline for the diagnosis of pulmonary embolism: an outcome study. *Acad Emerg Med* 2005;12:20–25.
34. Pauker SG, Kassirer JP. The threshold approach to diagnostic decision making. *N Engl J Med* 1980;302:1109–1117.
35. Hayden SR, Brown MD. Likelihood ratio: a powerful tool for incorporating the results of a diagnostic test into clinical decision making. *Ann Emerg Med* 1999;33:5.
36. Value of the ventilation/perfusion scan in acute pulmonary embolism. Results of the prospective investigation of pulmonary embolism diagnosis (PIOPED). The PIOPED Investigators. *JAMA* 1990;263:2753–2759.

37. Anderson RE et al. Diagnostic value of disease history, clinical presentation, and inflammatory parameters of appendicitis. *World J Surg* 1999;23:133–140.
38. Snyder BK, Hayden SR. Accuracy of leukocyte count in the diagnosis of acute appendicitis. *Ann Emerg Med* 1999;33:565–574.
39. Brown MD, Reeves MJ. Evidence-based emergency medicine/skills for evidence-based emergency care. Interval likelihood ratios: another advantage for the evidence-based diagnostician. *Ann Emerg Med* 2003;42:292–297.
40. Sackett DL, Richardson WS, Rosenberg W, Haynes RB. *Evidence-based Medicine: How to Practice and Teach EBM*. Churchill Livingstone, 2000.
41. Gallagher EJ. Clinical utility of likelihood ratios. *Ann Emerg Med* 1998; 31:391–397.
42. Choi BCK. Slopes of a receiver operating characteristic curve and likelihood ratios for a diagnostic test. *Am J Epidemiol* 1998;148:1127–1132.
43. Wagner JM, McKinney WP, Carpenter JL. Does this patient have appendicitis? *JAMA* 1996;276:1589–1594.
44. Rozycki GS, Ballard RB. Feliciano DV et al. Surgeon-performed ultrasound for the assessment of truncal injuries: lessons learned from 1540 patients. *J Trauma* 1998;228:557–567.
45. Fagan TJ. Letter: Nomogram for Bayes' theorem. *N Engl J Med* 1975;293:257.
46. Kassirer JP, Kopelmn RI. Cognitive errors in diagnosis: instantiation, classification, and consequences. *Am J Med* 1989;86:433–441.
47. Kovacs G, Croskerry P. Clinical decision making; an emergency medicine perspective. *Acad Emerg Med* 1999;6:947–952.
48. Gruppen LD, Wolf FM, Billi JE. Information gathering and integration as sources of error in diagnostic decision making. *Med Decision Making* 1991;11:233–239.
49. Feied CF, Smith MS, Handler JA. Keynote Address: Medical informatics and emergency medicine. *Acad Emerg Med* 2004;11:1118–1126.
50. Tversky A, Kahneman D. Judgement under uncertainty, heuristics and biases. *Science* 1974;185:1124–1131.
51. Croskerry P. Cognitive forcing strategies in clinical decision making. *Ann Emerg Med* 2003;41:110–120.
52. Sackett DL. Bias in analytic research. *J Chron Dis* 1979;32:51–63.
53. McDonald CJ. Medical heuristics: the silent adjudicators of clinical practice. *Ann Intern Med* 1996;124(1 Pt 1):56–62.
54. Reason J. *Human Error*. Cambridge University Press, 1990.
55. Gilovich T, Griffin D, Kahneman, D. *Heuristics and Biases: The Psychology of Intuitive Judgment*. Cambridge University Press, 2002.
56. Heylighen F. *Principia Cybernetica Web*. http://pespmc1.vub.ac.be/OCCAM-RAZ.html. Acessed 8 January 2004.
57. Simons HA. *Models of Man: Social and Rational*. Taylor & Francis, 1987.
58. Christensen-Szalanski JJ, Beck DE et al. The effect of journal coverage on physicians' perceptions of risk. *J Appl Psych* 1983;68:278–284.
59. Thomas KE, Hasbun R, Jekel J, Quagliarello VJ. The diagnostic accuracy of Kernig's sign, Brudzinski's sign, and nuchal rigidity in adults with suspected meningitis. *Clin Infect Dis* 2002;35:46–52.

60. Ehrlich JE. Cost-effectiveness of treatment options for prevention of rheumatic heart disease from Group A streptococcal pharyngitis in a pediatric population. *Prev Med* 2002;35:250–257.

61. Oxford English Dictionary. http://dictionary.oed.com. Accessed 11 July 2004.

62. Flavell JH. Metacognition and cognitive monitoring: a new area of cognitive-developmental inquiry. *Am Psychol* 1979;34:906–911.

63. Wells PS, Anderson DR, Rodger M et al. Derivation of a simple clinical model to categorize patients' probability of pulmonary embolism: increasing the models utility with the SimpliRED D-dimer. *Thromb Haemost* 2000;83:416–420.

64. Stein PD, Dalen JE, McIntyre KM et al. The electrocardiogram in acute pulmonary embolism. *Prog Cardiovasc Dis* 1975;17:247–257.

65. Stein PD et al. Arterial blood gas analysis in the assessment of suspected acute pulmonary embolism. *Chest* 1996;109:78–81.

66. Schutgens RE, Haas FJ, Gerritsen WB et al. The usefulness of five D-dimer assays in the exclusion of deep venous thrombosis. *J Thromb Haemost* 2003; 1:976–981.

67. Pioped Investigators. Value of the ventilation/perfusion scan in acute pulmonary embolism. *JAMA* 1990;263:2753–2759.

68. Remy-Jardin M et al. Clinical value of thin collimation in the diagnostic workup of pulmonary embolism. *AJR* 2000;175:407–411.

69. Swensen SJ et al. Outcomes after withholding anticoagulation from patients with suspected acute pulmonary embolism and negative computed tomographic findings: a cohort study. *Mayo Clin Proc* 2002;77:130–138.

70. Goodman LR et al. Subsequent pulmonary embolism: risk after negative helical CT pulmonary angiogram. Prospective comparison with scintigraphy. *Radiology* 2000;215:535–542.

71. Schoepf UF et al. CT angiography for diagnosis of pulmonary embolism: state of the art. *Radiology* 2004;230:330–337.

72. British Thoracic Society Standards of Care Committee, Pulmonary Embolism Guideline Development Group. British Thoracic Society guidelines for the management of suspected acute pulmonary embolism. *Thorax* 2003;58:470–483.

73. "Are screening serum Cr levels necessary prior to outpatient CT examinations?" *Radiology* 2000;216:2.

74. Schwartz S, Griffin T. *Medical Thinking: The Psychology of Medical Judgment and Decision Making*. Springer Verlag, 1986.

75. Talfryn H, Davies O, Crombie IK. When can odds ratios mislead? *Br Med J* 1998;316:989–991.

76. Muizelaar JP, Marmarou A et al. Adverse effects of prolonged hyperventilation in patients with severe head injury: a randomized clinical trial. *J Neurosurg* 1991;75:731–739.

77. *Guidelines for the Management and Prognosis of Severe Traumatic Brain Injury*. The Brain Trauma Foundation. www2.braintrauma.org/guidelines. Accessed 19 March 2004.

78. Intravenous nesiritide vs nitroglycerin for treatment of decompensated congestive heart failure: a randomized controlled trial. *JAMA* 2002; 287:1531–1540.

79. Sackner-Bernstein JD, Kowalski M, Fox M et al. short-term risk of death after treatment with nesiritide for decompensated heart failure: a pooled analysis of randomized controlled trials. *JAMA* 2005;293:1900–1905.

80. Lightowler JV, Wedzicha JA, Elliott MW, Ram FS. Non-invasive positive pressure ventilation to treat respiratory failure resulting from exacerbations of chronic obstructive pulmonary disease: Cochrane systematic review and meta-analysis. *Br Med J* 2003;326:185.

81. Guyatt G, Montori V et al. Patients at the Center. In our practice, and in our use of language. *ACP Journal Club* 2004;140:A11.

82. Shaughnessy AF, Slawson DC. POEMs: patient-oriented evidence that matters. *Ann Intern Med* 1997;126:667.

83. Slawson DC, Shaughnessy AF, Bennett JH. Becoming a medical information master: feeling good about *not* knowing everything. *J Fam Practice* 1994; 38:505–512.

84. SAEM Online Emergency Evidence-based Medicine Course. Accessed 14 March 2004.

85. Ebell MH, Barry HC, Slawson DC, Shaughnessy AF. Finding POEMs in the medical literature. *J Fam Practice* 1999;48:350–355.

86. Arroll B, Kenealy T. Antibiotics for the common cold and acute purulent rhinitis. *Cochrane Database of Systematic Reviews* 2002;3:CD000247.

87. Bosch X, Marrugat J. Platelet glycoprotein IIb/IIIa blockers for percutaneous coronary revascularization, and unstable angina and non-ST-segment elevation myocardial infarction (Cochrane review). In: *The Cochrane Library*, Issue 1, 2004.

88. Vandycke C, Martens, P. High-dose versus standard-dose epinephrine in cardiac arrest: a meta-analysis. *Resuscitation* 2000;45:161–166.

89. Barratt A, Wyer PC. Tips for learners of evidence-based medicine: relative risk reduction, absolute risk reduction and number needed to treat. *CMAJ* 2004;171:353–358.

90. Rowe BH, Klassen T, Wyer PC. One is the only number that you'll ever need. *Ann Emerg Med* 2000;36:520–523.

91. Gross R. *Decisions and Evidence in Medical Practice*. Mosby, 2001.

92. Merrer J, De Jonghe B, Golliot F et al. for the French Catheter Study Group in Intensive Care. Complications of femoral and subclavian venous catheterization in critically ill patients: a randomized controlled trial. *JAMA* 2001;286:700–707.

93. Lorente L, Villegas J, Martin MM, Jimenez A, Mora ML. Catheter-related infection in critically ill patients. *Intens Care Med* 2004;30:1681–1684.

94. van Zwieten K, Mullins ME, Jang T. Droperidol and the black box warning. *Ann Emerg Med* 2004;43:139–140.

95. Topol EJ. Failing the public's health: rofecoxib, Merck, and the FDA. *N Engl J Med* 2004;351:1707–1708.

96. Kitman JL. The secret history of lead. *Nation* 20 March 2000.

97. Altman DG, Bland JM. Absence of evidence is not evidence of absence. *Br Med J* 1995;311:485.

98. Martuzzi M, Bertollini R. The precautionary principle: science and human health protection. *Int J Occup Med Environ Health* 2004;17(1):43–46.

99. Smithline HA, Mader TJ, Crenshaw BJ. Do patients with acute medical conditions have capacity to give informed consent for emergency medicine research? *Acad Emerg Med* 1999;6:776–780.

100. Corke CF, Stow PJ, Green DT et al. How doctors discuss major interventions with high risk patients: an observational study. *Br Med J* 2005;330:182.

101. Rosenthal MM, Sutcliffe KM. *Medical Error: What Do We Know? What Do We Do?* Jossey-Bass, 2002.

102. Institute for Safe Medication Practices. www.ismp.org. Accessed 21 October 2004.

103. Davis D, Evans M, Jadad A. The case for knowledge translation: shortening the journey from evidence to effect. *Br Med J* 2003;327:33–35.

104. Meara J. Getting the message across: is communicating risk to the public worth it? *J Radiol Prot* 2002;22:79–85.

105. Picano E. Informed consent and communication of risk from radiological and nuclear medicine examinations: how to escape from a communication inferno. *Br Med J* 2004;329:849–851.

106. Rao AC, Naeem N, John C et al. Direct current cardioversion does not cause cardiac damage: evidence from cardiac troponin T estimation. *Heart* 1998; 80:229–230.

107. Greaves K, Crake T. Cardiac troponin T does not increase after electrical cardioversion for atrial fibrillation or atrial flutter. *Heart* 1998;80:226–228.

108. Available free of charge at www.ferne.org/ferne_storke_handheld.htm. Accessed 23 October 2004.

109. Shapiro J et al. HandiStroke: A handheld tool for the emergent evaluation of acute stroke patients *Acad Emerg Med* 2003;10:1325–1328.

110. The National Institute of Neurological Disorders and Stroke. Tissue plasminogen activator for acute ischemic stroke. *N Engl J Med* 1995;333: 1581–7.

111. Marler JR, Tilley BC, Lu M et al. Early stroke treatment associated with better outcome: the NINDS rt-PA stroke study. *Neurology* 2000;55:1649–1655.

112. Christakis NA, Lamont EB. Extent and determinants of error in doctors' prognoses in terminally ill patients: prospective cohort study. *Br Med J* 2000; 320:469–473.

113. Glare P, Virik K, Jones M et al. A systematic review of physicians' survival predictions in terminally ill cancer patients. *Br Med J* 2003;327:195.

114. Fine, MJ, Auble TE, Yealy DM et al. A prediction rule to identify low-risk patients with community-acquired pneumonia. *NEJM* 1997;336:243–250.

PART II

1. Sackett DL, Richardson WS, Rosenberg W, Haynes RB. *Evidence-based Medicine*. Churchill Livingstone, 1997.

2. DeAngelis CD. Conflict of interest and the public trust. *JAMA* 2000;284:2237.

3. Montori VM, Jaeschke R et al. Users' guide to detecting misleading claims in clinical research reports. *Br Med J* 2004;329:1093–1096.

4. Lijmer JG et al. Empirical evidence of design-related bias in studies of diagnostic tests. *JAMA* 1999;282:1061–1066.

5. Yadav D, Agarwal N, Pitchumoni CS. A critical evaluation of laboratory tests in acute pancreatitis. *Am J Gastroenterol* 2002;97:1309–1318.

6. Hoffman JR, Schriger DL, Mower WR et al. Low-risk criteria for cervical spine radiography in blunt trauma: a prospective study. *Ann Emerg Med* 1992; 12:1454–1460.

7. Stiell IG, Clement CM, McKnight RD et al. The Canadian C-spine rule versus the NEXUS low-risk criteria in patients with trauma. *N Engl J Med*. 2003; 349:2510–2518.

8. Ogawa, K. et al. Clinical significance of blood brain natriuretic peptide level measurement in the detection of heart disease in untreated outpatients: comparison of electrocardiography, chest radiography and echocardiography. *Circ J* 2002;66:122.

9. Commentary in *Emergency Medical Abstracts*. Abstract 4, 2000.

10. Maisel AS, Krishnaswamy P, Nowak RM et al. Breathing Not Properly Multinational Study Investigators. Rapid measurement of B-type natriuretic peptide in the emergency diagnosis of heart failure. *N Engl J Med* 2002; 347:161–167.

11. McCullough PA, Nowak RM, McCord J et al. B-type natriuretic peptide and clinical judgment in emergency diagnosis of heart failure: analysis from Breathing Not Properly (BNP) Multinational Study. *Circulation* 2002; 106.416–422.

12. Hohl CM, Mitelman BY, Wyer P, Lang E. Should emergency physicians use B-type natriuretic peptide testing in patients with unexplained dyspnea? *Can J Emerg Med* 2003;5(3):162–165.

13. Mulherin SA, Miller WC. Spectrum bias or spectrum effect? Subgroup variation in diagnostic test evaluation *Ann Intern Med* 2002;137:598–602.

14. Reid et al. Use of methodological standards in diagnostic test research. *JAMA* 1995;274:645–651.

15. McLaughlin SA, Crandall CS, McKinney PE. Octreotide: an antidote for sulfonylurea-induced hypoglycemia. *Ann Emerg Med* 2000;36:133–138.

16. Benson K, Hartz AJ. A comparison of observational studies and randomized, controlled trials. *N Engl J Med* 2000;342:1878–1886.

17. Concato J, Shah N, Horwitz RI. Randomized controlled trials, observational studies, and the hierarchy of research designs. *N Engl J Med* 2000; 342:1887–1892.

18. Recovery of a patient from clinical rabies, Wisconsin, 2004. *MMWR* 2004; 53:1171–1173.

19. Mailia, JJ et al. Nifedipine-associated myocardial ischemia or infarction in the treatment of hypertensive urgencies. *Ann Intern Med* 1987;107(2):185.

20. Reed JF. Analysis of two-treatment, two-period crossover trials in emergency medicine. *Ann Emerg Med* 2004;43:54–58.

21. Sackett DL. Bias in analytic research. *J Chron Dis* 1979;32:51-63.

22. Schulz KF. Blinding in randomized trials: hiding who got what. *Lancet* 2002;359:696–700.

23. Moher D, Schultz KF, Altman DG. The CONSORT statement: revised recommendations for improving the quality of reports of parallel-group randomised trials. *Lancet* 2001;357:1191–1194.
24. Hall CB, McBride JT, Walsh EE et al. Aerosolized ribavirin treatment of infants with respiratory syncytial viral infection: a randomized double-blind study. *N Engl J Med* 1983;308:1443–1447.
25. Siffredi M, Mastropasqua B et al. Effect of inhaled furosemide and cromolyn on bronchoconstriction induced by ultrasonically nebulized distilled water in asthmatic subjects. *Ann Allergy Asthma Immunol* 1997;78:238–243.
26. The fallacy files. www.fallacyfiles.org/strawman.html. Accessed 18 May 2004.
27. Scheinkestel CD, Bailey M, Myles PS et al. Hyperbaric or normobaric oxygen for acute carbon monoxide poisoning: a randomised controlled clinical trial. *MJA* 1999;170:203–210.
28. National Institute of Neurological Disorders and Stroke. Tissue plasminogen activator for acute ischemic stroke. *N Engl J Med* 1995;333:1581.
29. Lopez-Yunez AM et al. T-PA stroke treatments are associated with symptomatic intracerebral hemorrhage. *Stroke* 2001;32:12.
30. Katzan IL et al. The use of tissue-type plasminogen activator for acute ischemic stroke: the Cleveland area experience *JAMA* 2000;283:1151.
31. Todd K, Funk K, Funk J, Bonacci R. Clinical significance of reported changes in pain severity. *Ann Emerg Med* 1996;27:485–489.
32. Bracken MB, Shepard MJ et al. A randomized, controlled trial of methylprednisolone or naloxone in the treatment of acute spinal-cord injury: results of the Second National Acute Spinal Cord Injury Study. *N Engl J Med* 1990; 322:1405–1411.
33. Guyatt G, Montori V, Devereaux PJ, Schunemann H, Bhandari M. Patients at the center: in our practice, and in our use of language. *ACP J Club* 2004; 140:A11–A12.
34. www.consort-statement.org. Accessed 15 December 2004.
35. Johnston SC, Gress DR, Browner WS et al. Short-term prognosis after emergency department diagnosis of TIA. *JAMA* 2000;284:2901–2906.
36. Worster A, Haines T. Advanced statistics: understanding medical record review (MRR) studies. *Acad Emerg Med* 2004;11:187–192.
37. Gilbert EH, Lowenstein SR. Chart reviews in emergency medicine research: where are the methods? *Ann Emerg Med* 1996;27:305–308.
38. Gallagher EJ. $P < 0.05$ threshold for decerebrate genuflection. *Acad Emerg Med* 1999;6:1084–1087.
39. Guyatt G, Rennie D. *Users' guide to the medical literature.* JAMA 2002.
40. Greenhalgh T. How to read a paper: assessing the methodological quality of published papers. *Br Med J* 1997;315:305–308.
41. Oxman AD, Guyatt GH. A consumer's guide to subgroup analyses. *Ann Intern Med* 1992;116:78–84.
42. Assmann SF et al. Subgroup analysis and other (mis)uses of baseline data in clinical trials. *Lancet* 2000;355:1064–1066.
43. Oxman A, Guyatt G. Summarizing the evidence: when to believe a subgroup analysis. In: Guyatt G, Rennie D (eds) *Users' Guides to the Medical*

Literature: A Manual for Evidence-Based Clinical Practice. AMA Press, 2002:553–565.

44. Freemantle N. Interpreting the results of secondary end points and subgroup analyses in clinical trials: should we lock the crazy aunt in the attic? *Br Med J* 2001;322:989–991.

45. Sankoh AJ, Huque MF, Dubey SD. Some comments on frequently used multiple endpoint adjustment methods in clinical trials. *Statist Med* 1997; 16:2529–2542.

46. DeMets DL, Califf RM. Lessons learned from recent cardiovascular clinical trials: part I. *Circulation* 2002;106:746–751.

47. Montori VM, Permanyer-Miralda G, Ferreira-González I et al. Validity of composite endpoints in clinical trials. *Br Med J* 2005;330;594–596.

48. Freemantle N, Calvert M, Wood J et al. Composite outcomes in randomized trials: greater precision but with greater uncertainty? *JAMA* 2003; 289;2554–2559.

49. Ludbrook J. Interim analyses of data as they accumulate in laboratory experimentation. *BMC Med Res Methodol* 2003;3(1):15.

50. Zed PJ et al. Systematic reviews in emergency medicine. *Can J Emerg Med* 2003;5:5.

51. McKibbon A. *PDQ Evidence-based Principles and Practice.* Decker, 1999.

52. Easterbrook PJ et al. Publication bias in clinical research. *Lancet* 1991; 337:867–872.

53. Callaham MI, Weare RL et al. Positive-outcome bias and other limitations in outcome of research abstracts submitted to a scientific meeting. *JAMA* 1998;280:254–257.

54. Lee J. The power of negative thinking. *Can J Emerg Med* 2004;6:359–361.

55. Chan A, Hrobjartsson A, Haahr MT et al. Empirical evidence for selective reporting of outcomes in randomized trials. *JAMA* 2004;291:2457–2465.

56. Gregoire G et al. Selecting the language of the publications included in a meta-analysis: is there a Tower of Babel bias? *J Clin Epidemiol* 1995;48:159–163.

57. Tang A, Frazee B. Evidence-based emergency medicine/systematic review abstract. Antibiotic treatment for acute maxillary sinusitis. *Ann Emerg Med* 2003;42:705–708.

58. Egger M, Davey Smith G, Schneider M, Minder C. Bias in meta-analysis detected by a simple, graphical test. *Br Med J* 1997;315:629–634.

59. Jadad AR, Moore RA, Carroll D et al. Assessing the quality of reports of randomized clinical trials: is blinding necessary? *Control Clin Trials* 1996;17:1–12.

60. Antman EM, Lau J, Kupelnick B, Mosteller F, Chalmers TC. A comparison of results of meta-analyses of randomized control trials and recommendations of clinical experts: treatments for myocardial infarction. *JAMA* 1992; 268:240–248.

61. Juni P et al. The hazards of scoring the quality of clinical trials for meta-analysis. *JAMA* 1999;11:1054–1060

62. Balk EM, Bonis PA, Moskowitz H et al. Correlation of quality measures with estimates of treatment effect in meta-analyses of randomized controlled trials. *JAMA* 2002;287:2973–2982.

63. Ferreira OH, Ferreira ML et al. Effect of applying different "levels of evidence" criteria on conclusions of Cochrane reviews of intereventions for low back pain. *J Clin Epidem* 2002;55:1126–1129.
64. L'Abbe. Meta-analyses in clinical research. *Ann Intern Med* 1987;107:224–233.
65. Wears RL. Dueling meta-analyses. *Ann Emerg Med* 2000;36:233–236.
66. Moher D, Cook DJ, Eastwood S, Olkin I, Rennie D, Stroup DF. Improving the quality of reports of meta-analyses of randomised controlled trials: the QUOROM statement. Quality of Reporting of Meta-analyses. *Lancet* 1999; 354:1896–1900.
67. Counsell CE, Clarke M et al. The miracle of DICE therapy for acute stroke: fact or fictional product of subgroup analysis? *Br Med J* 1994;309:1677–1681.
68. www.abem.org. Accessed 24 December 2004.
69. Oxman AD, Guyatt GH. Guidelines for reading literature reviews. *CMAJ* 1988; 138:697–703.
70. http://jama.ama-assn.org/cgi/search?fulltext=rational+clinical+exam.
71. For methodology: www.bestbets.org.
72. Wyer PC et al. The clinician and the medical literature: when can we take a shortcut? *Ann Emerg Med* 2000;36:149–155.
73. Mackway-Jones K. Towards evidence based emergency medicine: best BETs from the Manchester Royal Infirmary. *Emerg Med J* 2003;20:169.
74. Field MJ, Lohr KN. *Guidelines for Clinical Practice: From Development to Use.* Institute of Medicine, 1992.
75. Shiffman RN, Shekelle P. Standardized reporting of clinical practice guidelines: a proposal from conference on guideline standardization. *Ann Intern Med* 2003;139:493–498.
76. Working group website: www.gradeworkinggroup.org. Accessed 10 November 2004.
77. GRADE Working Group. Grading quality of evidence and strength of recommendations. *Br Med J* 2004;328:1490.
78. Gallagher EJ. How well do clinical practice guidelines guide clinical practice? *Ann Emerg Med* 2002;40:394–398.
79. Laupacis A, Sekar N, Stiell IG. Clinical prediction rules: a review and suggested modifications of methodological standards. *JAMA* 1997;277:488–494.
80. Steyerberg EW, Harrell FE et al. Internal validation of predictive models: efficiency of some procedures for logistic regression analysis. *J Clin Epidemiol* 2001;54:774–781.
81. Fine MJ, Auble TE, Yealy DM et al. A prediction rule to identify low-risk patients with community-acquired pneumonia. *N Engl J Med* 1997;336:243–250.
82. Jefferson T, Demicheli V, Mugford M. *Elementary Economic Evaluation in Health Care.* BMJ Publishing Group, 1996.
83. Taylor C, Benger JR. Patient satisfaction in emergency medicine. *Emerg Med J* 2004;21:528–532.
84. Jenicek, M. *Foundations of Evidence-based Medicine.* Parthenon, 2003.
85. Klein G. *Sources of Power: How People Make Decisions.* MIT Press, 1999.
86. Smith R. "Publication ethics: an embarrassing amount of room for improvement." Talks at BMJ.com; see http://bmj.bmjjournals.com/talks. Accessed 21 December 2004.

87. Bennett DM, Taylor DM. Unethical practices in authorship of scientific papers. *Emerg Med* 2003;15:263–270.
88. Popp, Smith JR. ACCF/AHA Consensus Conference Report on Professionalism and Ethics. *JACC* 2004;44:1718–1721.
89. Rees ST. Who actually wrote the research paper? How to find out. *BMJ eletters*; see http://bmj.bmjjournals.com/cgi/eletters/326/7400/1202. Accessed 15 December 2004.
90. Abdulla S. UK fraud verdict prompts moves on ethics. *Nature* 1995;375:529.
91. Holmes DR, Firth BG, James A et al. Conflict of interest. *Am Heart J* 2004; 147:228–237.
92. Willman D. The National Institutes of Health: public servant or private marketer? *LA Times*, 22 December 2004.
93. International Committee of Medical Journal Editors. Uniform requirements for manuscripts submitted to biomedical journals. Available from www.icmjc.org/index.html#author. Accessed 15 December 2004.
94. Guidelines on Good Publication Practice. www.publicationethics.org.uk. Accessed 29 January 2005.
95. Abboud, L. Drug makers seek to bar 'placebo responders' from trials. *Wall Street J*, 18 June 2004.
96. Smith R. Medical journals and pharmaceutical companies: uneasy bedfellows. *Br Med J* 2003;326:1202–1205.
97. Lexchin J, Bero LA, Djulbegovic B, Clark O. Pharmaceutical industry sponsorship and research outcome and quality: systematic review. *Br Med J* 2003;326:1167–1177.
98. Als-Nielsen B, Chen W, Gluud C, Kjaergard LL. Association of funding and conclusions in randomized drug trials: a reflection of treatment effect or adverse events? *JAMA* 2003;290:921–928.
99. Campbell EG, Weissman, JS, Clarridge B et al. Characteristics of medical school faculty members serving on Institutional Review Boards: results of a national survey. *Acad Med* 2003;78:831–836.
100. Dyer C. Cardiologist admits research misconduct. *Br Med J* 1997;314:1501.
101. Campbell D. Medicine needs its MI5. *Br Med J* 1997;315:1677–1680.
102. Juni P, Rutjes AW, Dieppe PA. Are selective COX-2 inhibitors superior to traditional non steroidal anti-inflammatory drugs? *Br Med J* 2002; 324:1287–1288.
103. Sackett DL. Bias in analytic research. *J Chron Dis* 1979;32:51–63.
104. Melander H, Ahlqvist-Rastad J, Meijer G, Beerman B. Evidence b(i)ased medicine: selective reporting from studies sponsored by pharmaceutical industry. Review of studies in new drug applications. *Br Med J* 2003;326:1171–1175.
105. Chan A, Hrobjartsson A, Haahr MT et al. Empirical evidence for selective reporting of outcomes in randomized trials. *JAMA* 2004;291:2457–2465.
106. Kahn JO, Cherng DW, Mayer K et al. Evaluation of HIV-1 immunogen, an immunologic modifier, administered to patients infected with HIV having 300 to 549 x 106/L CD4 cell counts. *JAMA* 2000;284:2193–2202.
107. Forrow L et al. Absolutely relative: how research results are summarized can affect treatment decisions. *Am J Med* 1992;92:121–124.

108. Naylor CD et al. Measured enthusiasm: does the method of reporting trial results alter perceptions of therapeutic effectiveness? *Ann Intern Med* 1992; 117:916–921.
109. Nuovo J et al. Reporting Number needed to treat and absolute risk reduction in randomized controlled trials. *JAMA* 2002;287:2813.
110. Horton R. The dawn of McScience. *New York Review of Books* 2004;51(4).
111. Wilcken NR, Stockler MR. Fulvestrant: spreading the word, but not too thinly. *Lancet* 2003;362:1254.
112. Evans T et al. Registering clinical trials: an essential role for WHO. *Lancet* 2004;363:1413.
113. Mayor S. Drug companies agree to make clinical trial results public. *Br Med J* 2005;330:109.
114. Wilkes MS, Doblin BH, Shapiro MF. Pharmaceutical advertisements in leading medical journals: experts' assessments. *Ann Intern Med* 1992; 1116:912–919.
115. Gottlieb S. Congress criticizes drug industry for misleading advertising. *Br Med J* 2002;325:137.
116. Sackett DL, Oxman AD. HARLOT plc: an amalgamation of world's two oldest professions. *Br Med J* 2003;327:1442–1445.
117. Hodgkin P. Medicine, postmodernism, and the end of certainty. *Br Med J* 1996;313:1568–1569.
118. Sackett DL et al. Evidence-based medicine: how to practice and teach EBM, 2nd edn. Churchill Livingstone, 2000.
119. Jagoda AS, Cantrill SV et al. Clinical policy: neuroimaging and decision making in adult mild traumatic brain injury in the acute setting. *Ann Emerg Med* August 2002;40:231–249.

PART III

1. Presidential Committee on Information Literacy, final report, Association of College & Research Libraries. Available at www.ala.org/ala/acrlpubs/whitepapers/presidential.htm. Accessed 18 September 2004.
2. McKibbon A, Hunt D, Richardson WS et al. Finding the evidence. In: Guyatt G, Rennie D (eds) *Users' Guides to the Medical Literature: A Manual for Evidence-based Clinical Practice.* AMA Press, 2002:13–47.
3. Evidence Based Medicine Working Group. Evidence-based medicine: a new approach to teaching the practice of medicine. *JAMA* 1992;268:2420–2425.
4. Richardson WS, Wilson M, Williams J, Moyer V, Naylor CD. Diagnosis: clinical manifestations of disease. In: Guyatt G, Rennie D (eds) *Users' Guides to the Medical Literature: A Manual for Evidence-based Clinical Practice.* AMA Press, 2002:449–459.
5. Richardson WS, Wilson M, Lijmer J, Guyatt G, Cook D. Differential diagnosis. In: Guyatt G, Rennie D (eds) *Users' Guides to the Medical Literature: A Manual for Evidence-based Clinical Practice.* AMA Press, 2002:109–119.

6. McCrory P. Should we treat concussion pharmacologically? *Br J Sports Med* 2002;36:3–5.

7. CRASH Trial Collaborators X. Effect of intravenous corticosteroids on death within 14 days in 10,008 adults with clinically significant head injury (MRC CRASH trial): randomised placebo-controlled trial. *Lancet* 2004; 364:1321–1328.

8. Bucher H, Guyatt G, Cook D, Holbrook A, McAlister F. Therapy and applying the results: surrogate outcomes. In: Guyatt G, Rennie D (eds) *Users' Guides to the Medical Literature: A Manual for Evidence-based Clinical Practice.* AMA Press, 2002:393–413.

9. Wyer PC, Allen TY, Corrall CJ. Skills for evidence-based emergency care. How to find evidence when you need it: 4. Matching clinical questions to appropriate databases. *Ann Emerg Med* 2003;42:136–149.

10. Gallagher PE, Allen TY, Wyer PC. How to find evidence when you need it: 2. A clinician's guide to MEDLINE: The basics. *Ann Emerg Med* 2002; 39:436–440.

11. Corrall CJ, Wyer PC, Zick LS, Bockrath CR. How to find evidence when you need it: 1. Databases, search programs and strategies. *Ann Emerg Med* 2002; 39:302–306.

12. McCullough PA, Nowak RM, McCord J et al. B-type natriuretic peptide and clinical judgement in emergency diagnosis of heart failure: analysis from the Breathing Not Properly (BNP) Multinational Study. *Circulation* 2002;106·416–422.

13. Maisel AS, Krishnaswamy P, Nowak RM et al. Rapid measurement of B-type natriuretic peptide in the emergency diagnosis of heart failure. *N Engl J Med* 2002;347:161–167.

14. Hohl CM, Mitelman BY, Wyer P, Lang E. Should emergency physicians use B-type natriuretic peptide testing in patients with unexplained dyspnea? *Can J Emerg Med* 2003;5:162–165.

15. Brown MD, Reeves MJ. Interval likelihood ratios: another advantage for the evidence-based diagnostician. *Ann Emerg Med* 2003;42:292–297.

16. Rennie D, Guyatt GH. Users' guides to the medical literature (editorial). *JAMA* 1993;270:2096–2097.

17. Oxman A, Sackett DL, Guyatt GH, for the Evidence Based Medicine Working Group X. Users' guides to the medical literature: 1. How to get started. *JAMA* 1993;270:2093–2095.

18. Smith GCS, Pell JP. Parachute use to prevent death and major trauma related to gravitational challenge: systematic reviewe of randomised controlled trials. *Br Med J* 2003;327:1459–1461.

19. Stroup DF, Berlin JA, Morton SC et al. Meta-analysis of observational studies in epidemiology: a proposal for reporting. *JAMA* 2000;283:2008–2012.

20. Haynes RB. How to read clinical journals: II. To learn about a diagnostic test. *CMAJ* 1981;124:703–710.

21. Jaeschke R, Guyatt G, Lijmer J. Diagnostic tests. In: Guyatt G, Rennie D (eds) *Users' Guides to the Medical Literature: A Manual for Evidence-based Clinical Practice.* AMA Press, 2002:121–140.

22. Richardson WS, Wilson M, Guyatt G. The process of diagnosis. In: Guyatt G, Rennie D (eds) *Users' Guides to the Medical Literature: A Manual for Evidence-based Clinical Practice.* AMA Press, 2002:101–108.

23. Sackett DL, Haynes RB. The architecture of diagnostic research. In: Knottnerus JA (ed) *The Evidence Base of Clinical Diagnosis.* BMJ Books, 2002:19–38.

24. Sackett DL, Haynes RB. Evidence base of clinical diagnosis: the architecture of diagnostic research. *Br Med J* 2002;324:539–541.

25. Lijmer JG, Mol BW, Heisterkamp S et al. Empirical evidence of design-related bias in studies of diagnostic tests. *JAMA* 1999;282:1061–1066.

26. Deville WL, Buntinx F. Guidelines for conducting systematic reviews of studies evaluating the accuracy of diagnostic tests. In: Knottnerus JA (ed) *The Evidence Base of Clinical Diagnosis.* BMJ Books, 2002:145–166.

27. Rowe B, Alderson P. The Cochrane Library: A resource for clinical problem solving in emergency medicine. *Ann Emerg Med* 1999;34:86–90.

28. Wyer PC, Allen T, Corrall CJ. Finding evidence when you need it. *Evidence-Based Cardiovasc Med* 2004;8:2–7.

29. Rowe BH, Travers AH, Holroyd BR, Kelly KD, Bota GW. Nebulized ipratropium bromide in acute pediatric asthma: does it reduce hospital admissions among children presenting to the emergency department? *Ann Emerg Med* 1999;34:75–85.

30. Guyatt GH, Meade MO, Jaeschke RZ, Haynes RB. Practitioners of evidence based care: not all clinicians need to appraise evidence from scratch but all need some skills. *Br Med J* 2000;320:954–955.

31. Guyatt G, Rennie D (eds) *Users' Guides to the Medical Literature: A Manual For Evidence-based Clinical Practice.* AMA Press, 2002.

32. Emond SD, Wyer PC, Brown MD et al. How relevant are the systematic reviews in the Cochrane Library to emergency medical practice? *Ann Emerg Med* 2002;39:153–159.

33. Guyatt G, Montori V, Devereaux PJ, Schunemann H, Bhandari M. Patients at the center: in our practice, and in our use of language. *ACP J Club* 2004;140:A11–A12.

34. McKibbon KA, Haynes RB, Dilks CJW et al. How good are clinical MEDLINE searches? A comparative study of clinical end-user and librarian searches. *Comput Biomed Res* 1990;23:583–593.

35. Haynes RB, Wilczynski N, McKibbon A, Walker CJ, Sinclair JC. Developing optimal search strategies for detecting clinically sound studies in MEDLINE. *J Am Med Informatics Assoc* 1994;1:447–458.

36. Wells PS, Ginsberg JS, Anderson DR et al. Use of a clinical model for safe management of patients with suspected pulmonary embolism. *Ann Intern Med* 1998;129:997–1005.

37. McKibbon A, Eady A, Marks S. *PDQ Evidence-based Principles and Practice.* Decker, 1999.

38. Gallagher PE, Allen TY, Wyer PC. How to find evidence when you need it: 3. A clinician's guide to MEDLINE: Tricks and special skills. *Ann Emerg Med* 2002;39:547–551.

39. Katz MH, Nicholson BW, Singer DE et al. The triage decision in pulmonary edema. *J Gen Intern Med* 1988;3:533–539.

40. Sackett DL, Straus SE. Finding and applying evidence during clinical rounds: the "evidence cart." *JAMA* 1998;280:1336–1338.

41. Marchetti A, Magar R, Fischer J, Sloan E, Fischer P. A pharmacoeconomic evaluation of intravenous fosphenytoin (Cerebyx®) versus intravenous phenytoin (Dilantin®) in hospital emergency departments. *Clin Therapeut* 1996;18:953–966.

42. Touchette DR, Rhoney DH. Cost-minimization analysis of phenytoin and fosphenytoin in the emergency department. *Pharmacotherapy* 2000;20: 908–916.

43. Coplin WM, Rhoney DH, Rebuck JA et al. Randomized evaluation of adverse events and length-of-stay with routine emergency department use of phenytoin or fosphenytoin. *Neurol Res* 2002;24:842–848.

44. Rudis MI, Touchette DR, Swadron SP, Chiu AP, Orlinsky M. Cost-effectiveness of oral phenytoin, intravenous phenytoin, and intravenous fosphenytoin in the emergency department. *Ann Emerg Med* 2004;43:386–397.

45. Holliday SM, Benfield P, Plosker GL. Fosphenytoin: pharmacoeconomic implications of therapy. *Pharmacoeconomics* 1998;14:685–690.

46. Silberg WM, Lundberg GD, Musacchio RA. Assessing, controlling, and assuring the quality of medical information on the Internet: *caveant lector et viewor* (Let the reader and viewer beware). *JAMA* 1997;277:1244–1245.

47. Sauve S, Lee HN, Meade MO et al. The critically appraised topic: a practical approach to learning critical appraisal. *Ann Roy Coll Phys Surg Can* 1995; 28:396–398.

48. Dong P, Mondry A. Enhanced quality and quantity of retrieval of critically appraised topics using the CAT crawler. *Med Inform* 2004;29:43–55.

49. Wyer PC. The critically appraised topic: closing the evidence-transfer gap. *Ann Emerg Med* 1997;30:639–640.

50. Wyer PC, Rowe BH, Guyatt GH, Cordell WH. The clinician and the medical literature: when can we take a shortcut? *Ann Emerg Med* 2000;36: 149–155.

51. Oxman AD, Guyatt GH. Guidelines for reading literature reviews. *CMAJ* 1988;138:697–703.

52. Wyer PC, Allen TY, Corrall CJ. How to find evidence when you need it, Part 4. *Ann Emerg Med* 2003;42(1):136–149.

53. Durack DT. The weight of medical knowledge. *N Engl J Med* 1978;298(14): 773–775.

54. Maisel AS, Krishnaswamy P, Nowak RM et al. for the Breathing Not Properly Multinational Study Investigators. Rapid measurement of B-type natriuretic peptide in the emergency diagnosis of heart failure. *N Engl J Med* 2002;347: 161–167.
    McCullogh PA, Nowak RM, McCord J et al. B-type natriuretic peptide and clinical judgment in emergency diagnosis of heart failure: analysis from Breathing Not Properly (BNP) multinational study. *Circulation* 2002;106: 416–422.

55. Lader E. BNP levels had high sensitivity but moderate specificity for detecting congestive heart failure in the emergency department. *ACP Journal Club* 2003;138:23.
Hohl CM, Mitelman BV, Wyer P, Lang E. Should emergency physicians use B-type natriuretic peptide testing in patients with unexplained dyspnea? *CJEM* 2003;5:162–165.
Schwam E. B-type natriuretic peptide for diagnosis of heart failure in emergency department patients: a critical appraisal. *Acad Emerg Med* 2004;11:686–691.

INDEX

ABEM. *See* American Board of
  Emergency Medicine.
Absolute parameters, 86–87, 90–91
  absolute risk reduction, 86
  number needed to treat (NNT), 86–87
Absolute risk increase, 105
Absolute risk reduction (ARR),
  86, 100–102
Absolute treatment parameters, 91
Abstract, use of in clinical study evaluation,
  146–147
Accept threshold, 28–30
Access packages, databases and, 308–310
Accuracy, diagnostic testing characteristics
  and, 34
Action thresholds, confidence intervals and,
  194–197
Aggregate method, of meta-analyses, 215
Algorithms, cognitive error and, 71
American Board of Emergency Medicine
  (ABEM), 217
APC Journal Club, 291–292
Applicability of diagnostic tests, 51–55
  clinical scenarios, 53–54
  equipment and resources, 53
  external validity and, 150
  interpretation of, 52–53
  patients and, 52
  prognostic evidence and, 132–133
  treatment effects and, 99–104
ARR. *See* absolute risk reduction.
Attrition bias, 180
Availability bias, 62

Background knowledge, clinical study
  evaluation and, 146
Background questioning
  PICO, 268–276

question analyzing and, 266–268
  refinement of, 268–276
Backward vs. forward reasoning, 15–16
  pattern matching, 15–16
  recognition-primed decision model, 16
Base rate neglect, 64–65
Baseline group similarity, randomization
  and, 166
Baseline mismatching
  confounders, 167
  randomization and, 167
Baseline prognostic factors, randomization
  and, 164
Bayesian analysis, 20–23
Benefit parameters, treatment parameters
  and, 90
BestBETs, 314
Bias
  attrition, 180
  confirmation, 62
  evidence evaluation, 141–142
  misclassification, 179
  recall, 181
Blinding, 155–156
  assessors and, 169–170
  authors and, 170
  clinicians and, 169
  cointervention bias, 169
  interim analysis, 170
  internal validity and, 168–169
  investigators and researchers, 248
  performance bias, 169
  placebo effect, 168
  results section, 170
  review bias, 155–156
  statisticians and, 170
Boolean operators, 305–306
Built-in limits, 306